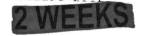

Stroke
SOURCEBOOK

Fourth Edition

Health Reference Series

Fourth Edition

Stroke

SOURCEBOOK

Basic Consumer Health Information about Ischemic Stroke, Hemorrhagic Stroke, Transient Ischemic Attack, and Other Forms of Brain Attack, with Information about Stroke Risk Factors and Prevention, Diagnostic Tests, Poststroke Complications, and Acute and Rehabilitative Treatments, Such as Stroke Medications, Surgeries, and Therapies

Along with Tips on Regaining Independence, Restoring Cognitive Function, and Dealing with Depression after Stroke, a Glossary of Related Medical Terms, and a Directory of Resources for Further Help and Information

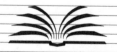

OMNIGRAPHICS

615 Griswold, Ste. 901, Detroit, MI 48226

Bibliographic Note

Because this page cannot legibly accommodate all the copyright notices, the Bibliographic Note portion of the Preface constitutes an extension of the copyright notice.

* * *

Health Reference Series
Keith Jones, *Managing Editor*
***

OMNIGRAPHICS
A PART OF RELEVANT INFORMATION
***

Library of Congress Cataloging-in-Publication Data

Names: Omnigraphics, Inc., issuing body.

Title: Stroke sourcebook: basic consumer health information about ischemic stroke, hemorrhagic stroke, transient ischemic attack, and other forms of brain attack, with information about stroke risk factors and prevention, diagnostic tests, post-stroke complications, and acute and rehabilitative treatments, such as stroke medications, surgeries, and therapies; along with tips on regaining independence, restoring cognitive function, and dealing with depression after stroke, a glossary of related medical terms, and a directory of resources for further help and information.

Description: Fourth edition. | Detroit, MI: Omnigraphics, [2017] | Series: Health reference series | Includes bibliographical references and index.

Identifiers: LCCN 2017010859 (print) | LCCN 2017012241 (ebook) | ISBN 9780780815629 (eBook) | ISBN 9780780815612 (hardcover: alk. paper)

Subjects: LCSH: Cerebrovascular disease--Popular works.

Classification: LCC RC388.5 (ebook) | LCC RC388.5 .S8566 2017 (print) | DDC 616.8/1--dc23

LC record available at https://lccn.loc.gov/2017010859

Table of Contents

Preface xiii

Part I: Introduction to Stroke

Chapter 1 — What Is Stroke? 3

Chapter 2 — Stroke Symptoms and What You
Should Do If Someone Has Them 21

Chapter 3 — Perinatal and Childhood Stroke 25

Chapter 4 — Strokes in Women and Men 29

    Section 4.1 — Women and Stroke 30

    Section 4.2 — Contraceptive Use and
    Stroke Risk................................... 33

    Section 4.3 — Menopausal Hormone
    Therapy (MHT) and Stroke
    Risk... 35

    Section 4.4 — Men and Stroke.......................... 38

Chapter 5 — Strokes in Older Adults.. 41

Chapter 6 — Racial and Ethnic Stroke Disparities 51

Chapter 7 — Geography and Stroke: The Stroke Belt............... 57

Chapter 8 — Statistics on Stroke in the United States............. 63

Chapter 9 — Recent Research on Stroke...................................... 69

Section 9.1 — Researchers Investigate
Genes Involved in Brain
Repair after Stroke 70

Section 9.2 — Stem Cell Therapy and
Stroke 72

Section 9.3 — Amplatzer PFO Occluder
Device for Prevention of
Recurrent Strokes 74

Chapter 10—Clinical Trials on Stroke 77

Section 10.1—What Are Clinical Trials? 78

Section 10.2—Rehabilitation Treatment
Following Stroke 83

Section 10.3—Vitamin D and Stroke 85

Section 10.4—Heart and Brain Interfaces
in Acute Ischemic Stroke 86

Section 10.5—Quality of Life after Stroke 88

Section 10.6—Carotid Plaque Imaging in
Acute Stroke 89

Section 10.7—The Effect of Aerobic
Exercise in Patients with
Minor Stroke 91

Part II: Types of Stroke

Chapter 11—Ischemic Stroke 95

Section 11.1—What Is Ischemic Stroke? 96

Section 11.2—Carotid Artery Dissection 98

Chapter 12—Hemorrhagic Stroke 103

Section 12.1—Intracerebral and
Subarachnoid Hemorrhagic
Stroke 104

Section 12.2—Cerebral Aneurysm 108

Chapter 13—Mini-Stroke: Transient Ischemic
Attack (TIA) 115

Chapter 14—Recurrent Stroke 119

Part III: Stroke Risk Factors and Prevention

Chapter 15—Stroke Risks 125

Chapter 16—Atherosclerosis and Carotid Artery
Disease 131

    Section 16.1—Atherosclerosis........................... 132

    Section 16.2—Carotid Artery Disease............. 144

Chapter 17—Atrial Fibrillation and Stroke 157

Chapter 18—Blood Clotting Disorders and Stroke.................. 167

Chapter 19—Peripheral Artery Disease................................... 171

Chapter 20—Diabetes and Stroke Risk................................... 181

Chapter 21—High Blood Pressure and High
Cholesterol 189

    Section 21.1—High Blood Pressure................. 190

    Section 21.2—High Blood Cholesterol............. 202

Chapter 22—Overweight, Obesity, and Stroke Risk 213

Chapter 23—Other Stroke Risk Factors 229

    Section 23.1—Inactivity, Exercise, and
        Stroke 230

    Section 23.2—Migraine and Stroke Risk 235

    Section 23.3—Sleep Apnea Increases
        Risk of Stroke............................ 239

    Section 23.4—Stress and Stroke Risk............. 244

    Section 23.5—Stress at Work and Stroke
        Risk... 246

    Section 23.6—Alcohol and Stroke.................... 248

    Section 23.7—Smoking and Stroke 251

    Section 23.8—Illegal Substance Use and
        Stroke 254

    Section 23.9—Traumatic Brain
        Injury (TBI) and Stroke............ 257

Chapter 24—Stroke Prevention 267

Section 24.1—Preventing and Managing
Diabetes...................................... 268

Section 24.2—Preventing and Managing
High Blood Pressure................ 270

Section 24.3—Preventing and Managing
High Cholesterol....................... 273

Section 24.4—Healthy Living Reduces
Stroke Risk............................... 276

Section 24.5—Quitting Smoking Reduces
Stroke Risk............................... 277

Section 24.6—Even Modest Weight Loss
Produces Health Benefits......... 281

Part IV: Diagnosis and Treatment of Stroke

Chapter 25—After a Stroke: The First 24 Hours...................... 287

Chapter 26—Working with a Neurologist................................. 291

Chapter 27—Diagnosing Stroke 297

Section 27.1—How a Stroke Is Diagnosed...... 298

Section 27.2—Blood Tests for Stroke.............. 301

Section 27.3—Cerebral Angiography.............. 305

Section 27.4—Echocardiogram........................ 308

Section 27.5—Electrocardiogram (EKG)......... 312

Section 27.6—Computerized Tomography
(CT) Scan.................................... 313

Section 27.7—Magnetic Resonance
Imaging (MRI)............................ 316

Section 27.8—Ultrasound 319

Chapter 28—Stroke Treatment 323

Chapter 29—Surgical Procedures Used in the
Treatment of Stroke 327

Section 29.1—Brain Aneurysm Repair........... 328

Section 29.2—Carotid Artery Angioplasty
and Stent Placement 337

Section 29.3—Carotid Endarterectomy.......... 346

Chapter 30—Medications Used to Treat Stroke 351

    Section 30.1—Tissue Plasminogen
              Activator (tPA) and
              Thrombolytic Therapy 352

    Section 30.2—Antiplatelets and
              Anticoagulants 355

    Section 30.3—Blood Pressure-Lowering
              Drugs 357

    Section 30.4—Taking Statins after Stroke
              Reduces Risk of Death 369

Chapter 31—Stroke Recovery 373

Part V: Poststroke Complications and Rehabilitation

Chapter 32—Cognitive Problems Caused by Stroke 379

    Section 32.1—Agnosia 380

    Section 32.2—Right Hemisphere Brain
              Damage 382

    Section 32.3—Vascular Dementia 385

    Section 32.4—Multi-Infarct
              Dementia (MID) 391

Chapter 33—Communication Problems after Stroke 395

Chapter 34—Swallowing Problems (Dysphagia)
              after Stroke 403

Chapter 35—Muscle Spasticity and Weakness
              after Stroke 409

    Section 35.1—Overview of Spasticity 410

    Section 35.2—Foot Drop 413

    Section 35.3—Constraint-Induced
              Movement Therapy 414

Chapter 36—Balance Problems after Stroke 417

Chapter 37—Pain and Fatigue after Stroke 423

    Section 37.1—Pain after Stroke 424

    Section 37.2—Fatigue after Stroke 429

Chapter 38—Bowel Control Problems and Stroke.................... 431

Chapter 39—Bladder Control Problems and Stroke................ 435

Chapter 40—Vision Problems after Stroke 443

Chapter 41—Poststroke Rehabilitation Facilities 447

    Section 41.1—Overview of Poststroke
            Rehabilitation and Types
            of Poststroke Therapies............ 448

    Section 41.2—How to Choose a
            Rehabilitation Facility.............. 458

    Section 41.3—Tips for Choosing a
            Rehabilitation Facility.............. 461

Part VI: Life after Stroke

Chapter 42—Recovering from Stroke 467

Chapter 43—Making the Home Safer for Stroke
    Survivors 471

Chapter 44—Rehabilitative and Assistive
    Technology 475

Chapter 45—Driving after Stroke... 481

Chapter 46—Nutrition and Exercise Tips for
    Poststroke Patients... 485

    Section 46.1—Advice for People with
            Swallowing Difficulties............ 486

    Section 46.2—Nutrition and Exercise
            after Stroke 488

Chapter 47—Skin Care after Stroke.. 493

Chapter 48—Sleep after Stroke 497

Chapter 49—Sexuality after Stroke 501

Chapter 50—Dealing with Depression after Stroke 505

Chapter 51—Caring for Someone with Memory
    Problems after Stroke... 509

Chapter 52—Tips for Caregivers of Stroke Patients 513

Chapter 53—Stroke Support Group 519

Chapter 54—Health Insurance and Disability
Concerns after Stroke 523

    Section 54.1—Affordable Care Act (ACA) 524

    Section 54.2—Health Insurance
Information for Stroke
Patients 526

    Section 54.3—Social Security Disability
Benefits...................................... 529

Chapter 55—Choosing Long-Term Care for Those
Disabled by Stroke... 539

    Section 55.1—Long-Term Care...................... 540

    Section 55.2—Assisted Living........................ 555

Chapter 56—Advance Care Planning.. 559

Part VII: Additional Help and Information

Chapter 57—Glossary of Terms Related to Stroke.................. 569

Chapter 58—Directory of Organizations That Help
Stroke Patients and Their Families 579

Index.. 591

Preface

About This Book

According to the Centers for Disease Control and Prevention (CDC), stroke kills more than 130,000 Americans each year – one out of every 20 deaths – making it the fifth leading cause of death for Americans. Stroke costs the United States an estimated $33 billion each year. This total includes the cost of healthcare services, medicines to treat stroke, and missed days of work. Stroke is also a leading cause of serious, long-term disability. Its effects include a broad range of cognitive and physical problems, such as speech and communication difficulties, dementia, muscle spasticity and weakness, balance problems, and incontinence. Early recognition of stroke symptoms and prompt medical attention can help patients achieve better outcomes. In addition, many strokes can be prevented through lifestyle changes that address underlying risk factors.

Stroke Sourcebook, Fourth Edition, provides updated information about the causes, diagnosis, treatment, and prevention of stroke. Readers will learn about ischemic stroke, hemorrhagic stroke, and transient ischemic attacks (TIAs, also known as mini-strokes), as well as stroke risk factors. Stroke risk factors include atherosclerosis, diabetes, heart disease, blood disorders, high cholesterol, high blood pressure, and obesity. Information on stroke diagnosis, acute and rehabilitative treatment, and poststroke complications is also included, along with tips for living with poststroke challenges, a glossary of related terms, and a directory of organizations that provide information to stroke patients and their caregivers.

How to Use This Book

This book is divided into parts and chapters. Parts focus on broad areas of interest. Chapters are devoted to single topics within a part.

Part I: Introduction to Stroke identifies the symptoms of stroke and discusses the incidence of stroke in children, men, women, and older adults. It also examines the impact of stroke in specific geographic regions and stroke-related health disparities among racial and ethnic populations. The part concludes with statistical information on stroke in the United States, in addition to recent findings and clinical trials in stroke research.

Part II: Types of Stroke discusses the two major types of stroke, ischemic and hemorrhagic. It also describes transient ischemic attacks, which are often called mini-strokes, and it addresses concerns about risk factors for recurrent strokes.

Part III: Stroke Risk Factors and Prevention provides information about conditions that predispose a person to having a stroke, including atherosclerosis, carotid artery disease, atrial fibrillation, and peripheral artery disease. It also discusses the role that diabetes, high blood pressure, high cholesterol, obesity, inactivity, stress, smoking, and substance abuse play in stroke risk, and it offers strategies for stroke prevention through lifestyle changes.

Part IV: Diagnosis and Treatment of Stroke offers information about common medical tests used to identify stroke. This part also discusses life-saving stroke treatments, including angioplasty, stent placement, carotid endarterectomy, and medications such as tissue plasminogen activator (tPA).

Part V: Poststroke Complications and Rehabilitation discusses the numerous cognitive and physical problems that stroke often causes, including brain damage, dementia, and difficulties with speech and communication. It also provides information about poststroke rehabilitation for physical disabilities, including swallowing problems, muscle spasticity and weakness, balance problems, pain, bowel and continence issues, and vision problems. The part concludes with facts about therapies used to help patients with activities of daily living during the poststroke period.

Part VI: Life after Stroke identifies common concerns of stroke patients and their families after hospitalization or rehabilitation, such as kitchen, bathroom, and living room modifications that can improve home safety and mobility. The part also examines skin care, sleep, sex, and depression issues often experienced after stroke. Tips for caregivers and a discussion about choosing long-term care facilities are also provided.

Part VII: Additional Help and Information provides a glossary of important terms related to stroke and a directory of organizations that offer information to stroke patients and their families and caregivers.

Bibliographic Note

This volume contains documents and excerpts from publications issued by the following U.S. government agencies: Administration for Community Living (ACL); Agency for Healthcare Research and Quality (AHRQ); Centers for Disease Control and Prevention (CDC); Centers for Medicare and Medicaid Services (CMS); Drug Enforcement Administration (DEA); *Eunice Kennedy Shriver* National Institute of Child Health and Human Development (NICHD); Genetic and Rare Diseases Information Center (GARD); LiverTox®, National Institutes of Health (NIH); National Cancer Institute (NCI); National Heart, Lung, and Blood Institute (NHLBI); National Highway Traffic Safety Administration (NHTSA); National Institute of Biomedical Imaging and Bioengineering (NIBIB); National Institute of Diabetes and Digestive and Kidney Diseases (NIDDK); National Institute of Neurological Disorders and Stroke (NINDS); National Institute on Aging (NIA); National Institute on Alcohol Abuse and Alcoholism (NIAAA); National Institute on Deafness and Other Communication Disorders (NIDCD); National Institute on Drug Abuse (NIDA); National Institutes of Health (NIH); Office of Minority Health (OMH); Office on Women's Health (OWH); U.S. Administration on Aging (AOA); U.S. Department of Veterans Affairs (VA); U.S. Food and Drug Administration (FDA); U.S. National Institutes of Health (NIH); and U.S. Social Security Administration (SSA).

In addition, this volume contains copyrighted documents from the following organizations: American Migraine Foundation; American Speech-Language-Hearing Association (ASHA); Cleveland Clinic; and Rehabilitation Institute of Chicago (renamed as Shirley Ryan AbilityLab).

It may also contain original material produced by Omnigraphics and reviewed by medical consultants.

About the Health Reference Series

The *Health Reference Series* is designed to provide basic medical information for patients, families, caregivers, and the general public. Each volume takes a particular topic and provides comprehensive coverage. This is especially important for people who may be dealing with a newly diagnosed disease or a chronic disorder in themselves or in a family member. People looking for preventive guidance, information about disease warning signs, medical statistics, and risk factors for health problems will also find answers to their questions in the *Health Reference Series*. The *Series*, however, is not intended to serve as a tool for diagnosing illness, in prescribing treatments, or as a substitute for the physician/patient relationship. All people concerned about medical symptoms or the possibility of disease are encouraged to seek professional care from an appropriate healthcare provider.

A Note about Spelling and Style

Health Reference Series editors use *Stedman's Medical Dictionary* as an authority for questions related to the spelling of medical terms and the *Chicago Manual of Style* for questions related to grammatical structures, punctuation, and other editorial concerns. Consistent adherence is not always possible, however, because the individual volumes within the *Series* include many documents from a wide variety of different producers, and the editor's primary goal is to present material from each source as accurately as is possible. This sometimes means that information in different chapters or sections may follow other guidelines and alternate spelling authorities.

Medical Review

Omnigraphics contracts with a team of qualified, senior medical professionals who serve as medical consultants for the *Health Reference Series*. As necessary, medical consultants review reprinted and originally written material for currency and accuracy. Citations including the phrase, "Reviewed (month, year)" indicate material reviewed by this team. Medical consultation services are provided to the *Health Reference Series* editors by:

Dr. Vijayalakshmi, MBBS, DGO, MD
Dr. Senthil Selvan, MBBS, DCH, MD
Dr. K. Sivanandham, MBBS, DCH, MS (Research), PhD

Our Advisory Board

Health Reference Series *Update Policy*

The inaugural book in the *Health Reference Series* was the first edition of *Cancer Sourcebook* published in 1989. Since then, the *Series* has been enthusiastically received by librarians and in the medical community. In order to maintain the standard of providing high-quality health information for the layperson the editorial staff at Omnigraphics felt it was necessary to implement a policy of updating volumes when warranted.

Medical researchers have been making tremendous strides, and it is the purpose of the *Health Reference Series* to stay current with the most recent advances. Each decision to update a volume is made on an individual basis. Some of the considerations include how much new information is available and the feedback we receive from people who use the books. If there is a topic you would like to see added to the update list, or an area of medical concern you feel has not been adequately addressed, please write to:

Managing Editor
Health Reference Series
Omnigraphics
615 Griswold, Ste. 901
Detroit, MI 48226

Part One

Introduction to Stroke

Chapter 1

What Is Stroke?

A stroke occurs if the flow of oxygen-rich blood to a portion of the brain is blocked. Without oxygen, brain cells start to die after a few minutes. Sudden bleeding in the brain also can cause a stroke if it damages brain cells. If brain cells die or are damaged because of a stroke, symptoms occur in the parts of the body that these brain cells control. Examples of stroke symptoms include sudden weakness; paralysis or numbness of the face, arms, or legs (paralysis is an inability to move); trouble speaking or understanding speech; and trouble seeing.

A stroke is a serious medical condition that requires emergency care. A stroke can cause lasting brain damage, long-term disability, or even death. If you think you or someone else is having a stroke, call 9-1-1 right away. Do not drive to the hospital or let someone else drive you. Call an ambulance so that medical personnel can begin life-saving treatment on the way to the emergency room. During a stroke, every minute counts.

Types of Stroke

Ischemic Stroke

An ischemic stroke occurs if an artery that supplies oxygen-rich blood to the brain becomes blocked. Blood clots often cause the blockages that lead to ischemic strokes.

This chapter contains text excerpted from the following sources: Text in this chapter begins with excerpts from "Stroke," National Heart, Lung, and Blood Institute (NHLBI), January 27, 2017; Text under the heading "Stroke in United States" is excerpted from "Questions and Answers about Stroke," National Institute of Neurological Disorders and Stroke (NINDS), March 29, 2016.

The two types of ischemic stroke are thrombotic and embolic. In a thrombotic stroke, a blood clot (thrombus) forms in an artery that supplies blood to the brain. In an embolic stroke, a blood clot or other substance (such as plaque, a fatty material) travels through the bloodstream to an artery in the brain. (A blood clot or piece of plaque that travels through the bloodstream is called an embolus.)

With both types of ischemic stroke, the blood clot or plaque blocks the flow of oxygen-rich blood to a portion of the brain.

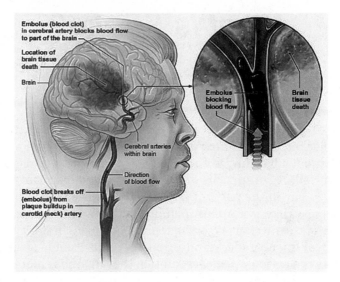

Figure 1.1. *Ischemic Stroke*

The illustration shows how an ischemic stroke can occur in the brain. If a blood clot breaks away from plaque buildup in a carotid (neck) artery, it can travel to and lodge in an artery in the brain. The clot can block blood flow to part of the brain, causing brain tissue death.

Hemorrhagic Stroke

A hemorrhagic stroke occurs if an artery in the brain leaks blood or ruptures (breaks open). The pressure from the leaked blood damages brain cells.

The two types of hemorrhagic stroke are intracerebral and subarachnoid. In an intracerebral hemorrhage, a blood vessel inside the brain leaks blood or ruptures. In a subarachnoid hemorrhage, a blood vessel on the surface of the brain leaks blood or ruptures. When this happens, bleeding occurs between the inner and middle layers of the membranes that cover the brain.

In both types of hemorrhagic stroke, the leaked blood causes swelling of the brain and increased pressure in the skull. The swelling and pressure damage cells and tissues in the brain.

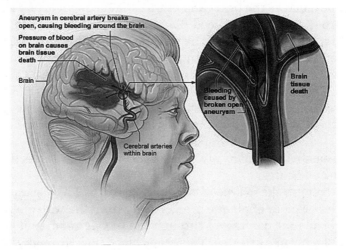

Figure 1.2. *Hemorrhagic Stroke*

The illustration shows how a hemorrhagic stroke can occur in the brain. An aneurysm in a cerebral artery breaks open, which causes bleeding in the brain. The pressure of the blood causes brain tissue death.

Other Names for a Stroke

- Brain attack
- Cerebrovascular accident (CVA)
- Hemorrhagic stroke (includes intracerebral hemorrhage and subarachnoid hemorrhage)
- Ischemic stroke (includes thrombotic stroke and embolic stroke)

A transient ischemic attack sometimes is called a TIA or mini-stroke. A TIA has the same symptoms as a stroke, and it increases your risk of having a stroke.

What Causes a Stroke?

Ischemic Stroke and Transient Ischemic Attack

An ischemic stroke or TIA occurs if an artery that supplies oxygen-rich blood to the brain becomes blocked. Many medical conditions can increase the risk of ischemic stroke or TIA.

For example, atherosclerosis is a disease in which a fatty substance called plaque builds up on the inner walls of the arteries. Plaque hardens and narrows the arteries, which limits the flow of blood to tissues and organs (such as the heart and brain). Plaque in an artery can crack or rupture (break open). Blood platelets, which are disc-shaped cell fragments, stick to the site of the plaque injury and clump together to form blood clots. These clots can partly or fully block an artery.

Plaque can build up in any artery in the body, including arteries in the heart, brain, and neck. The two main arteries on each side of the neck are called the carotid arteries. These arteries supply oxygen-rich blood to the brain, face, scalp, and neck. When plaque builds up in the carotid arteries, the condition is called carotid artery disease. Carotid artery disease causes many of the ischemic strokes and TIAs that occur in the United States.

An embolic stroke (a type of ischemic stroke) or TIA also can occur if a blood clot or piece of plaque breaks away from the wall of an artery. The clot or plaque can travel through the bloodstream and get stuck in one of the brain's arteries. This stops blood flow through the artery and damages brain cells.

Heart conditions and blood disorders also can cause blood clots that can lead to a stroke or TIA. For example, atrial fibrillation, or AF, is a common cause of embolic stroke.

In AF, the upper chambers of the heart contract in a very fast and irregular way. As a result, some blood pools in the heart. The pooling increases the risk of blood clots forming in the heart chambers.

An ischemic stroke or TIA also can occur because of lesions caused by atherosclerosis. These lesions may form in the small arteries of the brain, and they can block blood flow to the brain.

Hemorrhagic Stroke

Sudden bleeding in the brain can cause a hemorrhagic stroke. The bleeding causes swelling of the brain and increased pressure in the skull. The swelling and pressure damage brain cells and tissues.

Examples of conditions that can cause a hemorrhagic stroke include high blood pressure, aneurysms, and arteriovenous malformations (AVMs).

"Blood pressure" is the force of blood pushing against the walls of the arteries as the heart pumps blood. If blood pressure rises and stays high over time, it can damage the body in many ways.

Aneurysms are balloon-like bulges in an artery that can stretch and burst. AVMs are tangles of faulty arteries and veins that can rupture within the brain. High blood pressure can increase the risk of hemorrhagic stroke in people who have aneurysms or AVMs.

Who Is at Risk for a Stroke?

Certain traits, conditions, and habits can raise your risk of having a stroke or TIA. These traits, conditions, and habits are known as risk factors. The more risk factors you have, the more likely you are to have a stroke. You can treat or control some risk factors, such as high blood pressure and smoking. Other risk factors, such as age and gender, you can't control.

The major risk factors for stroke include:

- **High blood pressure.** High blood pressure is the main risk factor for stroke. Blood pressure is considered high if it stays at or above 140/90 millimeters of mercury (mmHg) over time. If you have diabetes or chronic kidney disease, high blood pressure is defined as 130/80 mmHg or higher.

- **Diabetes.** Diabetes is a disease in which the blood sugar level is high because the body doesn't make enough insulin or doesn't use its insulin properly. Insulin is a hormone that helps move blood sugar into cells where it's used for energy.

- **Heart diseases.** Coronary heart disease, cardiomyopathy, heart failure, and atrial fibrillation can cause blood clots that can lead to a stroke.

- **Smoking.** Smoking can damage blood vessels and raise blood pressure. Smoking also may reduce the amount of oxygen that reaches your body's tissues. Exposure to secondhand smoke also can damage the blood vessels.

- **Age and gender.** Your risk of stroke increases as you get older. At younger ages, men are more likely than women to have strokes. However, women are more likely to die from strokes. Women who take birth control pills also are at slightly higher risk of stroke.

- **Race and ethnicity.** Strokes occur more often in African-American, Alaska Native, and American-Indian adults than in white, Hispanic, or Asian-American adults.

- **Personal or family history of stroke or TIA.** If you've had a stroke, you're at higher risk for another one. Your risk of having a repeat stroke is the highest right after a stroke. A TIA also increases your risk of having a stroke, as does having a family history of stroke.

- **Brain aneurysms or AVMs.** Aneurysms are balloon-like bulges in an artery that can stretch and burst. AVMs are tangles of faulty arteries and veins that can rupture (break open) within the brain. AVMs may be present at birth, but often aren't diagnosed until they rupture.

Other risk factors for stroke, many of which of you can control, include:

- Alcohol and illegal drug use, including cocaine, amphetamines, and other drugs
- Certain medical conditions, such as sickle cell disease, vasculitis (inflammation of the blood vessels), and bleeding disorders
- Lack of physical activity
- Overweight and obesity
- Stress and depression
- Unhealthy cholesterol levels
- Unhealthy diet
- Use of nonsteroidal anti-inflammatory drugs (NSAIDs), but not aspirin, may increase the risk of heart attack or stroke, particularly in patients who have had a heart attack or cardiac bypass surgery. The risk may increase the longer NSAIDs are used. Common NSAIDs include ibuprofen and naproxen.

Following a heart-healthy lifestyle can lower the risk of stroke. Some people also may need to take medicines to lower their risk. Sometimes strokes can occur in people who don't have any known risk factors.

What Are the Signs and Symptoms of a Stroke?

The signs and symptoms of a stroke often develop quickly. However, they can develop over hours or even days. The type of symptoms depends on the type of stroke and the area of the brain that's affected. How long symptoms last and how severe they are vary among different people.

Signs and symptoms of a stroke may include:

- Sudden weakness

- Paralysis (an inability to move) or numbness of the face, arms, or legs, especially on one side of the body

- Confusion

- Trouble speaking or understanding speech

- Trouble seeing in one or both eyes

- Problems breathing

- Dizziness, trouble walking, loss of balance or coordination, and unexplained falls

- Loss of consciousness

- Sudden and severe headache

A TIA has the same signs and symptoms as a stroke. However, TIA symptoms usually last less than 1–2 hours (although they may last up to 24 hours). A TIA may occur only once in a person's lifetime or more often.

At first, it may not be possible to tell whether someone is having a TIA or stroke. All stroke-like symptoms require medical care.

If you think you or someone else is having a TIA or stroke, call 9-1-1 right away. Do not drive to the hospital or let someone else drive you. Call an ambulance so that medical personnel can begin life-saving treatment on the way to the emergency room. During a stroke, every minute counts.

What Are Stroke Complications?

After you've had a stroke, you may develop other complications, such as:

- **Blood clots and muscle weakness.** Being immobile (unable to move around) for a long time can raise your risk of developing blood clots in the deep veins of the legs. Being immobile also can lead to muscle weakness and decreased muscle flexibility.

- **Problems swallowing and pneumonia.** If a stroke affects the muscles used for swallowing, you may have a hard time eating or drinking. You also may be at risk of inhaling food or drink into your lungs. If this happens, you may develop pneumonia.

- **Loss of bladder control.** Some strokes affect the muscles used to urinate. You may need a urinary catheter (a tube placed into the bladder) until you can urinate on your own. Use of these catheters can lead to urinary tract infections. Loss of bowel control or constipation also may occur after a stroke.

How Is a Stroke Diagnosed?

Your doctor will diagnose a stroke based on your signs and symptoms, your medical history, a physical exam, and test results. Your doctor will want to find out the type of stroke you've had, its cause, the part of the brain that's affected, and whether you have bleeding in the brain.

If your doctor thinks you've had a TIA, he or she will look for its cause to help prevent a future stroke.

Medical History and Physical Exam

Your doctor will ask you or a family member about your risk factors for stroke. Examples of risk factors include high blood pressure, smoking, heart disease, and a personal or family history of stroke. Your doctor also will ask about your signs and symptoms and when they began.

During the physical exam, your doctor will check your mental alertness and your coordination and balance. He or she will check for numbness or weakness in your face, arms, and legs; confusion; and trouble speaking and seeing clearly.

Your doctor will look for signs of carotid artery disease, a common cause of ischemic stroke. He or she will listen to your carotid arteries with a stethoscope. A whooshing sound called a bruit may suggest changed or reduced blood flow due to plaque buildup in the carotid arteries.

Diagnostic Tests and Procedures

Your doctor may recommend one or more of the following tests to diagnose a stroke or TIA.

Brain Computed Tomography

A brain computed tomography scan, or brain CT scan, is a painless test that uses X-rays to take clear, detailed pictures of your brain. This test often is done right after a stroke is suspected. A brain CT scan can show bleeding in the brain or damage to the brain cells from a stroke. The test also can show other brain conditions that may be causing your symptoms.

Magnetic Resonance Imaging

Magnetic resonance imaging (MRI) uses magnets and radio waves to create pictures of the organs and structures in your body. This test can detect changes in brain tissue and damage to brain cells from a stroke. An MRI may be used instead of, or in addition to, a CT scan to diagnose a stroke.

Computed Tomography Arteriogram and Magnetic Resonance Arteriogram

A CT arteriogram (CTA) and magnetic resonance arteriogram (MRA) can show the large blood vessels in the brain. These tests may give your doctor more information about the site of a blood clot and the flow of blood through your brain.

Carotid Ultrasound

Carotid ultrasound is a painless and harmless test that uses sound waves to create pictures of the insides of your carotid arteries. These arteries supply oxygen-rich blood to your brain. Carotid ultrasound shows whether plaque has narrowed or blocked your carotid arteries. Your carotid ultrasound test may include a Doppler ultrasound. Doppler ultrasound is a special test that shows the speed and direction of blood moving through your blood vessels.

Carotid Angiography

Carotid angiography is a test that uses dye and special X-rays to show the insides of your carotid arteries. For this test, a small tube called a catheter is put into an artery, usually in the groin (upper thigh). The tube is then moved up into one of your carotid arteries. Your doctor will inject a substance (called contrast dye) into the carotid artery. The dye helps make the artery visible on X-ray pictures.

Heart Tests

Electrocardiogram (EKG)

An EKG is a simple, painless test that records the heart's electrical activity. The test shows how fast the heart is beating and its rhythm (steady or irregular). An EKG also records the strength and timing of electrical signals as they pass through each part of the heart. An EKG can help detect heart problems that may have led to a stroke.

For example, the test can help diagnose atrial fibrillation or a previous heart attack.

Echocardiography

Echocardiography, or echo, is a painless test that uses sound waves to create pictures of your heart. The test gives information about the size and shape of your heart and how well your heart's chambers and valves are working. Echo can detect possible blood clots inside the heart and problems with the aorta. The aorta is the main artery that carries oxygen-rich blood from your heart to all parts of your body.

Blood Tests

Your doctor also may use blood tests to help diagnose a stroke. A blood glucose test measures the amount of glucose (sugar) in your blood. Low blood glucose levels may cause symptoms similar to those of a stroke. A platelet count measures the number of platelets in your blood. Blood platelets are cell fragments that help your blood clot. Abnormal platelet levels may be a sign of a bleeding disorder (not enough clotting) or a thrombotic disorder (too much clotting).

Your doctor also may recommend blood tests to measure how long it takes for your blood to clot. Two tests that may be used are called Prothrombin Time (PT) and Partial Thromboplastin Time (PTT) tests. These tests show whether your blood is clotting normally.

How Is a Stroke Treated?

Treatment for a stroke depends on whether it is ischemic or hemorrhagic. Treatment for a TIA depends on its cause, how much time has passed since symptoms began, and whether you have other medical conditions.

Strokes and TIAs are medical emergencies. If you have stroke symptoms, call 9-1-1 right away. Do not drive to the hospital or let someone else drive you. Call an ambulance so that medical personnel can begin lifesaving treatment on the way to the emergency room. During a stroke, every minute counts.

Once you receive immediate treatment, your doctor will try to treat your stroke risk factors and prevent complications by recommending heart-healthy lifestyle changes.

Treating an Ischemic Stroke or Transient Ischemic Attack

An ischemic stroke or TIA occurs if an artery that supplies oxygen-rich blood to the brain becomes blocked. Often, blood clots cause the blockages that lead to ischemic strokes and TIAs. Treatment for an ischemic stroke or TIA may include medicines and medical procedures.

Medicines

If you have a stroke caused by a blood clot, you may be given a clot-dissolving, or clot-busting, medication called tissue plasminogen activator (tPA). A doctor will inject tPA into a vein in your arm. This type of medication must be given within 4 hours of symptom onset. Ideally, it should be given as soon as possible. The sooner treatment begins, the better your chances of recovery. Thus, it's important to know the signs and symptoms of a stroke and to call 9-1-1 right away for emergency care.

If you can't have tPA for medical reasons, your doctor may give you antiplatelet medicine that helps stop platelets from clumping together to form blood clots or anticoagulant medicine (blood thinner) that keeps existing blood clots from getting larger. Two common medicines are aspirin and clopidogrel.

Medical Procedures

If you have carotid artery disease, your doctor may recommend a carotid endarterectomy or carotid artery angioplasty. Both procedures open blocked carotid arteries.

Researchers are testing other treatments for ischemic stroke, such as intra-arterial thrombolysis and mechanical clot removal in cerebral ischemia (MERCI).

In intra-arterial thrombolysis, a long flexible tube called a catheter is put into your groin (upper thigh) and threaded to the tiny arteries of the brain. Your doctor can deliver medicine through this catheter to break up a blood clot in the brain.

MERCI is a device that can remove blood clots from an artery. During the procedure, a catheter is threaded through a carotid artery to the affected artery in the brain. The device is then used to pull the blood clot out through the catheter.

Treating a Hemorrhagic Stroke

A hemorrhagic stroke occurs if an artery in the brain leaks blood or ruptures. The first steps in treating a hemorrhagic stroke are to find the cause of bleeding in the brain and then control it. Unlike ischemic strokes, hemorrhagic strokes aren't treated with antiplatelet medicines and blood thinners because these medicines can make bleeding worse.

If you're taking antiplatelet medicines or blood thinners and have a hemorrhagic stroke, you'll be taken off the medicine. If high blood pressure is the cause of bleeding in the brain, your doctor may prescribe medicines to lower your blood pressure. This can help prevent further bleeding.

Surgery also may be needed to treat a hemorrhagic stroke. The types of surgery used include aneurysm clipping, coil embolization, and AVM repair.

Aneurysm Clipping and Coil Embolization

If an aneurysm (a balloon-like bulge in an artery) is the cause of a stroke, your doctor may recommend aneurysm clipping or coil embolization.

Aneurysm clipping is done to block off the aneurysm from the blood vessels in the brain. This surgery helps prevent further leaking of blood from the aneurysm. It also can help prevent the aneurysm from bursting again. During the procedure, a surgeon will make an incision (cut) in the brain and place a tiny clamp at the base of the aneurysm. You'll be given medicine to make you sleep during the surgery. After the surgery, you'll need to stay in the hospital's intensive care unit for a few days.

Coil embolization is a less complex procedure for treating an aneurysm. The surgeon will insert a tube called a catheter into an artery in the groin. He or she will thread the tube to the site of the aneurysm. Then, a tiny coil will be pushed through the tube and into the aneurysm. The coil will cause a blood clot to form, which will block blood flow through the aneurysm and prevent it from bursting again. Coil embolization is done in a hospital. You'll be given medicine to make you sleep during the surgery.

Arteriovenous Malformation Repair

If an AVM is the cause of a stroke, your doctor may recommend an AVM repair. (An AVM is a tangle of faulty arteries and veins that can rupture within the brain.) AVM repair helps prevent further bleeding in the brain.

Doctors use several methods to repair AVMs. These methods include:

• Injecting a substance into the blood vessels of the AVM to block blood flow

- Surgery to remove the AVM
- Using radiation to shrink the blood vessels of the AVM

Treating Stroke Risk Factors

After initial treatment for a stroke or TIA, your doctor will treat your risk factors. He or she may recommend heart-healthy lifestyle changes to help control your risk factors.

Heart-healthy lifestyle changes may include:

- Heart-healthy eating
- Aiming for a healthy weight
- Managing stress
- Physical activity
- Quitting smoking

If heart-healthy lifestyle changes aren't enough, you may need medicine to control your risk factors.

How Can a Stroke Be Prevented?

Taking action to control your risk factors can help prevent or delay a stroke. If you've already had a stroke. Talk to your doctor about whether you may benefit from aspirin primary prevention, or using aspirin to help prevent your first stroke. The following heart-healthy lifestyle changes can help prevent your first stroke and help prevent you from having another one.

- **Be physically active.** Physical activity can improve your fitness level and health. Talk with your doctor about what types and amounts of activity are safe for you.

- **Don't smoke, or if you smoke or use tobacco, quit.** Smoking can damage and tighten blood vessels and raise your risk of stroke. Talk with your doctor about programs and products that can help you quit. Also, secondhand smoke can damage the blood vessels.

- **Aim for a healthy weight.** If you're overweight or obese, work with your doctor to create a reasonable weight-loss plan. Controlling your weight helps you control risk factors for stroke.

- **Make heart-healthy eating choices.** Heart-healthy eating can help lower your risk or prevent a stroke.

- **Manage stress.** Use techniques to lower your stress levels.

If you or someone in your family has had a stroke, be sure to tell your doctor. By knowing your family history of stroke, you may be able to lower your risk factors and prevent or delay a stroke. If you've had a TIA, don't ignore it. TIAs are warnings, and it's important for your doctor to find the cause of the TIA so you can take steps to prevent a stroke.

Life after a Stroke

The time it takes to recover from a stroke varies—it can take weeks, months, or even years. Some people recover fully, while others have long-term or lifelong disabilities.

Ongoing care, rehabilitation, and emotional support can help you recover and may even help prevent another stroke.

If you've had a stroke, you're at risk of having another one. Know the warning signs and what to do if a stroke or TIA occurs. Call 9-1-1 as soon as symptoms start.

Do not drive to the hospital or let someone else drive you. By calling an ambulance, medical personnel can begin lifesaving treatment on the way to the emergency room. During a stroke, every minute counts.

Ongoing Care

Heart-Healthy Lifestyle Changes

Heart-healthy lifestyle changes can help you recover from a stroke and may help prevent another one. Examples of these changes include heart-healthy eating, aiming for a healthy weight, managing stress, physical activity, and quitting smoking.

Medicines

Your doctor also may prescribe medicines to help you recover from a stroke or control your stroke risk factors. Take all of your medicines as your doctor prescribes. Don't cut back on the dosage unless your doctor tells you to do so. If you have side effects or other problems related to your medicines, talk with your doctor.

Medicines called anticoagulants or blood thinners, which prevent blood clots or keep existing blood clots from getting larger, are the main treatment for people who have known carotid artery disease, which can lead to a stroke. Two common medicines are aspirin and clopidogrel.

You'll likely need routine blood tests to check how well these medicines are working.

The most common side effect of blood thinners is bleeding. This happens if the medicine thins your blood too much. This side effect can be life-threatening. Bleeding can occur inside your body cavities (internal bleeding) or from the surface of your skin (external bleeding).

Know the warning signs of bleeding so you can get help right away. They include:

- Blood in your urine, bright red blood in your stools, or black tarry stools

- Bright red vomit or vomit that looks like coffee grounds

- Increased menstrual flow

- Pain in your abdomen or severe pain in your head

- Unexplained bleeding from the gums and nose

- Unexplained bruising or tiny red or purple dots on the skin

A lot of bleeding after a fall or injury or easy bruising or bleeding also may mean that your blood is too thin. Call your doctor right away if you have any of these signs. If you have severe bleeding, call 9-1-1.

Your doctor also may discuss beginning statin treatment. Doctors recommend statin medications for many people because they help lower or control blood cholesterol levels and decrease the chance for stroke and heart attack. Doctors usually prescribe statins for people who have:

- Diabetes

- Heart disease or have had a stroke

- High low-density lipoprotein (LDL) cholesterol levels

You should still follow a heart-healthy lifestyle, even if you take medicines to control your risk factors for stroke. Take all medicines regularly, as your doctor prescribes. Don't change the amount of your medicine or skip a dose unless your doctor tells you to.

Talk with your doctor about how often you should schedule follow-up visits or tests. These visits and tests can help your doctor monitor your stroke risk factors and adjust your treatment as needed.

Rehabilitation

After a stroke, you may need rehabilitation (rehab) to help you recover. Rehab may include working with speech, physical, and occupational therapists.

Language, Speech, and Memory

You may have trouble communicating after a stroke. You may not be able to find the right words, put complete sentences together, or put words together in a way that makes sense. You also may have problems with your memory and thinking clearly. These problems can be very frustrating.

Speech and language therapists can help you learn ways to communicate again and improve your memory.

Muscle and Nerve Problems

A stroke may affect only one side of the body or part of one side. It can cause paralysis (an inability to move) or muscle weakness, which can put you at risk for falling. Physical and occupational therapists can help you strengthen and stretch your muscles. They also can help you relearn how to do daily activities, such as dressing, eating, and bathing.

Bladder and Bowel Problems

A stroke can affect the muscles and nerves that control the bladder and bowels. You may feel like you have to urinate often, even if your bladder isn't full. You may not be able to get to the bathroom in time. Medicines and a bladder or bowel specialist can help with these problems.

Swallowing and Eating Problems

You may have trouble swallowing after a stroke. Signs of this problem are coughing or choking during eating or coughing up food after eating. A speech therapist can help you with these issues. He or she may suggest changes to your diet, such as eating puréed (finely chopped) foods or drinking thick liquids.

Mental Healthcare and Support

After a stroke, you may have changes in your behavior or judgment. For example, your mood may change quickly. Because of these and other changes, you may feel scared, anxious, and depressed. Recovering from a stroke can be slow and frustrating.

Talk about how you feel with your healthcare team. Talking to a professional counselor also can help. If you're very depressed, your doctor may recommend medicines or other treatments that can improve your quality of life.

Joining a patient support group may help you adjust to life after a stroke. You can see how other people have coped with having strokes. Talk with your doctor about local support groups, or check with an area medical center.

Support from family and friends also can help relieve fear and anxiety. Let your loved ones know how you feel and what they can do to help you.

Stroke in United States

Stroke is a leading cause of serious, long-term adult disability. Four million Americans are living with the effects of stroke. The length of time to recover from a stroke depends on its severity. Fifty to 70 percent of stroke survivors regain functional independence, but 15 to 30 percent are permanently disabled.

Cost of Stroke

Stroke places a major health burden on our society in terms of mortality, morbidity, and economic costs. The National Stroke Association estimates stroke costs the United States about $43 billion a year. Direct costs for medical care and therapy average $28 billion a year. The average cost per patient for the first 90 days after a stroke is $15,000 although 10 percent of those cases exceed $35,000.

Chapter 2

Stroke Symptoms and What You Should Do If Someone Has Them

Symptoms of Stroke in Men and Women[1]

During a stroke, every minute counts! Fast treatm1ent can lessen the brain damage that stroke can cause. By knowing the signs and symptoms of stroke, you can take quick action and perhaps save a life—maybe even your own.

- Sudden numbness or weakness in the face, arm, or leg, especially on one side of the body

- Sudden confusion, trouble speaking, or difficulty understanding speech

- Sudden trouble seeing in one or both eyes

- Sudden trouble walking, dizziness, loss of balance, or lack of coordination

This chapter includes text excerpted from documents published by two public domain sources. Text under headings marked 1 are excerpted from "Stroke—Signs and Symptoms," Centers for Disease Control and Prevention (CDC), January 17, 2017; Text under heading marked 2 is excerpted from "Questions and Answers about Stroke," National Institute of Neurological Disorders and Stroke (NINDS), March 29, 2016.

- Sudden severe headache with no known cause

Call 9-1-1 right away if you or someone else has any of these symptoms.

What Should a Bystander Do?[1]

Acting F.A.S.T. can help stroke patients get the treatments they desperately need. The stroke treatments that work best are available only if the stroke is recognized and diagnosed within 3 hours of the first symptoms. Stroke patients may not be eligible for these if they don't arrive at the hospital in time.

If you think someone may be having a stroke, act F.A.S.T. and do the following simple test:

- **F—Face:** Ask the person to smile. Does one side of the face droop?

- **A—Arms:** Ask the person to raise both arms. Does one arm drift downward?

- **S—Speech:** Ask the person to repeat a simple phrase. Is the speech slurred or strange?

- **T—Time:** If you see any of these signs, call 9-1-1 right away.

Note the time when any symptoms first appear. This information helps healthcare providers determine the best treatment for each person. Do not drive to the hospital or let someone else drive you. Call an ambulance so that medical personnel can begin life-saving treatment on the way to the emergency room.

Act in Time[2]

Ischemic strokes, the most common strokes, can be treated with a drug called tPA which dissolves artery-obstructing clots. The window of opportunity to use tPA to treat stroke patients is three hours, but to be evaluated and receive treatment, patients need to get to the hospital within 60 minutes. A five-year clinical trial conducted by NINDS found that selected stroke patients who received tPA within three hours of the onset of stroke symptoms were at least 30 percent more likely than placebo patients to recover from their stroke with little or no disability after three months.

Treating a Transient Ischemic Attack (TIA)[1]

If your symptoms go away after a few minutes, you may have had a transient ischemic attack (TIA). Although brief, a TIA is a sign of a serious condition that will not go away without medical help.

Unfortunately, because TIAs clear up, many people ignore them. But paying attention to a TIA can save your life. Tell your healthcare team about your symptoms right away.

Risk Factors for Stroke[2]

There are things you can do to prevent stroke. High blood pressure increases your risk of stroke four to six times. Heart disease, especially a condition known as atrial fibrillation or AF, can double your risk of stroke. Your risk also increases if you smoke, have diabetes, sickle cell disease, high cholesterol, or a family history of stroke.

Chapter 3

Perinatal and Childhood Stroke

Perinatal Stroke

Perinatal stroke is defined as an acute syndrome due to cerebrovascular injury occurring from 20 weeks gestation to 28 days postnatal life. Specific disease states include arterial ischemic stroke, cerebral sinus venous thrombosis, arterial presumed perinatal ischemic stroke, periventricular venous infarction, and neonatal hemorrhagic stroke. The majority of affected children are born at term and about 15 percent are preterm. It is an important cause of chronic neurologic and cognitive disability including cerebral palsy, epilepsy, neuropsychological impairment, and behavioral disorders.

Perinatal stroke etiologies are often non-neurologic in nature and injury/repair processes rely on complex signaling in multiple cell types. Maternal and/or fetal /neonatal vascular, hemostatic, hematopoietic, and immune cell systems are of particular import as they are intricately involved in the origins and consequences of perinatal stroke.

This chapter contains text excerpted from the following sources: Text under the heading "Perinatal Stroke" is excerpted from "Perinatal Stroke (R01)," National Institutes of Health (NIH), September 23, 2016; Text under the heading "Childhood Stroke" is excerpted from "Recognition and Treatment of Stroke in Children," National Institute of Neurological Disorders and Stroke (NINDS), September 10, 2008. Reviewed April 2017.

Causes of Perinatal Stroke

Adult and perinatal stroke etiologies are different. Disorders such as hypertension, hyperlipidemia, and diabetes increase adult stroke risk. In contrast, perinatal stroke has been primarily linked to maternal, placental, and/or fetal and neonatal conditions. Complications of pregnancy, such as gestational diabetes, hypertension, and preeclampsia, have been associated with perinatal stroke, as has pregnancy's naturally occurring prothrombotic state. Placental pathologies such as poor perfusion or chorioamnionitis have also been implicated. Genetic prothrombotic factors in the newborn, congenital heart disease, and acute systemic illness and inflammation are among the conditions that increase risk. The impact of these states on the developing neurovascular unit and the mechanisms by which they increase stroke incidence have not been comprehensively investigated.

Perinatal Stroke Consequences

Perinatal stroke is an important cause of chronic neurologic and cognitive disability and, as problems often persist over a lifetime, is associated with a significant global burden of disease. The incidence is high, more than 1 in 3,000 live births, and similar to stroke incidence in the elderly. Underlying mechanisms of disease are poorly understood and as a consequence, there are few specific treatments, prevention strategies, and rehabilitative approaches for this disorder.

Childhood Stroke

Probably the most fundamental difference between cerebrovascular diseases in children and adults is the wide array of risk factors seen in children versus adults. Congenital heart disease and sickle cell disease, for example, are common causes of stroke in children, while atherosclerosis is rare in children. No cause can be detected in about a fifth of the children with ischemic infarction, yet many of these children seem to do well. The recognized causes of cerebrovascular disorders in children are numerous, and the probability of identifying the cause depends on the thoroughness of the evaluation. A probable cause of cerebral infarction was identified in 184 of 228 (79%) children in the Canadian Pediatric Ischemic Stroke Registry (CPISR). The source of an intracranial hemorrhage is even more likely to be found.

The most common cause of stroke in children is probably congenital or acquired heart disease. In the Canadian Pediatric Ischemic Stroke Registry, heart disease was found in 40 of 228 (19%) of the children with arterial thrombosis. Many of these children are already known to have heart disease prior to their stroke, but in other instances a less obvious cardiac lesion is discovered only after a stroke. Complex cardiac anomalies involving both the valves and chambers are collectively the biggest problem, but virtually any cardiac lesion can sometimes lead to a stroke. Of particular concern are cyanotic lesions with polycythemia, which increase the risk of both thrombosis and embolism.

Both the frequency and the cause of pediatric stroke may depend somewhat on both the geographic location and the specific hospital setting. The Canadian Pediatric Ischemic Stroke Registry, for example, lists only 5 children (2%) with cerebral infarction due to sickle cell anemia. A large metropolitan hospital in the United States might care for this many patients in a year, but early estimates that cerebral infarction occurred in 17 percent of people with sickle cell disease proved far higher than the 4–5 percent figure derived from more representative samples in Jamaica and in Africa.

Prehospital Emergency Care

Lack of general awareness of cerebrovascular disorders in children probably delays medical attention for children with cerebrovascular disorders. It is not unusual, for example, for children with a cerebral infarction to be brought to a physician several days after the onset of symptoms. In contrast, family members are usually well aware of the significance of an acute neurological impairment in older individuals, and these patients are typically seen by a physician earlier than children with a similar lesion.

Data from the Canadian Pediatric Ischemic Stroke Registry indicate that 48–72 hours often elapse between the onset of symptoms of arterial occlusion and a child's diagnosis. Venous occlusion was discovered a bit more quickly than arterial occlusion, at least in younger children, perhaps because of the common occurrence of epileptic seizures in children with venous thrombosis. This seems to be fairly typical of the pattern seen in the United States as well. The typical adult with a new onset neurological deficit from cerebrovascular disease undoubtedly sees a physician much sooner. It is likely that this delay in the diagnosis of children reflects a lack of awareness by both physicians and families that cerebrovascular disease occurs in children. To the extent that treatment might be improved by earlier evaluation and treatment, prompt recognition and treatment could improve management.

Treatment and Rehabilitation

No randomized controlled treatment trials have been completed in children with stroke; many of the procedures increasingly used in children with cerebrovascular disease have been adapted from studies in adults. Accumulating experience with antithrombotic and anticoagulant treatment in children suggests that these agents can be safely used in children, though their efficacy and proper dose still need to be established by controlled trials. Thrombolytic agents should be as effective in children as in adults, but the safety data are inadequate for children and the timing and dosage need to be determined for children and adolescents.

Chapter 4

Strokes in Women and Men

Chapter Contents

Section 4.1—Women and Stroke 30

Section 4.2—Contraceptive Use and Stroke Risk 33

Section 4.3—Menopausal Hormone Therapy (MHT)
and Stroke Risk 35

Section 4.4—Men and Stroke 38

Section 4.1

Women and Stroke

This section includes text excerpted from documents published
by two public domain sources. Text under headings marked 1 are
excerpted from "Women and Stroke," Centers for Disease Control
and Prevention (CDC), October 30, 2015; Text under heading marked
2 is excerpted from "Stroke: Hope through Research," *Know Stroke*,
National Institute of Neurological Disorders and Stroke (NINDS),
November 23, 2016.

Stroke in Women[1]

One in five women in the United States will have a stroke in her
lifetime. Nearly 60 percent of stroke deaths are in women, and stroke
kills twice as many women as breast cancer. Surprised? You're not
alone. Stroke is the third leading cause of death for women, yet most
women do not know their risk of having a stroke. These facts are
alarming, but there is some good news: Up to 80 percent of strokes can
be prevented. This means it is important to know your risk of having
a stroke and to take action to reduce that risk.

What Is a Stroke?[1]

A stroke, sometimes called a brain attack, occurs when blood flow to
an area of the brain is cut off. When brain cells are starved of oxygen,
they die. Stroke is a medical emergency. It's important to get treatment as soon as possible. A delay in treatment increases the risk of
permanent brain damage or death.

Common Risk Factors for Stroke[1]

- **High blood pressure** is a main risk factor for stroke, yet nearly
  one in three women with high blood pressure does not know she
  has it.

- Stroke risk increases with **age**, and women live longer than
  men. This is why 6 in 10 people who die from stroke are women.
  Also, the percentage of strokes in women aged 45 or younger

is increasing. Younger women may have different symptoms of stroke, such as dizziness or headache, than women age 46 and older do.

• Women are twice as likely as men to experience depression and anxiety, and women often report higher stress levels than men do. These **mental health issues** all raise a person's risk for stroke.

Not all women are equally affected by stroke. African-American women are nearly twice as likely to have a stroke as white women, mainly because of having high blood pressure, being overweight, and having diabetes.

Pregnancy and Childbirth Related Risk Factors[2]

Some risk factors for stroke apply only to women. Primary among these are pregnancy, childbirth, and menopause. These risk factors are tied to hormonal fluctuations and changes that affect a woman in different stages of life. Research in the past few decades has shown that high-dose oral contraceptives, the kind used in the 1960s and 1970s, can increase the risk of stroke in women. Fortunately, oral contraceptives with high doses of estrogen are no longer used and have been replaced with safer and more effective oral contraceptives with lower doses of estrogen. Some studies have shown the newer low-dose oral contraceptives may not significantly increase the risk of stroke in women.

Other studies have demonstrated that pregnancy and childbirth can put a woman at an increased risk for stroke. Pregnancy increases the risk of stroke as much as three to 13 times. Of course, the risk of stroke in young women of childbearing years is very small to begin with, so a moderate increase in risk during pregnancy is still a relatively small risk. Pregnancy and childbirth cause strokes in approximately eight in 100,000 women. Unfortunately, 25 percent of strokes during pregnancy end in death, and hemorrhagic strokes, although rare, are still the leading cause of maternal death in the United States. Subarachnoid hemorrhage, in particular, causes one to five maternal deaths per 10,000 pregnancies.

A study sponsored by the National Institute of Neurological Disorders and Stroke (NINDS) showed that the risk of stroke during pregnancy is greatest in the postpartum period—the 6 weeks following childbirth. The risk of ischemic stroke after pregnancy is about nine times higher and the risk of hemorrhagic stroke is more than 28 times higher for postpartum women than for women who are not pregnant or postpartum. The cause is unknown.

In the same way that the hormonal changes during pregnancy and childbirth are associated with increased risk of stroke, hormonal changes at the end of the childbearing years can increase the risk of stroke. Several studies have shown that menopause, the end of a woman's reproductive ability marked by the termination of her menstrual cycle, can increase a woman's risk of stroke. Fortunately, some studies have suggested that hormone replacement therapy can reduce some of the effects of menopause and decrease stroke risk.

How Can I Prevent Stroke?[1]

Most strokes can be prevented by keeping medical conditions under control and making lifestyle changes. A good place to start is to know your ABCS of heart health:

- **Aspirin:** Aspirin may help reduce your risk for stroke. But you should check with your doctor before taking aspirin because it can make some types of stroke worse. Before taking aspirin, talk with your doctor about whether aspirin is right for you.

- **Blood Pressure:** Control your blood pressure.

- **Cholesterol:** Manage your cholesterol.

- **Smoking:** Quit smoking or don't start.

  Make lifestyle changes:

- **Eat healthy and stay active.** Choose healthy foods most of the time, including foods with less salt, or sodium, to lower your blood pressure, and get regular exercise. Being overweight or obese raises your risk of stroke.

- **Talk to your doctor about your chances of having a stroke,** including your age and whether anyone in your family has had a stroke.

- **Get other health conditions under control,** such as diabetes or heart disease.

Section 4.2

Contraceptive Use and Stroke Risk

This section contains text excerpted from the following sources:
Text under the heading "Birth Control Methods" is excerpted from
"Birth Control Methods," Office on Women's Health (OWH), U.S.
Department of Health and Human Services (HHS), October 15, 2015;
Text beginning with the heading "Does Taking Birth Control Pills
Increase My Risk for Stroke?" is excerpted from "Stroke Fact Sheet,"
Office on Women's Health (OWH), U.S. Department of Health and
Human Services (HHS), July 16, 2012. Reviewed April 2017.

Birth Control Methods

Birth control (contraception) is any method, medicine, or device
used to prevent pregnancy. Women can choose from many different
types of birth control. Some work better than others at preventing
pregnancy. The type of birth control you use depends on your health,
your desire to have children now or in the future, and your need to
prevent sexually transmitted infections. Your doctor can help you
decide which type is best for you right now.

Combination birth control pills (birth control with both estrogen
and progesterone) and some other forms of hormonal birth control,
such as the vaginal ring or skin patch, may raise your risk for blood
clots and high blood pressure. Blood clots and high blood pressure can
cause a stroke or heart attack. A blood clot in the legs can also go to
your lungs, causing serious damage or even death. These are serious
side effects of hormonal birth control, but they are rare.

Does Taking Birth Control Pills Increase My Risk for Stroke?

Taking birth control pills is generally safe for young, healthy
women. But birth control pills can raise the risk of stroke for some
women, especially women over 35; women with high blood pressure,
diabetes, or high cholesterol; and women who smoke. Talk with your
doctor if you have questions about the pill.

If you are taking birth control pills, and you have any of the symptoms listed below, call 9-1-1:

- Eye problems such as blurred or double vision

- Pain in the upper body or arm

- Bad headaches

- Problems breathing

- Spitting up blood

- Swelling or pain in the leg

- Yellowing of the skin or eyes

- Breast lumps

- Unusual (not normal) heavy bleeding from your vagina

Does Using the Birth Control Patch Increase My Risk for Stroke?

The patch is generally safe for young, healthy women. The patch can raise the risk of stroke for some women, especially women over 35; women with high blood pressure, diabetes, or high cholesterol; and women who smoke.

Studies show that women who use the patch may be exposed to more estrogen (the female hormone in birth control pills and the patch that keeps users from becoming pregnant) than women who use the birth control pill. Research is underway to see if the risk for blood clots (which can lead to stroke or heart attack) is higher in patch users. Talk with your doctor if you have questions about the patch.

How Is Stroke Treated?

Strokes caused by blood clots can be treated with clot-busting drugs such as tPA, or tissue plasminogen activator. tPA must be given within three hours of the start of a stroke to work, and tests must be done first. This is why it is so important for a person having a stroke to get to a hospital fast.

Other medicines are used to treat and to prevent stroke. Anticoagulants, such as warfarin, and antiplatelet agents, such as aspirin, block the blood's ability to clot and can help prevent a stroke in patients with high risk, such as a person who has atrial fibrillation (a kind of irregular heartbeat).

Surgery is sometimes used to treat or prevent stroke. Carotid end-arterectomy is a surgery to remove fatty deposits clogging the carotid artery in the neck, which could lead to a stroke. For hemorrhagic stroke, a doctor may perform surgery to place a metal clip at the base of an aneurysm (a thin or weak spot in an artery that balloons out and can burst) or remove abnormal blood vessels.

Section 4.3

Menopausal Hormone Therapy (MHT) and Stroke Risk

This section contains text excerpted from the following sources: Text in this section begins with excerpts from "Menopausal Hormone Therapy and Cancer," National Cancer Institute (NCI), December 5, 2011. Reviewed April 2017; Text under the heading "Effects of Menopausal Hormone Therapy (MHT)" is excerpted from "Menopausal Hormone Therapy (MHT)," Office on Women's Health (OWH), U.S. Department of Health and Human Services (HHS), September 22, 2010. Reviewed April 2017.

Menopausal hormone therapy (MHT) is a treatment that doctors may recommend to relieve common symptoms of menopause and to address long-term biological changes, such as bone loss, that result from declining levels of the natural hormones estrogen and progesterone in a woman's body during and after the completion of menopause.

MHT usually involves treatment with estrogen alone, estrogen plus progesterone, or estrogen plus progestin, which is a synthetic hormone with effects similar to those of progesterone. Women who have had a hysterectomy are generally prescribed estrogen alone. Women who have not had this surgery are prescribed estrogen plus progestin, because estrogen alone is associated with an increased risk of endometrial cancer, whereas research has suggested that estrogen plus progestin may not be.

Effects of Menopausal Hormone Therapy (MHT)

Some women can use menopausal hormone therapy (MHT) to help control the symptoms of menopause. MHT, which used to be called hormone replacement therapy (HRT), involves taking the hormones estrogen and progesterone. (Women who don't have a uterus anymore take just estrogen.)

MHT can be very good at helping with moderate to severe symptoms of the menopausal transition and preventing bone loss. But MHT also has some risks, especially if used for a long time.

MHT can help with menopause by:

- Reducing hot flashes, night sweats, and related problems such as poor sleep and irritability

- Treating vaginal symptoms, such as dryness and discomfort, and related effects, such as pain during sex

- Slowing bone loss

- Possibly easing mood swings and mild depressive symptoms (MHT is not an antidepressant medication—talk to your doctor if you are having signs of depression.)

For some women, MHT may increase their chances of:

- Stroke
- Blood clots
- Heart attack
- Breast cancer
- Gallbladder disease

Research into the risks and benefits of MHT continues. For example, a study suggests that the low-dose patch form of MHT may not have the possible risk of stroke that other forms can have. Talk with your doctor about the positives and negatives of MHT based on your medical history and age. Keep in mind, too, that you may have symptoms when you stop MHT. You also can talk with your doctor about treatments other than MHT that can help deal with specific symptoms or prevent bone loss.

Keep in mind when considering MHT that:

- Once a woman reaches menopause, MHT is recommended only as a short-term treatment.

- Doctors very rarely recommend MHT to prevent certain chronic diseases like osteoporosis.
- Women who have gone through menopause should not take MHT to prevent heart disease.
- MHT should not be used to prevent memory loss, dementia, or Alzheimer disease.

You should not use menopausal hormone therapy (MHT) if you:

- Have had a stroke
- Have had a heart attack
- Have had blood clots
- May be pregnant
- Have problems with vaginal bleeding
- Have had certain kinds of cancers (such as breast and uterine cancer)
- Have liver disease
- Have heart disease

If you choose MHT, experts recommend that you:

- Use it at the lowest dose that helps
- Use it for the shortest time needed

MHT can cause side effects. Call your doctor if you develop any of these problems:

- Vaginal bleeding
- Bloating
- Breast tenderness or swelling
- Headaches
- Mood changes
- Nausea

Section 4.4

Men and Stroke

This section includes text excerpted from "Men and Stroke," Centers for Disease Control and Prevention (CDC), October 29, 2015.

Stroke is the fifth leading cause of death in men, killing almost the same number of men each year as prostate cancer and Alzheimer disease combined. Stroke is a leading cause of long-term disability among American men. In addition, men have strokes at younger ages than women. These facts are alarming, but there is some good news: Up to 80 percent of strokes can be prevented. This means it is important to know your risk of having a stroke and taking action to reduce that risk.

What Is a Stroke?

A stroke, sometimes called a brain attack, occurs when blood flow to an area of the brain is cut off. When brain cells are starved of oxygen, they die. Stroke is a medical emergency. It's important to get treatment as soon as possible. A delay in treatment increases the risk of permanent brain damage or death.

What Puts Men at Risk of Stroke?

- High blood pressure is a main risk factor for stroke, yet nearly one in three men with high blood pressure does not know he has it.

- Smoking damages blood vessels, which can cause a stroke. Men are more likely to be smokers than women.

- Being overweight or obese increases your risk of stroke. Almost 3 in 4 American men are in weight ranges that increase their risk for stroke.

- More men than women have been diagnosed with diabetes, which increases your risk of stroke because it can cause disease of blood vessels in the brain.

- Men are more likely than women to drink too much alcohol, increasing the risk for stroke.

- Being inactive can increase the risk of stroke. Only 1 in 4 men gets enough physical activity, even though exercising only 30 minutes a day can decrease the risk of stroke.

How Can I Prevent Stroke?

Most strokes can be prevented by keeping medical conditions under control and making lifestyle changes. A good place to start is to know your ABCS of heart health:

- **Aspirin:** Aspirin may help reduce your risk for stroke. But you should check with your doctor before taking aspirin because it can make some types of stroke worse. Before taking aspirin, talk with your doctor about whether aspirin is right for you.

- **Blood Pressure:** Control your blood pressure.

- **Cholesterol:** Manage your cholesterol.

- **Smoking:** Quit smoking or don't start.

Make lifestyle changes:

- **Eat healthy and stay active.** Choose healthy foods most of the time, including foods with less salt, or sodium, to lower your blood pressure, and get regular exercise. Being overweight or obese raises your risk of stroke.

- **Talk to your doctor about your risk factors for stroke,** including your age and whether anyone in your family has had a stroke.

- **Get other health conditions under control,** such as diabetes or heart disease.

Chapter 5

Strokes in Older Adults

Stroke[1]

A stroke is sometimes called a "brain attack." Most often, stroke occurs when blood flow to the brain stops because it is blocked by a clot. When this happens, the brain cells in the immediate area begin to die.

Some brain cells die because they stop getting the oxygen and nutrients they need to function. Other brain cells die because they are damaged by sudden bleeding into or around the brain. The brain cells that don't die immediately remain at risk for death. These cells can linger in a compromised or weakened state for several hours. With timely treatment, these cells can be saved.

New treatments are available that greatly reduce the damage caused by a stroke. But you need to arrive at the hospital as soon as possible after symptoms start to prevent disability and to greatly improve your chances for recovery. Knowing stroke symptoms, calling 911 immediately, and getting to a hospital as quickly as possible are critical.

This chapter includes text excerpted from documents published by two public domain sources. Text under headings marked 1 are excerpted from "Stroke," NIHSeniorHealth, National Institute on Aging (NIA), February 2013. Reviewed April 2017; Text under heading marked 2 is excerpted from "Stroke Fact Sheet," Centers for Disease Control and Prevention (CDC), June 16, 2016.

Ischemic Stroke

There are two kinds of stroke. The most common kind of stroke is called ischemic stroke. It accounts for approximately 80 percent of all strokes. An ischemic stroke is caused by a blood clot that blocks or plugs a blood vessel supplying blood to the brain. Blockages that cause ischemic strokes stem from three conditions:

- The formation of a clot within a blood vessel of the brain or neck, called thrombosis.

- The movement of a clot from another part of the body, such as from the heart to the neck or brain, called an embolism.

- A severe narrowing of an artery (stenosis) in or leading to the brain, due to fatty deposits lining the blood vessel walls.

Hemorrhagic Stroke

The other kind of stroke is called hemorrhagic stroke. A hemorrhagic stroke is caused by a blood vessel that breaks and bleeds into the brain.

One common cause of a hemorrhagic stroke is a bleeding aneurysm. An aneurysm is a weak or thin spot on an artery wall. Over time, these weak spots stretch or balloon out due to high blood pressure. The thin walls of these ballooning aneurysms can rupture and spill blood into the space surrounding brain cells.

Artery walls can also break open because they become encrusted, or covered with fatty deposits called plaque, eventually lose their elasticity and become brittle, thin, and prone to cracking. Hypertension, or high blood pressure, increases the risk that a brittle artery wall will give way and release blood into the surrounding brain tissue.

Stroke Facts[2]

- Stroke is the fifth leading cause of death in the United States, killing more than 130,000 Americans each year—that's 1 of every 20 deaths.

- Someone in the United States has a stroke every 40 seconds. Every four minutes, someone dies of stroke.

- Every year, about 795,000 people in the United States have a stroke. About 610,000 of these are first or new strokes; 185,000 are recurrent strokes.

- Stroke is an important cause of disability. Stroke reduces mobility in more than half of stroke survivors age 65 and over.

- Stroke costs the nation $33 billion annually, including the cost of healthcare services, medications, and lost productivity.

- You can't control some stroke risk factors, like heredity, age, gender, and ethnicity. Some medical conditions—including high blood pressure, high cholesterol, heart disease, diabetes, overweight or obesity, and previous stroke or transient ischemic attack (TIA)—can also raise your stroke risk. Avoiding smoking and drinking too much alcohol, eating a balanced diet, and getting exercise are all choices you can make to reduce your risk.

Effects of a Stroke[1]

The brain is the most complex organ in the human body. It is the seat of intelligence, interpreter of the senses, initiator of all movement, and the controller of behavior. How a stroke affects us depends on which part of the brain is damaged.

Stroke damage in the brain can affect the entire body—resulting in mild to severe disabilities. These include paralysis, problems with thinking, trouble speaking, and emotional problems.

Movement Problems

A common disability that results from stroke is complete paralysis on one side of the body, called hemiplegia. A related disability that is not as debilitating as paralysis is one-sided weakness, or hemiparesis. The paralysis or weakness may affect only the face, an arm, or a leg, or it may affect one entire side of the body and face.

A stroke patient may have problems with the simplest of daily activities, such as walking, dressing, eating, and using the bathroom. Movement problems can result from damage to the part of the brain that controls balance and coordination. Some stroke patients also have trouble swallowing, called dysphagia.

Thinking Problems

Stroke may cause problems with thinking, awareness, attention, learning, judgment, and memory.

In some cases of stroke, the patient suffers a "neglect" syndrome. The neglect syndrome means that the stroke patient has no knowledge of one side of his or her body, or one side of the visual field, and is unaware of the problem. A stroke patient may be unaware of his or her surroundings, or may be unaware of the mental problems that resulted from the stroke.

Speech Problems

Stroke victims often have a problem forming or understanding speech. This problem is called aphasia. Aphasia usually occurs along with similar problems in reading and writing. In most people, language problems result from damage to the left hemisphere of the brain.

Slurred speech due to weakness or incoordination of the muscles involved in speaking is called dysarthria, and is not a problem with language. Because it can result from any weakness or incoordination of the speech muscles, dysarthria can arise from damage to either side of the brain.

Emotional Problems

A stroke can also lead to emotional problems. Stroke patients may have difficulty controlling their emotions or may express inappropriate emotions in certain situations. One common disability that occurs with many stroke patients is depression.

Poststroke depression may be more than a general sadness resulting from the stroke incident. It is a serious behavioral problem that can hamper recovery and rehabilitation and may even lead to suicide. Poststroke depression is treated as any depression is treated, with antidepressant medications and therapy.

Stroke patients may experience pain, uncomfortable numbness, or strange sensations after a stroke. These sensations may be due to many factors, including damage to the sensory regions of the brain, stiff joints, or a disabled limb.

Pain

An uncommon type of pain resulting from stroke is called central stroke pain or central pain syndrome or CPS. CPS results from damage to an area called the thalamus. The pain is a mixture of sensations, including heat and cold, burning, tingling, numbness, and sharp stabbing and underlying aching pain.

The pain is often worse in the hands and feet and is made worse by movement and temperature changes, especially cold temperatures. Unfortunately, since most pain medications provide little relief from these sensations, very few treatments or therapies exist to combat CPS.

Brainstem Stroke

The brainstem controls vital bodily functions such as breathing, blood pressure and heart beat. A stroke in the brainstem can be fatal or can leave someone in a "locked-in" state in which the person cannot control anything below the neck. As with other types of stroke, early treatment is crucial.

Prevention and Diagnosis[1]

Stroke is preventable and treatable. A better understanding of the causes of stroke has helped people make lifestyle changes that have cut the stroke death rate nearly in half in the last two decades.

Preventing Stroke

While family history of stroke plays a role in your risk, there are many risk factors you can control:

- **If you have high blood pressure,** work with your doctor to get it under control.

- **If you smoke,** quit.

- **If you have diabetes,** learn how to manage it. Many people do not realize they have diabetes, which is a major risk factor for heart disease and stroke.

- **If you are overweight,** start maintaining a healthy diet and exercising regularly.

- **If you have high cholesterol,** work with your doctor to lower it. A high level of total cholesterol in the blood is a major risk factor for heart disease, which raises your risk of stroke.

Diagnosing Stroke

Physicians have several diagnostic techniques and imaging tools to help diagnose stroke quickly and accurately. The first step in diagnosis is a short neurological examination, or an evaluation of the nervous system.

When a possible stroke patient arrives at a hospital, a health-care professional, usually a doctor or nurse, will ask the patient or a companion what happened and when the symptoms began. Blood tests, an electrocardiogram, and a brain scan such as computed tomography or CT, or magnetic resonance imaging or MRI, will often be done.

Measuring Stroke Severity

One test that helps doctors judge the severity of a stroke is the standardized NIH Stroke Scale, developed by the National Institute of Neurological Disorders and Stroke (NINDS) at the National Institutes of Health, or NIH. Healthcare professionals use the NIH Stroke Scale to measure a patient's neurological deficits by asking the patient to answer questions and to perform several physical and mental tests.

Other scales include the Glasgow Coma Scale, the Hunt and Hess Scale, the Modified Rankin Scale, and the Barthel Index.

Diagnostic Imaging: CT Scan

Healthcare professionals also use a variety of imaging techniques to evaluate acute stroke patients. The most widely used is computed tomography or CT scan, sometimes pronounced "CAT" scan, which is comprised of a series of cross-sectional images of the head and brain.

CT scans are sensitive for detecting hemorrhage and are therefore useful for differentiating hemorrhagic stroke, caused by bleeding in the brain, from ischemic stroke, caused by a blockage of blood flow to the brain.

Hemorrhage is the primary reason for avoiding thrombolytic therapy (drugs that break up or dissolve blood clots), the only proven therapy for acute ischemic stroke.

Because thrombolytic therapy might make a hemorrhagic stroke worse, doctors must confirm that the acute symptoms are not due to hemorrhage prior to giving the drug.

A CT scan may show evidence of early ischemia—an area of tissue that is dead or dying due to a loss of blood supply. Ischemic strokes generally show up on a CT scan about six to eight hours after the start of stroke symptoms. Though not as common in practice, CT scans also can be performed with a contrast agent to help visualize a blockage in the large arteries supplying the brain, or detect areas of decreased blood flow to the brain.

Because CT is readily available at all hours at most major hospitals, produces images quickly, and is good for ruling out hemorrhage prior to starting thrombolytic therapy, CT is the most widely used diagnostic imaging technique for acute stroke.

Diagnostic Imaging: MRI Scan

Another imaging technique used in acute stroke patients is the magnetic resonance imaging or MRI scan. MRI uses magnetic fields to detect a variety of changes in the brain and blood vessels caused by a stroke. One effect of ischemic stroke is the slowing of water movement through the injured brain tissue. Because MRI can show this type of injury very soon after stroke symptoms start, MRI has proven useful for diagnosing acute ischemic stroke before it is visible on CT. MRI also allows doctors to visualize blockages in the arteries, identify sites of prior stroke, and create a stroke treatment and prevention plan.

Medications[1]

With stroke, treatment depends on the stage of the disease. There are three treatment stages for stroke: prevention, therapy immediately after stroke, and rehabilitation after stroke. Stroke therapies include medications, surgery, and rehabilitation.

Medication or drug therapy is the most common treatment for stroke. The most popular kinds of drugs to prevent or treat stroke are antithrombotics—which include antiplatelet agents and anticoagulants—and thrombolytics.

Thrombolytics

In treating a stroke that has just occurred, every minute counts. Ischemic strokes—the most common kind—can be treated with thrombolytic drugs. These drugs halt the stroke by dissolving the blood clot that is blocking blood flow to the brain. But a person needs to be at the hospital as soon as possible after stroke symptoms start to be evaluated and receive treatment.

A thrombolytic drug known as tissue plasminogen activator (tPA) can be effective if a person receives it intravenously (in a vein) within 3 hours after his or her stroke symptoms have started. Because there is such a narrow time window for giving tPA, it is important to note the time any stroke symptoms appear. Since thrombolytic drugs can increase bleeding, tPA should be used only after the doctor is certain that the patient has suffered an ischemic and not a hemorrhagic stroke.

Antithrombotics

Antithrombotics prevent the formation of blood clots that can become stuck in an artery of the brain and cause strokes. Antiplatelet drugs prevent clotting by decreasing the activity of platelets, which are blood cells that help blood clot. By reducing the risk of blood clots, these drugs lower the risk of ischemic stroke.

In the case of stroke, doctors prescribe antiplatelet drugs mainly for prevention. The most widely known and used antiplatelet drug is aspirin. Other antiplatelet drugs include clopidogrel, ticlopidine, and dipyridamole.

Other Drugs

Anticoagulants reduce the risk of stroke by reducing the clotting property of the blood. The most commonly used oral anticoagulants include warfarin, also known as Coumadin®, dabigatran (Pradaxa) and rivaroxaban (Xarelto). Injectable anticoagulants include heparin, enoxaparin (Lovenox), and dalteparin (Fragmin).

Neuroprotectants are medications or other treatments that protect the brain from secondary injury caused by stroke. Although the U.S. Food and Drug Administration (FDA) has not approved any neuro-protectants for use in stroke at this time, many have been tested or are being tested in clinical trials. Cooling of the brain (hypothermia) is beneficial for improving neurological function after a cardiac arrest.

Rehabilitation after Stroke[1]

Stroke is the number one cause of serious adult disability in the United States. Stroke disability is devastating to the stroke patient and family, but therapies are available to help rehabilitate patients after stroke.

Physical Therapy

For most stroke patients, rehabilitation mainly involves physical therapy. The aim of physical therapy is to have the stroke patient relearn simple motor activities such as walking, sitting, standing, lying down, and the process of switching from one type of movement to another.

To achieve this, stroke patients work with physical therapists who use training, exercises, and physical manipulation of the stroke patient's body to restore movement, balance, and coordination.

Occupational Therapy

Another type of therapy to help patients relearn daily activities is occupational therapy. This type of therapy also involves exercise and training. Its goal is to help the stroke patient relearn everyday activities such as eating, drinking and swallowing, dressing, bathing, cooking, reading and writing, and toileting. Occupational therapists seek to help the patient become independent or semi-independent.

Speech Therapy

Speech and language problems arise when brain damage occurs in the language centers of the brain. Due to the brain's great ability to learn and change, which is called brain plasticity, other areas can adapt to take over some of the lost functions.

Speech therapy helps stroke patients relearn language and speaking skills, or learn other forms of communication. Speech therapy is appropriate for patients who have no problems with cognition or thinking, but have problems understanding speech or written words, or problems forming speech.

Besides helping with language skills, speech therapy also helps stroke patients develop coping skills to deal with the frustration of not being able to communicate fully. With time and patience, a stroke survivor should be able to regain some, and sometimes all, language and speaking abilities.

Therapy for Mental Health

Many stroke patients require psychological or psychiatric help after a stroke. Psychological problems such as depression, anxiety, frustration, and anger are common disabilities in people who have suffered a stroke.

Talk therapy, along with the right medication, can help ease some of the mental and emotional problems that result from stroke. Sometimes it is helpful for family members of the stroke patient to seek psychological help for themselves as well.

Chapter 6

Racial and Ethnic Stroke Disparities

African-American Women and Stroke

African-American women are more likely to have a stroke than any other group of women in the United States. African-American women are twice as likely to have a stroke as white women. They also are more likely to have strokes at younger ages and to have more severe strokes.

This chapter contains text excerpted from the following sources: Text under the heading "African-American Women and Stroke" is excerpted from "African-American Women and Stroke," Centers for Disease Control and Prevention (CDC), November 18, 2015; Text under the heading "African-American Men and Stroke" is excerpted from "African-American Men and Stroke," Centers for Disease Control and Prevention (CDC), November 18, 2015; Text under the heading "Hispanic Women and Stroke" is excerpted from "Hispanic Women and Stroke," Centers for Disease Control and Prevention (CDC), December 26, 2015; Text under the heading "Hispanic Men and Stroke" is excerpted from "Hispanic Men and Stroke," Centers for Disease Control and Prevention (CDC), December 26, 2015; Text under the heading "Asian Americans and Stroke" is excerpted from "Stroke and Asian Americans," Office of Minority Health (OMH), U.S. Department of Health and Human Services (HHS), November 19, 2015; Text under the heading "American Indian and Alaska Natives and Stroke" is excerpted from "American Indian and Alaska Native Heart Disease and Stroke Fact Sheet," Centers for Disease Control and Prevention (CDC), June 16, 2016.

Why Are African-American Women at Higher Risk?

- **High blood pressure,** a main risk factor for stroke, often starts at a younger age and is more severe in African-American women than in white women.

- Eating too much **salt or sodium** can raise your blood pressure, putting you at higher risk of stroke. Some researchers think African Americans may be more sensitive to the effects of salt, which in turn increases the risk for developing high blood pressure. African Americans should reduce their sodium intake to 1,500 milligrams per day.

- **Sickle cell anemia** is the most common genetic disorder in African Americans and can lead to a stroke. Strokes can occur when sickle-shaped cells block blood vessels to the brain.

- African-American women tend to have higher rates of **obesity and diabetes,** which increases the risk for high blood pressure and stroke.

As an African-American woman, you may have some of the health problems that can lead to a stroke without even knowing it.

African-American Men and Stroke

African-American men are at greater risk of having a stroke than any other group of men in the United States. Compared to white men, they are twice as likely to have a stroke, have strokes at younger ages, die from stroke, or have stroke-related disability that affects their daily activities.

Why are African-American Men at Higher Risk?

- Two out of five African-American men have **high blood pressure**—a main risk factor for stroke. High blood pressure often starts at a younger age and is more severe in African-American men than in white men. African-American men with high blood pressure are also less likely to have it under control.

- People with **diabetes** are at higher risk of stroke. One out of seven African-American men has been diagnosed with diabetes; and many more have the disease but do not know it.

- **Sickle cell anemia** is the most common genetic disorder in African Americans and can lead to a stroke. Strokes can occur when sickle-shaped cells block blood vessels to the brain.

- **Smoking** doubles your risk of stroke. About one out of five African-American men smokes cigarettes.

- Being **overweight** or obese increases your risk of stroke. Seventy percent of African-American men are overweight.

- **Eating too much salt**, or sodium, can raise your blood pressure, putting you at higher risk of stroke. Researchers think there may be a gene that makes African Americans more sensitive to the effects of salt, which in turn increases the risk of developing high blood pressure. African Americans should limit their sodium intake to 1,500 milligrams per day.

American Indians and Alaska Natives and Stroke

Heart disease is the leading cause of death among American Indians and Alaska Natives. In 2014, heart disease caused 3,288 deaths. Stroke is the seventh leading cause of death among American Indians and Alaska Natives. In 2014, stroke caused 649 deaths among American Indians and Alaska Natives. Heart disease and stroke are also major causes of disability and can decrease a person's quality of life.

- Heart disease is the first and stroke the sixth leading cause of death Among American Indians and Alaska Natives.

- The heart disease death rate was 20 percent greater and the stroke death rate 14 percent greater among American Indians and Alaska Natives (1996–1998) than among all U.S. races (1997) after adjusting for misreporting of American Indian and Alaska Native race on state death certificates.

- The highest heart disease death rates are located primarily in South Dakota and North Dakota, Wisconsin, and Michigan.

- Counties with the highest stroke death rates are primarily in Alaska, Washington, Idaho, Montana, Wyoming, South Dakota, Wisconsin, and Minnesota.

- American Indians and Alaska Natives die from heart diseases at younger ages than other racial and ethnic groups in the United States. Thirty–six percent of those who die of heart disease die before age 65.

- Diabetes is an extremely important risk factor for cardiovascular disease among American Indians.

- Cigarette smoking, a risk factor for heart disease and stroke, is highest in the Northern Plains (44.1%) and Alaska (39%) and lowest in the Southwest (21.2%) among American Indians and Alaska Natives.

Asian Americans and Stroke

Overall, Asians Americans adults are less likely than white adults to die from a stroke. In general, Asian Americans adults have lower rates of being overweight or obese, lower rates of hypertension, and they are less likely to be current cigarette smokers.

At a Glance—Diagnosed Cases of Stroke:

Table 6.1. Age-Adjusted Percentages of Stroke among Persons 18 Years of Age and Over, 2012

Asian	Non-Hispanic White	Asian/ Non-Hispanic White Ratio
1.8	2.4	0.8

Source: Summary Health Statistics for U.S. Adults: 2014. Table 2, Centers for Disease Control and Prevention (CDC), 2014.

At a Glance—Death Rate:

Table 6.2. Age-Adjusted Stroke Death Rates per 100,000 (2013)

	Asians/Pacific Islanders	Non-Hispanic White	Asians/Pacific Islanders/Non-Hispanic White Ratio
Men	31.2	34.9	0.9
Women	27.9	34.5	0.8
Total	29.4	35	0.8

Source: National Vital Statistics Report. Vol. 64, No. 02. Table 16–17, Centers for Disease Control and Prevention (CDC), 2014.

Hispanic Women and Stroke

Hispanic women have some of the highest rates of diabetes and obesity, which are two risk factors for stroke. Stroke is the third leading cause of death for Hispanic women—and it affects Hispanic women at younger ages than non-Hispanic white women.

Why Are Hispanic Women at Higher Risk?

- **High blood pressure** is one of the main risk factors for a stroke. About 3 out of 10 Hispanic women have high blood pressure, and many do not know it.

- People with **diabetes** are at higher risk of stroke. About 1 out of 6 Hispanic women has diabetes—including many who don't know they have the disease. Diabetes is more common in people of Mexican, Dominican, Puerto Rican, and Central American ancestry.

- Being **overweight or obese** increases your risk of stroke. About 4 out of 5 Hispanic women are overweight or obese.

- **Smoking** doubles your stroke risk. About 1 out of 10 Hispanic women smokes.

Scientists don't know exactly why Hispanic women have a higher risk for high blood pressure, obesity, and diabetes, but they believe lifestyle and social factors may play a role.

Hispanic Men and Stroke

In the United States, 1 out of 4 Hispanic men dies of stroke or heart disease. Hispanics are also more likely to have strokes at younger ages than non-Hispanic whites: The average age for a stroke among non-Hispanic whites is 80, but among Hispanics, it's 67.

Why Are Hispanic Men at Higher Risk?

- **High blood pressure** is one of the main risk factors for stroke. About 3 out of 10 Hispanic men have high blood pressure, and many do not know it.

- People with **diabetes** are at higher risk of stroke. About 1 out of 6 Hispanic men has diabetes—including many who don't know they have the disease. Diabetes is more in people of Mexican, Dominican, Puerto Rican, and Central American ancestry.

- Being **overweight or obese** increases your risk of stroke. About 4 out of 5 Hispanic men are overweight or obese.

- **Smoking** doubles your stroke risk. About 1 out of 5 Hispanic men smokes.

Scientists don't know exactly why Hispanic men have a higher risk for high blood pressure, obesity, and diabetes, but they believe lifestyle and social factors may play a role.

Chapter 7

Geography and Stroke: The Stroke Belt

About 795,000 strokes occur in the United States each year, causing more than 130,000 fatalities and making it the fifth leading cause of death in the country. Although in most cases it's difficult to predict or prevent a stroke, there are a number of risk factors that are known to contribute to the likelihood of having one, including high blood pressure, age, obesity, and smoking. But in the 1950s medical researchers began to document another factor: Geography.

What Is the Stroke Belt?

It's been found that people living in a region generally comprising the southeastern part of the United States have about an 18 percent higher risk of experiencing a stroke than people with similar traits (age, sex, race, etc.) living in other areas. Since the initial findings in the 1950s, additional research has been conducted by a number of organizations, and most, including studies by the Centers for Disease Control (CDC) and the National Institutes of Health (NIH), have confirmed that geography does, indeed, appear to be a factor in the risk of stroke. The exact statistics and individual states involved have varied with time and sources, but the following states have been included in what's become known as the "Stroke Belt":

- Alabama
- Arkansas
- Georgia
- Indiana
- Kentucky
- Louisiana

- Mississippi
- North Carolina
- South Carolina
- Tennessee
- Virginia

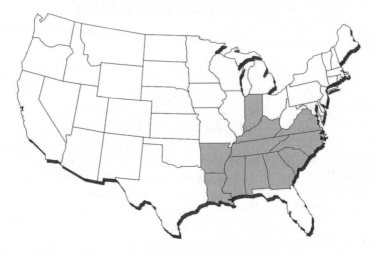

Figure 7.1. *Map Showing 11 States in the Stroke Belt*

(Source: "Stroke Belt Initiative," National Heart, Lung, and Blood Institute (NHLBI).)

Some researchers have reported that individuals from Georgia, North Carolina, and South Carolina have an even higher stroke risk than those in the other Stroke Belt States, with the death rates for some age groups in those states being as much as twice as high as the rest of the country. And further study by the NIH has also demonstrated that those who lived in the Stroke Belt from childhood carry the elevated stroke risk with them even if they move out of the area, while people who move to the Stroke Belt as adults do not have an elevated risk.

East Texas and North Florida, which border on Stroke Belt states, have also been shown to have higher rates of stroke than the rest of the country. But since most statistical analysis only includes entire states with elevated stroke risk, these areas are not considered part of the Stroke Belt.

What Is the Explanation for the Stroke Belt?

Even though the existence of the Stroke Belt has been confirmed by a number of independent studies, the reason for its existence is not fully understood. Many theories have been proposed, but so far none has been definitively proven, although it's fairly certain that the reasons are regional, rather than state-specific. Researchers have examined ethnicity, access to healthcare, and even climate as possible contributing factors but have been unable to make a positive determination.

The NIH has concluded that the Stroke Belt is most likely the result of a combination of genetic and lifestyle factors, including smoking, a sedentary lifestyle, and a diet rich in saturated fats, all of which contribute to conditions like high blood pressure and high cholesterol, which can mean a higher risk of stroke. The so-called "Southern Diet" has been identified by several studies as one plausible explanation for the geographic trend. A study by the American Stroke Association found that this type of diet, characterized by "a high intake of foods such as fried chicken, fried fish, fried potatoes, bacon, ham, liver and gizzards, and sugary drinks such as sweet tea," resulted in a significantly higher risk of stroke. Those who ate these foods about six times per week had a 41 percent higher stroke risk compared to those who ate them just once a month. But it's worth pointing out that this nationwide study also concluded that people who maintain this type of diet are at higher risk for stroke no matter where they live, although the Southern cultural tradition may account for its prevalence in that region.

An NIH study showed that people who lived in the Stroke Belt from childhood carried the elevated stroke risk with them even if they moved out of the area. Although no reason for this has been established, it could be because of changes to the body caused by a childhood spent in the Stroke Belt, or it could be because of diet and exercise habits developed when these people were children.

Prevention

No matter where you live, some risk factors for stroke can't be changed, including age, gender, genetic makeup, and ethnicity. But there are a number of lifestyle changes you can make to help lessen your risk of stroke. These include:

- **Maintain a healthy diet.** Generally, this includes eating a variety of vegetables, fruits, whole grains, lean protein, and the "good fats," like certain oils, nuts, fatty fish, and cheese, while staying away from foods that contain saturated fats, trans fats, added sugars, and excess sodium.

- **Get enough physical activity.** The Centers for Disease Control recommends 150 minutes of moderate activity—such as brisk walking, water aerobics, or bicycling—plus at least two or more days of muscle-strengthening activities, per week. The alternative is 75 minutes of more vigorous activity—like jogging, running, or swimming laps—plus two or more days of muscle-strengthening activities per week.

- **Stop smoking.** If you smoke, quitting can cut your risk of stroke in half. Smoking can thicken blood, increase clot formation, and cause the buildup of plaque in the arteries, all of which can be contributing factors to stroke.

- **Drink alcohol in moderation.** A number of studies have shown that alcohol can increase blood pressure and therefore escalate the risk of stroke. Experts recommend no more than two drinks per day for men and one drink per day for women. One drink equates to approximately 1½ ounces of liquor, 5 ounces of wine, or 12 ounces of beer.

Stroke Risk Scorecard

The National Stroke Association has developed a Stroke Risk Scorecard, which can help you become more familiar with your personal risk for stroke. It can be downloaded at: www.stroke.org/stroke-resources/resource-library/stroke-risk-scorecard.

References

1. "Geography: The Stroke Belt," HeartHealthyWomen.org, n.d.

2. Lambert, Katie. "Loosening the Stroke Belt," Bestofatlanta. com, n.d.

3. "Prevalence of Stroke: United States, 2006–2010," Centers for Disease Control and Prevention (CDC), May 25, 2012.

4. "Southern Diet Could Raise Your Risk of Stroke," American Heart Association, February 7, 2013.

5. "Stroke," Centers for Disease Control and Prevention (CDC), December 28, 2016.

6. "Stroke: Challenges, Progress, and Promise," National Institutes of Health (NIH), February 2009.

7. "The Stroke Belt," Saebo.com, September 16, 2015.

Chapter 8

Statistics on Stroke in the United States

Stroke is the fifth leading cause of death in the United Sates. In 2014, stroke killed more than 133,000 people, accounting for about 1 of every 20 deaths in the United States. According to the American Heart Association (AHA), about 795,000 people in the United States suffer a stroke each year (about 610,000 first attacks and 185,000 recurrent attacks). Four million Americans who have survived a stroke are living with impairments and 15 percent to 30 percent are permanently disabled. The American Heart Association also estimates that stroke cost about $33 billion in both direct and indirect costs in 2011 in the United States alone.

Statistics

Despite steady decreases in U.S. stroke mortality over the past several decades, stroke remained the fourth leading cause of death during 2010–2012 and the fifth leading cause in 2013. Most studies have focused on the excess mortality experienced by black persons compared with white persons and by residents of the southeastern

---

This chapter contains text excerpted from the following sources: Text in this chapter begins with excerpts from "Know the Signs and Symptoms of a Stroke," Centers for Disease Control and Prevention (CDC), June 16, 2016; Text under the heading "Statistics" is excerpted from "Differences in Stroke Mortality among Adults Aged 45 and Over: United States, 2010–2013," Centers for Disease Control and Prevention (CDC), July 2015.

states, referred to as the Stroke Belt. Few stroke mortality studies have focused on Asian or Pacific Islander and Hispanic persons or have explored urban–rural differences.

Stroke mortality among adults aged 45 and over varied by race and Hispanic origin and sex during 2010–2013.

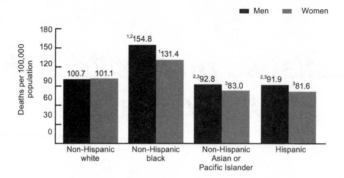

Figure 8.1. *Age-Adjusted Stroke Death Rates among Men and Women Aged 45 and over, by Race and Hispanic Origin: Average Annual, 2010–2013*

- The age-adjusted stroke death rate for non-Hispanic black men aged 45 and over (154.8 deaths per 100,000 population) was 54 percent higher than the rate for non-Hispanic white men, 67 percent higher than the rate for non-Hispanic Asian or Pacific Islander men, and 68 percent higher than the rate for Hispanic men of the same age.

- The rate for non-Hispanic black women (131.4 per 100,000 population) was 30 percent higher than the rate for non-Hispanic white women, 58 percent higher than the rate for non-Hispanic Asian or Pacific Islander women, and 61 percent higher than the rate for Hispanic women of the same age.

- Non-Hispanic Asian or Pacific Islander and Hispanic men and women had the lowest age-adjusted stroke death rates (men: 92.8 and 91.9 per 100,000 population; women: 83.0 and 81.6).

- Non-Hispanic white men and women aged 45 and over had similar age-adjusted stroke death rates (100.7 and 101.1 deaths per 100,000 population). Men in the other race-ethnicity groups had higher age-adjusted stroke death rates than women of the same race and ethnicity (12 percent to 18 percent higher).

The age distribution of stroke deaths varied by race and Hispanic origin during 2010–2013.

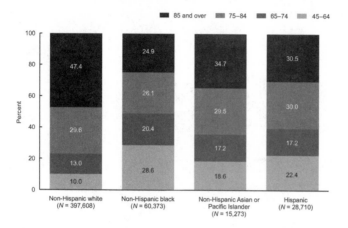

Figure 8.2. *Stroke Deaths, by Age Group and Race and Hispanic Origin: Average Annual, 2010–2013*

- More than one-fourth of the stroke deaths among non-Hispanic black persons aged 45 and over (28.6%) occurred to those in the youngest age group (45–64). By contrast, the portion of stroke deaths in this age group among the other race/ethnicity groups ranged from one-tenth among non-Hispanic white persons (10%) to less than one-fourth among Hispanic persons (22.4%).

- The portion of stroke deaths in the oldest age group (85 and over) was largest among non-Hispanic white persons (nearly one-half or 47.4%) and smallest among non-Hispanic black persons (one-fourth or 24.9%).

- The percent distribution of stroke deaths by age was similar among non-Hispanic Asian or Pacific Islander and Hispanic persons.

Stroke mortality among persons aged 45 and over decreased with increasing county median household income during 2010–2013.

- The age-adjusted stroke death rate for persons aged 45 and over decreased as county median household income increased.

- The age-adjusted stroke death rate for persons residing in counties in the lowest median household income quartile was 32 percent higher than the rate for persons residing in counties in the highest quartile (126.9 compared with 96.1 deaths per 100,000 population).

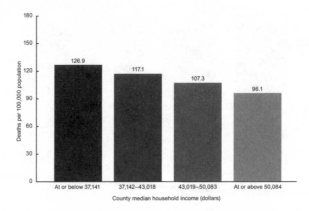

Figure 8.3. *Age-Adjusted Stroke Death Rates among Persons Aged 45 and over, by County Median Household Income Quartile: Average Annual, 2010–2013*

During 2010–2013, stroke mortality among persons aged 45 and over increased as place of residence became more rural.

- Among persons aged 45 and over, age-adjusted stroke death rates were highest in nonmetropolitan counties (micropolitan and noncore: 120.5 and 121.0 deaths per 100,000 population) and lowest in large central and large fringe metro counties (97.6 and 96.8).

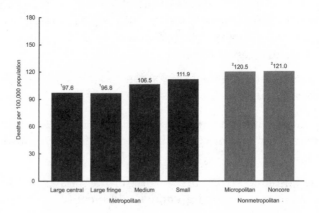

Figure 8.4. *Age-Adjusted Stroke Death Rates among Persons Aged 45 and over, by Urbanization Level of County of Residence: Average Annual, 2010–2013*

Among persons aged 45 and over, stroke mortality inside and outside the Stroke Belt varied by race and Hispanic origin during 2010–2013.

- Non-Hispanic black and non-Hispanic white persons aged 45 and over residing inside the Stroke Belt experienced excess stroke mortality compared with their counterparts residing outside the Stroke Belt (22 percent and 21 percent higher mortality).

- The age-adjusted stroke death rate for non-Hispanic Asian or Pacific Islander persons residing inside the Stroke Belt did not differ from the rate for those residing outside the Stroke Belt (88.0 compared with 87.4 deaths per 100,000 population).

- In contrast to the other population groups, Hispanic persons residing inside the Stroke Belt had substantially lower stroke mortality than Hispanic persons residing outside the Stroke Belt (50.8 compared with 87.6 deaths per 100,000 population).

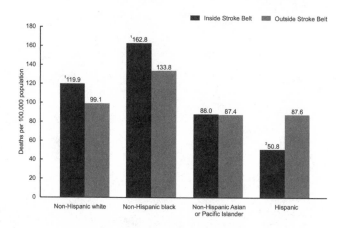

Figure 8.5. *Age-Adjusted Stroke Death Rates among Persons Aged 45 and over, by Residence inside or outside the Stroke Belt and Race and Hispanic Origin: Average Annual, 2010–2013*

Chapter 9

Recent Research on Stroke

Chapter Contents

Section 9.1—Researchers Investigate Genes
Involved in Brain Repair after Stroke 70

Section 9.2—Stem Cell Therapy and Stroke 72

Section 9.3—Amplatzer PFO Occluder Device for
Prevention of Recurrent Strokes 74

Section 9.1

Researchers Investigate Genes Involved in Brain Repair after Stroke

This section includes text excerpted from "Scientists Identify Main Component of Brain Repair after Stroke," National Institutes of Health (NIH), October 27, 2015.

Looking at brain tissue from mice, monkeys and humans, scientists have found that a molecule known as growth and differentiation factor 10 (GDF10) is a key player in repair mechanisms following stroke. The findings suggest that GDF10 may be a potential therapy for recovery after stroke. The study, published in *Nature Neuroscience*, was supported by the National Institute of Neurological Disorders and Stroke (NINDS), part of the National Institutes of Health (NIH).

"These findings help to elucidate the mechanisms of repair following stroke. Identifying this key protein further advances our knowledge of how the brain heals itself from the devastating effects of stroke, and may help to develop new therapeutic strategies to promote recovery," said Francesca Bosetti, Ph.D., stroke program director at NINDS.

Stroke can occur when a brain blood vessel becomes blocked, preventing nearby tissue from getting essential nutrients. When brain tissue is deprived of oxygen and nutrients, it begins to die. Once this occurs, repair mechanisms, such as axonal sprouting, are activated as the brain attempts to overcome the damage. During axonal sprouting, healthy neurons send out new projections ("sprouts") that re-establish some of the connections lost or damaged during the stroke and form new ones, resulting in partial recovery. Before this study, it was unknown what triggered axonal sprouting.

Previous studies suggested that GDF10 was involved in the early stages of axonal sprouting, but its exact role in the process was unclear. S. Thomas Carmichael, M.D., Ph.D., and his colleagues at the David Geffen School of Medicine at the University of California Los Angeles took a closer look at GDF10 to identify how it may contribute to axonal sprouting.

Examining animal models of stroke as well as human autopsy tissue, Dr. Carmichael's team found that GDF10 was activated very early after stroke. Then, using rodent and human neurons in a dish, the researchers tested the effect of GDF10 on the length of axons, the neuronal projections that carry messages between brain cells. They discovered that GDF10 stimulated axonal growth and increased the length of the axons.

"We found that GDF10 caused many different neurons in a dish to grow, including human neurons that were derived from stem cells," said Dr. Carmichael.

His group also found that GDF10 may be important for functional recovery after stroke. They treated mouse models of stroke with GDF10 and had the animals perform various motor tasks to test recovery. The results suggested that increasing levels of GDF10 were associated with significantly faster recovery after stroke. When the researchers blocked GDF10, the animals did not perform as well on the motor tasks, suggesting the repair mechanisms were impaired—and that the natural levels of GDF10 in the brain represent a signal for recovery.

"We were surprised by how consistently GDF10 caused new connections to form across all of the levels of analysis. We looked at rodent cortical neurons and human neurons in dish as well as in live animals. It's a demanding gauntlet to run, but the effects of GDF10 held up in all of the levels that we tested," said Dr. Carmichael.

It has been widely believed that mechanisms of brain repair are similar to those that occur during development. Dr. Carmichael's team conducted comprehensive analyses to compare the effects of GDF10 on genes related to stroke repair with genes involved in development and learning and memory, processes that result in connections forming between neurons.

Surprisingly, there was little similarity. The findings revealed that GDF10 affected entirely different genes following stroke than those involved in development or learning and memory.

"We found that regeneration is a unique program in the brain that occurs after injury. It is not simply Development 2.0, using the same mechanisms that take place when the nervous system is forming," said Dr. Carmichael.

More research is necessary to determine whether GDF10 can be a potential treatment for stroke recovery.

Section 9.2

Stem Cell Therapy and Stroke

This section contains text excerpted from the following sources:
Text in this section begins with excerpts from "Focus on Stem Cell
Research," National Institute of Neurological Disorders and Stroke
(NINDS), December 19, 2016; Text under the heading "Stem Cell
Therapy Heals Injured Mouse Brain" is excerpted from "Stem Cell
Therapy Heals Injured Mouse Brain," National Institutes of Health
(NIH), August 22, 2016.

Stem cells possess the unique ability to differentiate into many distinct cell types in the body, including brain cells, but they also retain the ability to produce more stem cells, a process termed self-renewal. There are multiple types of stem cell, such as embryonic stem (ES) cells, induced pluripotent stem (iPS) cells, and adult or somatic stem cells. While various types of stem cells share similar properties there are differences as well. For example, ES cells and iPS cells are able to differentiate into any type of cell, whereas adult stem cells are more restricted in their potential. The promise of all stem cells for use in future therapies is exciting, but significant technical hurdles remain that will only be overcome through years of intensive research.

Stem Cell Therapy Heals Injured Mouse Brain

Scientists and clinicians have long dreamed of helping the injured brain repair itself by creating new neurons, and an innovative National Institutes of Health (NIH)-funded study published on August 22, 2016 in *Nature Medicine* may bring this goal much closer to reality. A team of researchers has developed a therapeutic technique that dramatically increases the production of nerve cells in mice with stroke-induced brain damage.

The therapy relies on the combination of two methods that show promise as treatments for stroke-induced neurological injury. The first consists of surgically grafting human neural stem cells into the damaged area, where they mature into neurons and other brain cells. The second involves administering a compound called 3K3A-APC, which the scientists have shown helps neural stem cells grown in a petri dish develop into neurons. However, it was unclear what effect the molecule, derived from a human protein called activated protein-C (APC), would have in live animals.

A month after their strokes, mice that had received both the stem cells and 3K3A-APC performed significantly better on tests of motor and sensory functions compared to mice that received neither or only one of the treatments. In addition, many more of the stem cells survived and matured into neurons in the mice given 3K3A-APC.

"This University of Southern California (USC)-led animal study could pave the way for a potential breakthrough in how we treat people who have experienced a stroke," added Jim Koenig, Ph.D., a program director at the NIH's National Institute of Neurological Disorders and Stroke (NINDS), which funded the research. "If the therapy works in humans, it could markedly accelerate the recovery of these patients."

The researchers induced stroke-like brain damage in mice by disrupting blood flow to a specific part of their brains. One week later—the equivalent of several months in humans—the team inserted the stem cells next to the dead tissue and then gave the mice several infusions of either a placebo or 3K3A-APC.

"When you give these mice 3K3A-APC, it works much better than stem cells alone," said Berislav Zlokovic, M.D., Ph.D., the USC professor who led the research. "We showed that 3K3A-APC helps the cells convert into neurons and make structural and functional connections with the host's nervous system."

To confirm that the stem cells were responsible for the animals' improved function, the researchers used a targeted toxin to kill the neurons that had developed from them in another group of mice given the combination therapy. These mice showed the same improved performance on the tests of sensory and motor functions prior to being given the toxin but lost these gains afterwards, suggesting that the neurons that grew from the implanted cells were necessary for the improvements.

In a separate experiment, the team examined the connections between the neurons that developed from the stem cells in the damaged brain region and nerve cells in a nearby region called the primary motor cortex. The mice given the stem cells and 3K3A-APC had many more neuronal connections, called synapses, linking these areas than mice given the placebo. In addition, when the team stimulated the mice's paws with a mechanical vibration, the neurons that grew from the stem cells responded much more strongly in the treated animals.

"That means the transplanted cells are being functionally integrated into the host's brain after treatment with 3K3A-APC," Dr.

Zlokovic explained. "No one in the stroke field has ever shown this, so I believe this is going to be the gold standard for future studies."

3K3A-APC is currently being studied in a NINDS-funded Phase II clinical trial to determine if it can reduce the death of neurons deprived of blood flow immediately following a stroke. As a result of the mouse study, Dr. Zlokovic and his team, including co-first authors Yaoming Wang and Zhen Zhao, now hope to pursue another Phase II clinical trial to test whether the combination of neural stem cell grafts and 3K3A-APC can stimulate the growth of new neurons in human stroke patients to improve function. If that trial succeeds, it may be possible to test the treatment's effects on other neurological conditions, such as spinal cord injuries, for which stem cell therapies are being investigated.

Section 9.3

Amplatzer PFO Occluder Device for Prevention of Recurrent Strokes

This section includes text excerpted from "FDA Approves New Device for Prevention of Recurrent Strokes in Certain Patients," U.S. Food and Drug Administration (FDA), October 28, 2016.

The U.S. Food and Drug Administration (FDA) has approved the Amplatzer PFO Occluder device. The PFO Occluder reduces the risk of a stroke in patients who previously had a stroke believed to be caused by a blood clot that passed through a small hole in the heart, called a patent foramen ovale (PFO), and then traveled to the brain.

"The Amplatzer PFO Occluder provides a non-surgical method for doctors to close a PFO," said Bram Zuckerman, M.D., director of the Division of Cardiovascular Devices in the FDA's Center for Devices and Radiological Health. "But as the device labeling clearly states, patients need to be evaluated carefully by a neurologist and cardiologist to rule out other known causes of stroke and help ensure that PFO closure with the device is likely to assist in reducing the risk of a recurrent stroke."

About 25 to 30 percent of Americans have a PFO, which typically causes no health problems and does not require treatment. The cause of most strokes can be identified, such as poorly controlled high blood pressure, narrowed blood vessels due to cholesterol deposits and scar tissue (atherosclerosis), or a blood clot caused by an abnormal heart rhythm (atrial fibrillation). However, in some patients, medical tests cannot identify the cause of the stroke, which is referred to as a cryptogenic stroke. In a small percentage of these patients, it is believed that the PFO provided a path for a blood clot to travel to the brain where it blocked a blood vessel resulting in a stroke. Patients with a cryptogenic stroke and a PFO may be at an increased risk of having a second stroke.

The Amplatzer PFO Occluder is inserted through a catheter that is placed in a leg vein and advanced to the heart. It is then implanted close to the hole in the heart between the top right chamber (right atrium) and the top left chamber (left atrium). The device had been on the market more than a decade ago under a humanitarian device exemption (HDE), but was voluntarily withdrawn by the manufacturer in 2006 after the FDA concluded that the target population for this device was greater than 4,000 patients and that the device no longer qualified for an HDE approval. For the past 10 years, no FDA-approved heart occluder devices have been on the market specifically indicated to close PFOs to reduce the risk of a recurrent stroke in patients with a prior cryptogenic stroke.

In approving the Amplatzer PFO Occluder, the FDA concluded that the device demonstrated a reasonable assurance of safety and effectiveness. The safety and efficacy was assessed in a randomized study that evaluated 499 participants aged 18 to 60 years old who were treated with the Amplatzer PFO Occluder plus blood-thinning medications compared to 481 participants who were treated with blood-thinning medications alone. While the rate of new strokes in both treatment groups was very low, the study found a 50 percent reduction in the rate of new strokes in participants using the Amplatzer PFO Occluder plus blood-thinning medications compared to participants taking only blood-thinning medications.

Adverse effects associated with the device or the implantation procedure include injury to the heart, irregular and/or rapid heart rate (atrial fibrillation), blood clots in the heart, leg or lung, bleeding and stroke.

The Amplatzer PFO Occluder device should not be used in patients with a heart valve infection or other untreated infections, or a heart tumor or blood clot at the implant site. The device is also contraindicated in patients with other abnormal connections between the heart chambers or in whom the cardiovascular anatomy or blood clots would interfere with the ability to move the catheter used to deliver the device to the heart.

Patients should discuss with their medical team (consisting of a neurologist and a cardiologist) the risks and benefits of PFO closure in comparison to using medications alone.

The Amplatzer PFO Occluder device is manufactured by St. Jude Medical Inc. based in Plymouth, Minnesota.

Chapter 10

Clinical Trials on Stroke

Chapter Contents

Section 10.1—What Are Clinical Trials? 78

Section 10.2—Rehabilitation Treatment Following
Stroke 83

Section 10.3—Vitamin D and Stroke 85

Section 10.4—Heart and Brain Interfaces in Acute
Ischemic Stroke 86

Section 10.5—Quality of Life after Stroke 88

Section 10.6—Carotid Plaque Imaging in Acute
Stroke 89

Section 10.7—The Effect of Aerobic Exercise in
Patients with Minor Stroke 91

Section 10.1

What Are Clinical Trials?

This section includes text excerpted from "NIH Clinical Research Trials and You—The Basics," National Institutes of Health (NIH), January 18, 2017.

What Are Clinical Trials and Why Do People Participate?

Clinical trials are part of clinical research and at the heart of all medical advances. Clinical trials look at new ways to prevent, detect, or treat disease. Treatments might be new drugs or new combinations of drugs, new surgical procedures or devices, or new ways to use existing treatments. The goal of clinical trials is to determine if a new test or treatment works and is safe. Clinical trials can also look at other aspects of care, such as improving the quality of life for people with chronic illnesses.

People participate in clinical trials for a variety of reasons. Healthy volunteers say they participate to help others and to contribute to moving science forward. Participants with an illness or disease also participate to help others, but also to possibly receive the newest treatment and to have the additional care and attention from the clinical trial staff. Clinical trials offer hope for many people and an opportunity to help researchers find better treatments for others in the future.

Types of Clinical Trials

There are different types of clinical trials:

- **Natural history studies** provide valuable information about how disease and health progress.

- **Prevention trials** look for better ways to prevent a disease in people who have never had the disease or to prevent the disease from returning. Better approaches may include medicines, vaccines, or lifestyle changes, among other things.

- **Screening trials** test the best way to detect certain diseases or health conditions.

- **Diagnostic trials** determine better tests or procedures for diagnosing a particular disease or condition.

- **Treatment trials** test new treatments, new combinations of drugs, or new approaches to surgery or radiation therapy.

- **Quality of life trials** (or supportive care trials) explore and measure ways to improve the comfort and quality of life of people with a chronic illness.

Phases of Clinical Trials

Clinical trials are conducted in "phases." Each phase has a different purpose and helps researchers answer different questions.

- **Phase I trials:** Researchers test an experimental drug or treatment in a small group of people (20–80) for the first time. The purpose is to evaluate its safety and identify side effects.

- **Phase II trials:** The experimental drug or treatment is administered to a larger group of people (100–300) to determine its effectiveness and to further evaluate its safety.

- **Phase III trials:** The experimental drug or treatment is administered to large groups of people (1,000–3,000) to confirm its effectiveness, monitor side effects, compare it with standard or equivalent treatments, and collect information that will allow the experimental drug or treatment to be used safely.

- **Phase IV trials:** After a drug is approved by the U.S. Food and Drug Administration (FDA) and made available to the public, researchers track its safety, seeking more information about a drug or treatment's risks, benefits, and optimal use.

Who Participates in Clinical Trials?

Many different types of people participate in clinical trials. Some are healthy, while others may have illnesses. A healthy volunteer is a person with no known significant health problems who participates in clinical research to test a new drug, device, or intervention. Research procedures with healthy volunteers are designed to develop new knowledge, not to provide direct benefit to study participants. Healthy volunteers have always played an important role in research.

Healthy volunteers are needed for several reasons. When developing a new technique, such as a blood test or imaging device, healthy volunteers (formerly called "normal volunteers") help define the limits of "normal." These volunteers serve as controls for patient groups and are often matched to patients on characteristics such as age, gender, or family relationship. They receive the same test, procedure, or drug the patient group receives. Investigators learn about the disease process by comparing the patient group to the healthy volunteers.

Factors like how much of your time is needed, discomfort you may feel, or risk involved depends on the trial. While some require minimal amounts of time and effort, other studies may require a major commitment in time and effort on behalf of the volunteer, and may involve some discomfort. The research procedure may also carry some risk. The consent process for healthy volunteers includes a detailed discussion of the study's procedures and tests.

A patient volunteer has a known health problem and participates in research to better understand, diagnose, treat, or cure that disease or condition. Research procedures with a patient volunteer help develop new knowledge. These procedures may or may not benefit the study participants.

Patient volunteers may be involved in studies similar to those in which healthy volunteers participate. These studies involve drugs, devices, or interventions designed to prevent, treat, or cure disease. Although these studies may provide direct benefit to patient volunteers, the main aim is to prove, by scientific means, the effects and limitations of the experimental treatment. Consequently, some patients serve as controls by not taking the test drug, or by receiving test doses of the drug large enough only to show that it is present, but not at a level that can treat the condition. A study's benefits may be indirect for the volunteers but may help others.

All clinical trials have guidelines about who can participate, called Inclusion/Exclusion Criteria. Factors that allow someone to participate in a clinical trial are "inclusion criteria." Those that exclude or not allow participation are "exclusion criteria." These criteria are based on factors such as age, gender, the type and stage of a disease, previous treatment history, and other medical conditions. Before joining a clinical trial, a participant must qualify for the study. Some research studies seek participants with illnesses or conditions to be studied in the clinical trial, while others need healthy volunteers.

Some studies need both types. Inclusion and exclusion criteria are not used to reject people personally; rather, the criteria are used to identify appropriate participants and keep them safe, and to help ensure that researchers can find new information they need.

What Do I Need to Know If I Am Thinking about Participating?

Risks and Benefits

Clinical trials involve risks, just as routine medical care and the activities of daily living. When weighing the risks of research, you can consider two important factors:

1. the degree of harm that could result from participating in the study, and

2. the chance of any harm occurring.

Most clinical studies pose the risk of minor discomfort, which lasts only a short time. However, some study participants experience complications that require medical attention. In rare cases, participants have been seriously injured or have died of complications resulting from their participation in trials of experimental therapies. The specific risks associated with a research protocol are described in detail in the informed consent document, which participants are asked to sign before participating in research. Also, a member of the research team explains the major risks of participating in a study and will answer any questions you have about the study. Before deciding to participate, carefully consider possible risks and benefits.

Potential Benefits

Well-designed and well-executed clinical trials provide the best approach for participants to:

- Play an active role in their healthcare.

- Gain access to new research treatments before they are widely available.

- Receive regular and careful medical attention from a research team that includes doctors and other health professionals.

- Help others by contributing to medical research.

Potential Risks

Risks to participating in clinical trials include the following:

- There may be unpleasant, serious, or even life-threatening side effects to experimental treatment.

- The study may require more time and attention than standard treatment would, including visits to the study site, more blood tests, more treatments, hospital stays, or complex dosage requirements.

How Am I Protected?

Ethical Guidelines

The goal of clinical research is to develop knowledge that improves human health or increases understanding of human biology. People who participate in clinical research make it possible for this to occur. The path to finding out if a new drug is safe or effective is to test it on patient volunteers. By placing some people at risk of harm for the good of others, clinical research has the potential to exploit patient volunteers. The purpose of ethical guidelines is both to protect patient volunteers and to preserve the integrity of the science. Ethical guidelines in place today were primarily a response to past research abuses.

Informed Consent

Informed consent is the process of learning the key facts about a clinical trial before deciding whether to participate. The process of providing information to participants continues throughout the study. To help someone decide whether to participate, members of the research team explain details of the study. The research team provides an informed consent document, which includes such details about the study as its purpose, duration, required procedures, and who to contact for various purposes. The informed consent document also explains risks and potential benefits.

If the participant decides to enroll in the trial, the informed consent document will be signed. Informed consent is not a contract. Volunteers are free to withdraw from the study at any time.

Institutional Review Board (IRB) Review

Most, but not all, clinical trials in the United States are approved and monitored by an Institutional Review Board (IRB) in order to ensure that the risks are minimal and are worth any potential benefits. An IRB is an independent committee that consists of physicians, statisticians, and members of the community who ensure that clinical trials are ethical and that the rights of participants are protected. Potential research participants should ask the sponsor or research coordinator whether the research they are considering participating in was reviewed by an IRB.

Section 10.2

Rehabilitation Treatment Following Stroke

This section includes text excerpted from "A New Rehabilitation Treatment Following Stroke," ClinicalTrials.gov, National Institutes of Health (NIH), March 31, 2017.

Stroke is the number one cause of disability in the United Nations with about 1 million new cases each year. Following stroke, patients with perceptual and cognitive impairments have the worst prognostic outcomes. There is evidence to suggest that perceptual and cognitive symptoms can be alleviated by multisensory integration, which has the effect of enhancing motor, perceptual and cognitive processes.

This research project will investigate for the first time the functional benefits that stem from multisensory stimulation of attention in stroke patients with perceptual and cognitive impairments. The research project will involve multisensory learning paradigms with stimulus and environmental parameters that optimally enhance perceptual learning and cognitive function. Multisensory learning paradigms will be tailored for patients with stroke to determine the perceptual and cognitive symptoms that can be alleviated, and Functional magnetic resonance imaging or functional MRI (fMRI) will be used to evaluate the underlying neural substrates of the effects. The project will show whether multisensory stimulation provides an effective means of attentional rehabilitation after stroke and whether the effects generalize to everyday life, with long-term outcomes that improve functional independence in patients with stroke.

Eligibility

Ages Eligible for Study: 30 Years and older (Adult, Senior)
Sexes Eligible for Study: All
Accepts Healthy Volunteers: No

Criteria

Inclusion criteria:

- Participant is willing and able to give informed consent for participation in the study.

- Participants who have a history of stroke (within the last 2 days – 2 months) and demonstrate a clinical deficit in unilateral neglect and/ or extinction on the standardized measure from the Oxford Cognitive Screen (OCS) and/or extinction task from BCoS (Birmingham Cognitive Screen).

- Participants have sufficient comprehension and concentration to undergo cognitive screening lasting about 1 hour (BCoS subtests, and other neglect and extinction related tests).

- Participants are medically stable.

- Participants with no history of other neurological and psychiatric disorders with exception of stroke.

Exclusion criteria:

- Participants unwilling or unable to give consent.

- Participants without cognitive deficits and unilateral neglect or extinction.

- Participants who cannot concentrate sufficiently to undergo the screening and/or who are not medically stable.

- Participants with a history of other neurological and psychiatric disorders (with exception of stroke).

- Counter-indicators for fMRI (only relevant to the brain scanning portion of the study). Participants with counter-indicators for fMRI will still be invited to take part in the rehabilitation program.

Section 10.3

Vitamin D and Stroke

This section includes text excerpted from "Vitamin D
and Stroke," ClinicalTrials.gov, National Institutes of
Health (NIH), March 31, 2017.

Stroke remains one of the most devastating neurological diseases,
often causing death, or gross physical impairment. It is the second
most common cause of death worldwide and a major cause of acquired
disability in adults. Vitamin D deficiency has been reported to contribute to the risk of cardiovascular disease especially stroke.

Eligibility

Ages Eligible for Study: 18 Years to 80 Years (Adult, Senior)
Sexes Eligible for Study: All
Accepts Healthy Volunteers: No
Sampling Method: Probability Sample

Criteria

Inclusion criteria:

• Onset is within one week

• Confirmed stroke by brain CAT and / or MRI scan either haem-
orrhage or infarction

Exclusion criteria:

• Cognitive and mental changes

• Recurrent stroke

• Hepatic and renal impairment

• Endocrinal diseases

• Steroid therapy

• Vitamin D or Ca supplementation

- Previous fractures

- Bone diseases

- brain neoplasm

- Autoimmune diseases

- History of acute and chronic inflammatory diseases

- Malignancy

- Trauma

- Surgery

- Acute vascular diseases that occurred within four weeks prior the onset of stroke

- History myocardial infarction <3 months

Section 10.4

Heart and Brain Interfaces in Acute Ischemic Stroke

This section includes text excerpted from "HEart and BRain Interfaces in Acute Ischemic Stroke (HEBRAS)," ClinicalTrials.gov, National Institutes of Health (NIH), March 31, 2017.

The primary aim of this prospective observational study is to investigate whether an enhanced diagnostic MRI work-up (including cardiac MRI, angiography of the aortic arch and the brain-supplying arteries) combined with an in-hospital Holter-ECG of up to 5 days duration leads to a significant increase in relevant pathologic findings with respect to stroke aetiology as compared to the findings obtained by a routine diagnostic work-up (including stroke unit monitoring, 24h-Holter-ECG, echocardiography, Doppler-ultrasound of the brain-supplying arteries) in patients with acute ischemic stroke and no atrial fibrillation according to past medical history or baseline ECG. A better understanding of the stroke aetiology may improve secondary stroke prevention and long term outcome.

Eligibility

Ages Eligible for Study: 18 Years and older (Adult, Senior)
Sexes Eligible for Study: All
Accepts Healthy Volunteers: No
Sampling Method: Non-Probability Sample

Criteria

Inclusion criteria:

- Age ≥18 years

- Written informed consent by the patient

- Acute ischemic stroke, as confirmed by cerebral MRI or CT

- Admission to the stroke unit of the Department of Neurology, Charité, Campus Benjamin Franklin

Exclusion criteria:

- Atrial fibrillation known by past medical history or documented by routine electrocardiogram (ECG) on hospital admission

- Participation in an interventional clinical trial

- Pre-stroke life expectancy <1 year

- Mechanic heart valve, cardiac pacemaker or other contraindications to undergo MRI

- History of adverse response to MRI contrast agents

- Known Liver disease prior to stroke

- Mild to severe renal dysfunction (creatinine > 1.3 mg/dl (females); creatinine > 1,7 mg/dl (males))

- Severe congestive heart failure (NYHA III or IV).

Section 10.5

Quality of Life after Stroke

This section includes text excerpted from "Quality of Life after Stroke Using a Telemedicine-Based Stroke Network (STROKE TeleQOL)," ClinicalTrials.gov, National Institutes of Health (NIH), March 31, 2017.

To study the effect of a telemedicine model of stroke care on patient-based outcomes.

Approximately 750,000 patients suffer from acute ischemic stroke (AIS) annually in the United States. AIS is a leading cause of long-term disability and the third-leading cause of mortality. Effective therapies exist to ameliorate the disability associated with AIS, but implementation of these therapies is time-sensitive. Currently, there is a shortage in healthcare professionals with expertise in the treatment of stroke and such expertise tends to be concentrated in large community-based or academic medical centers. To respond to this shortage, stroke networks are being organized in a "hub-and-spoke" model to facilitate the rapid delivery of time-sensitive interventions such as intravenous (i.v.) tissue plasminogen activator (tPA) or rapid evaluation for AIS. Some networks are also using telemedicine to facilitate this approach and bring the needed expertise via robotic tele-presence (RTP). Though the accuracy of stroke diagnosis and i.v. tPA utilization may be higher in RTP based networks, the impact of this model on patient's outcomes has been difficult to elucidate. To this end, meaningful validated outcome assessments are crucial to understand the impact of stroke interventions including telemedicine or RTP based networks. The objective of this study is to translate evidence-based practice of healthcare, patient-centered outcome assessments, and patient-family perceptions of delivery of care into meaningful data. This will aid in the validation of the role of interventions such as "hub-and-spoke" RTP based models in stroke care.

Eligibility

Ages Eligible for Study: 18 Years and older (Adult, Senior)

Sexes Eligible for Study: All
Accepts Healthy Volunteers: No
Sampling Method: Non-Probability Sample

Criteria

Inclusion criteria:

- Patients with suspected acute ischemic stroke (AIS)

- Age >17 years

Exclusion criteria:

- Hemorrhagic strokes (ICH or SAH)

- Transient ischemic attacks (TIA)

- Trauma

- Inability to obtain informed consent

- Participation in another study

Section 10.6

Carotid Plaque Imaging in Acute Stroke

This section includes text excerpted from "Carotid Plaque Imaging in
Acute Stroke (CAPIAS)," ClinicalTrials.gov, National
Institutes of Health (NIH), March 31, 2017.

The purpose of this study is to determine the frequency, characteristics, and consequences of vulnerable carotid artery plaques ipsilateral to an acute ischemic stroke or TIA in the territory of the internal
carotid artery.

Even with extensive diagnostic workup the underlying etiol-
ogy remains unidentified in about 25% of patients with acute ischemic stroke (AIS) or transient ischemic attack (TIA). Non-invasive
high-resolution magnetic resonance imaging (HR-MRI) of the carotid
artery allows detecting vulnerable plaques (VP) and quantifying

single plaque components. The hypotheses behind this study are that i) a substantial proportion of cases of AIS and TIA within the anterior circulation and no identified cause (cryptogenic AIS or TIA) are caused by VP in the carotid artery; ii) that these patients are at a high risk of developing a recurrent stroke, TIA, or clinically silent lesions detectable by brain MRI; and iii) that VP in the carotid artery are associated with specific infarct patterns as detected by diffusion-weighted MR imaging. Finally, the investigators will search for biomarkers associated with vulnerable carotid artery plaques. Motivating this study are the following considerations: i) data on the frequency and characteristics of VP in patients with cryptogenic AIS or TIA will provide valuable insights into stroke mechanisms; ii) depending on the results this study may have implications for diagnostic decision making and provide the basis for the planning of targeted interventional studies.

Eligibility

Ages Eligible for Study: 50 Years and older (Adult, Senior)
Sexes Eligible for Study: All
Accepts Healthy Volunteers: No
Sampling Method: Probability Sample

Criteria

Inclusion criteria:

- Age > 49 years old

- Acute ischemic stroke or transient ischemic attack (TIA)

- Neurological symptoms compatible with a stroke or TIA in the anterior circulation (territory of the internal carotid artery)

- Onset of symptoms within the last 7 days

- 1 or more acute ischemic lesion(s) visible on MR diffusion-weighted imaging (DWI) in the territory of a single internal carotid artery

- Presence of carotid artery plaques in the ipsilateral or contralateral carotid artery as defined by ultrasound (criteria: plaque thickness at least 2mm; located within 1cm proximal or distal to the carotid bifurcation)

- Written informed consent

Exclusion criteria:

- Primary referral to an outside hospital (to avoid recruitment bias)

- DWI positive lesions outside the territory of a single internal carotid artery

- Carotid artery stenosis > 69% (North American Symptomatic Carotid Endarterectomy Trial (NASCET) criteria) ipsilateral to the stroke or TIA as defined by ultrasound (systolic peak flow velocity ≥ 300 cm/s)

- Standard contraindications for MRI

- Documented allergy to MRI contrast media

- History of radiation to the neck area

- Renal clearance < 30 ml/minute

- Creatinine levels > 2 times the upper limit of the standard range of the respective laboratory within the last 30 days prior to MRI

- Surgical procedure within 24 hours preceding the MRI

Section 10.7

The Effect of Aerobic Exercise in Patients with Minor Stroke

This section includes text excerpted from "The Effect of Aerobic Exercise in Patients with Minor Stroke (HITPALS)," ClinicalTrials. gov, National Institutes of Health (NIH), March 31, 2017.

In a randomized-controlled study the effect of high-intensity training, 5 days a week at home for 12 weeks is tested in patients with lacunar stroke.

Little is known about effect of exercise for patients with lacunar stroke, no studies have investigated the feasibility or effect of aerobic exercise in this subgroup of stroke. The patients have few and temporary symptoms and are therefore early discharged from the hospital. After an cerebral infarct the patients have increased risk of recurrent stroke and they are at risk of developing cognitive deficits or vascular dementia over time. Researchers want to investigate if high-intensity training at home in the acute phase has an effect on aerobic fitness, endothelial response and health profile in this potential fragile group of patients.

Eligibility

Ages Eligible for Study: 18 Years and older (Adult, Senior)
Sexes Eligible for Study: All
Accepts Healthy Volunteers: No

Criteria

Inclusion criteria:

- lacunar stroke verified by clinical examination and computerized tomography (CT)- or MRI-scans

- able to speak and read Danish

Exclusion criteria:

- previous large artery stroke,

- symptoms or comorbidities in the musculoskeletal system, which hinder bicycling,

- dyspnoea caused by heart or pulmonary disease,

- aphasia or dementia which hinder completion of the Talk Test.

Part Two

Types of Stroke

Chapter 11

Ischemic Stroke

Chapter Contents

Section 11.1—What Is Ischemic Stroke? 96
Section 11.2—Carotid Artery Dissection 98

Section 11.1

What Is Ischemic Stroke?

This section contains text excerpted from the following sources: Text in this section begins with excerpts from "Stroke—Types of Stroke," Centers for Disease Control and Prevention (CDC), January 26, 2017; Text beginning with the heading "Types of Ischemic Stroke" is excerpted from "Stroke," National Heart, Lung, and Blood Institute (NHLBI), January 27, 2017.

Most strokes (87%) are ischemic strokes. An ischemic stroke happens when blood flow through the artery that supplies oxygen-rich blood to the brain becomes blocked.

Blood clots often cause the blockages that lead to ischemic strokes.

Types of Ischemic Stroke

An ischemic stroke occurs if an artery that supplies oxygen-rich blood to the brain becomes blocked. Blood clots often cause the blockages that lead to ischemic strokes.

The two types of ischemic stroke are thrombotic and embolic.

1. In a **thrombotic stroke**, a blood clot (thrombus) forms in an artery that supplies blood to the brain.

2. In an **embolic stroke**, a blood clot or other substance (such as plaque, a fatty material) travels through the bloodstream to an artery in the brain. (A blood clot or piece of plaque that travels through the bloodstream is called an embolus.)

With both types of ischemic stroke, the blood clot or plaque blocks the flow of oxygen-rich blood to a portion of the brain.

Treating an Ischemic Stroke

An ischemic stroke occurs if an artery that supplies oxygen-rich blood to the brain becomes blocked. Often, blood clots cause the blockages that lead to ischemic strokes. Treatment for an ischemic stroke may include medicines and medical procedures.

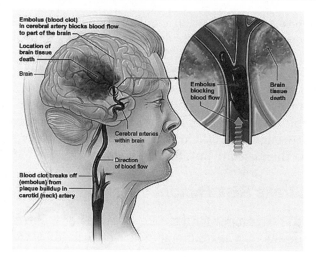

Figure 11.1. *Ischemic Stroke*

The illustration shows how an ischemic stroke can occur in the brain. If a blood clot breaks away from plaque buildup in a carotid (neck) artery, it can travel to and lodge in an artery in the brain. The clot can block blood flow to part of the brain, causing brain tissue death.

Medicines

If you have a stroke caused by a blood clot, you may be given a clot-dissolving, or clot-busting, medication called tissue plasminogen activator (tPA). A doctor will inject tPA into a vein in your arm. This type of medication must be given within 4 hours of symptom onset. Ideally, it should be given as soon as possible. The sooner treatment begins, the better your chances of recovery. Thus, it's important to know the signs and symptoms of a stroke and to call 9–1–1 right away for emergency care.

If you can't have tPA for medical reasons, your doctor may give you antiplatelet medicine that helps stop platelets from clumping together to form blood clots or anticoagulant medicine (blood thinner) that keeps existing blood clots from getting larger. Two common medicines are aspirin and clopidogrel.

Medical Procedures

If you have carotid artery disease, your doctor may recommend a carotid endarterectomy or carotid artery angioplasty. Both procedures open blocked carotid arteries.

Researchers are testing other treatments for ischemic stroke, such as intra-arterial thrombolysis and mechanical clot removal in cerebral ischemia (MERCI). In intra-arterial thrombolysis, a long flexible tube called a catheter is put into your groin (upper thigh) and threaded to the tiny arteries of the brain. Your doctor can deliver medicine through this catheter to break up a blood clot in the brain. MERCI is a device that can remove blood clots from an artery. During the procedure, a catheter is threaded through a carotid artery to the affected artery in the brain. The device is then used to pull the blood clot out through the catheter.

Treating Stroke Risk Factors

After initial treatment for a stroke, your doctor will treat your risk factors. He or she may recommend heart-healthy lifestyle changes to help control your risk factors.

Heart-healthy lifestyle changes may include:

- Heart-healthy eating

- Aiming for a healthy weight

- Managing stress

- Physical activity

- Quitting smoking

If heart-healthy lifestyle changes aren't enough, you may need medicine to control your risk factors.

Section 11.2

Carotid Artery Dissection

"Carotid Artery Dissection," © 2017 Omnigraphics.
Reviewed April 2017.

A carotid artery dissection is a tear in one of the carotid arteries, which supply blood to the brain and face. The tear allows blood to enter the artery's wall and separate its layers, which in turn can compress the artery and restrict blood flow to the brain. The condition is serious, with about half of the people who experience a carotid artery dissection subsequently suffering from a stroke. Although carotid artery dissection occurs across all age groups, it has been recognized as a leading cause of stroke in young adults. Although dissection causes just 0.4 percent of all strokes, it is responsible for 5 to 20 percent of strokes in younger patients.

Causes of Carotid Artery Dissection

Carotid artery dissection most often results from trauma to the neck, in which case it's called traumatic or secondary dissection. Its causes can include:

- sports injuries
- motor vehicle accidents
- hyperextension from turning the head
- activities such as yoga or exercise
- chiropractic neck manipulation
- medical procedures
- attempted strangulation

Other causes can be related to medical conditions. Here it's referred to as spontaneous carotid artery dissection, and it can result from such conditions as:

- atherosclerosis
- hypertension
- Marfan syndrome, Ehlers-Danlos syndrome, or other connective tissue disorders
- fibromuscular dysplasia
- respiratory tract infection
- artery wall inflammation
- kidney disease

Symptoms of Carotid Artery Dissection

Carotid artery dissection can sometimes be asymptomatic in its early stages, but in some instances it may progress to a major stroke.

Symptoms vary depending on what part of the brain experiences reduced blood flow, but they can include:

- headache, usually around the eyes
- sudden face or neck pain
- vision loss in one eye
- drooping eyelid
- small pupils
- weakness
- numbness
- difficulty with speech
- tinnitus (ringing in the ear)
- fainting

Diagnosis of Carotid Artery Dissection

In most cases a physical examination by a doctor does little to help diagnose carotid artery dissection, although sometimes the sound of turbulent blood flow can be heard through a stethoscope. Rather, advanced imaging techniques are required to confirm that a dissection has occurred. Some of the tests used in diagnosis include:

- **Duplex ultrasonography.** This is simple test in which sound waves are used to provide an image of the blood moving through arteries. It is not as accurate as some of the more sophisticated imaging techniques, but it is often used as a starting point.

- **Magnetic resonance angiography (MRA).** This is a type of magnetic resonance imaging (MRI) that uses a magnetic field and radio waves to record an accurate image of the blood vessels. Often, dye is injected prior to the test to increase contrast and provide more accurate results.

- **Computed tomography angiography.** Also called CT angiography, this procedure uses X-rays to display images of the inner workings of the blood vessels. Contrast dye is usually injected to increase image resolution.

- **Conventional angiography.** In this test, a catheter (thin tube) is inserted into an artery in the groin and threaded up to the neck for the injection of contrast dye. Then X-ray images are created to give doctors a view of the blood vessels. At the same time, the catheter might also be used for procedures to correct a dissection, if required.

Other tests that might be used to evaluate a patient with suspected carotid artery dissection include a complete blood workup, electrocardiogram (ECG), echocardiogram, and electroencephalogram (EEG).

Treatment of Carotid Artery Dissection

Initial treatment of traumatic carotid artery dissection, generally by an emergency medical technician (EMT) or in an emergency room, involves immobilizing the head and neck to help prevent further injury. Following diagnosis to confirm a dissection and its exact location, treatment for either type of dissection may proceed either with medication or surgery.

- **Treatment with medication.** Drugs used to treat carotid artery dissection usually include antiplatelet and anticoagulant medications. Antiplatelets, including aspirin, are a type of medication that slow the time it takes for blood to clot and also prevent existing clots from growing while the dissection heals. Anticoagulants, sometimes called blood thinners, are another type of drug that reduce or prevent clotting. They are considered more aggressive than antiplatelets, have more side effects, and generally cost more. Doctors decide what kind of medication to prescribe based on the type and severity of the damage, and in either case, additional angiography tests are needed to confirm that the dissection has healed before treatment can be discontinued.

- **Surgical procedures.** Some cases of carotid artery dissection require surgical intervention in order to affect a repair. This can include such procedures as stent implantation and carotid artery ligation. Carotid stent implantation, also called carotid angioplasty, involves threading a small tube called a stent through a catheter in the groin and placing it in the damaged artery to repair it. Sometimes more invasive procedures, such as a carotid ligation, are needed to fix a dissection. Here, the surgeon makes an incision in the patient's neck to gain access to the carotid artery and repairs it by ligating, or suturing, the blood vessel. Surgical procedures are generally followed up with a course of antiplatelet or anticoagulant drugs, as well as other medications.

Prognosis of Carotid Artery Dissection

Unsurprisingly, the prognosis for patients who have experienced a carotid artery dissection depends on the severity of the dissection, its location, complications from treatment, and the person's overall health. Overall, about 75 percent of those with a spontaneous dissection make a good recovery, and the mortality rate is around 5 percent. But the prognosis for patients with traumatic dissection are not as favorable, with 37 to 58 percent experiencing some degree of neurological dysfunction at the time of their discharge from the hospital and a higher mortality rate than those with spontaneous dissection. And, in some cases of either type of dissection, headaches and neck pain may continue for many years after the event, and all patients need to work with a vascular specialist for long-term care and monitoring.

References

1. "Carotid Artery Dissection," iTriagehealth.com, n.d.

2. "Carotid Artery Dissection," Mount Sinai Hospital, 2017.

3. "Carotid Dissection," UCLA Health, n.d.

4. Weinberg, Ido, MD. "Carotid Dissection," Angiologist.com, January 31, 2011

5. Zohrabian, David, MD, FAAEM, FACEP. "Carotid Artery Dissection," Medscape.com, December 14, 2016.

Chapter 12

Hemorrhagic Stroke

Chapter Contents

Section 12.1—Intracerebral and Subarachnoid
          Hemorrhagic Stroke... 104
Section 12.2—Cerebral Aneurysm... 108

Section 12.1

Intracerebral and Subarachnoid Hemorrhagic Stroke

There are two types of strokes, ischemic and hemorrhagic. The ischemic type results from a blockage in a blood vessel to the brain, while a hemorrhagic stroke occurs when a blood vessel either bursts or leaks, allowing blood to accumulate and compress the brain. And although hemorrhagic strokes are far less common, accounting for just 13 percent of all strokes, they are responsible for about 40 percent of stroke fatalities. They can be caused by a wide variety of conditions, including high blood pressure, atherosclerosis (hardened arteries), overtreatment with anticoagulants, and heavy alcohol or drug use, or they may be the result of a congenital condition (one present at birth). Hemorrhagic strokes are divided into two types, intracerebral and subarachnoid.

Intracerebral Hemorrhagic Stroke

Intracerebral hemorrhagic strokes occur when a blood vessel inside the brain bursts and allows blood to leak into the surrounding brain tissue, creating pressure, which damages brain cells and causes them to malfunction. This type of hemorrhagic stroke accounts for about 10 percent of all strokes but is responsible for a much higher percentage of fatalities. Intracerebral hemorrhagic strokes are most often caused by high blood pressure but may also result from trauma, malformed blood vessels, the overuse of anticoagulants, and other conditions.

Symptoms

Symptoms of intracerebral hemorrhagic stroke can include:

- sudden, severe headache, or a mild but long-lasting headache

- headache resulting from head trauma

- weakness or partial paralysis
- numbness
- vision impairment
- confusion
- drowsiness
- persistent vomiting
- seizure
- loss of consciousness

Diagnosis

Common tests used to diagnose intracerebral hemorrhagic stroke include:

- **Computed tomography (CT)**. This test uses specialized X-rays to confirm that a hemorrhagic stroke has taken place and show details of its location and impact.
- **Magnetic resonance imaging (MRI)**. An MRI uses a strong magnetic field to provide a detailed view of the brain and also confirm the diagnosis and provide additional details.
- **CT angiography**. This X-ray test can help determine whether the hemorrhage is spreading.
- **Blood sugar level.** This checks for low blood sugar, a condition whose symptoms can sometimes mimic those of a stroke.

Treatment

Intracerebral hemorrhagic stroke is a serious medical emergency. Almost half of patients with a large hemorrhage die within a few days, and those who survive may not recover all brain function. Treatment includes:

- **Surgery.** Usually a small hole is drilled into the skull to relieve pressure. In some cases more invasive surgery is required to remove blood and effect repairs, although this is very risky, since it can cause further damage.
- **Medication.** Typical medications used to treat intracerebral hemorrhagic stroke include anticoagulants to prevent clotting,

steroids to reduce swelling, and anticonvulsants if the patient had seizures. In some cases medication may be used to lower blood pressure, but only if it is very high, since parts of the brain have already been deprived of blood flow.

- **Follow-up therapy.** Physical, occupational, and speech therapies are often required after intracerebral hemorrhagic stroke to help patients recover or improve cognitive function and physical abilities.

Subarachnoid Hemorrhagic Stroke

Subarachnoid hemorrhagic strokes occur when a burst vessel in the brain causes blood to fill the space between the brain and the thin tissues that surround it, creating pressure that builds up and damages the brain. This condition makes up about 15 percent of all strokes, accounting for almost one-quarter of stroke fatalities. Women and middle-aged people are those most likely to be affected. Subarachnoid hemorrhagic strokes are most often the result of a burst aneurysm, a bulge in a blood vessel, but other causes can include malformed blood vessels, head injury, bleeding disorders, and the overuse of anticoagulants.

Symptoms

Aneurysms often cause no symptoms until they actually rupture, unless they happen to be pressing on a nerve or begin leaking. Subsequent symptoms can include:

- sudden, severe headache
- pain in the face or eyes
- vision problems
- vomiting
- loss of consciousness

Diagnosis

The diagnosis of subarachnoid hemorrhagic strokes is essentially the same as that for intracerebral hemorrhagic strokes, including CT and MRI scans and CT angiography. In some instances, a lumbar puncture (spinal tap) may also be performed, but this could be risky if the pressure in the skull is too great.

Treatment

Subarachnoid hemorrhagic strokes are also a serious medical emergency. About 35 percent of patients who arrive at a hospital die shortly thereafter. Among survivors, about half experience long-term neurological problems. And repeat hemorrhages can be a risk. Treatment may include:

- **Surgery.** A plastic tube called a shunt might be inserted into the skull to drain fluid and relieve pressure. To repair an aneurysm, a tiny coil may be threaded through an artery and into the affected blood vessel to effect a repair. In some instances, a metal clip might be placed around the aneurysm to prevent rupturing.

- **Medication.** Some of the medications used to treat subarachnoid hemorrhagic strokes include pain relievers, calcium blockers to prevent vasospasms—arterial spasms that can lead to ischemic stroke—and medication to adjust blood pressure to optimal levels.

- **Follow-up therapy.** Physical, occupational, and speech therapies are often required after subarachnoid hemorrhagic stroke to help patients recover or improve cognitive function and physical abilities.

References

1. Carey, Elea. "Intracranial Hemorrhages," Healthline.com, November 23, 2015.

2. Giraldo, Elias A., MD, MS. "Intracerebral Hemorrhage," Merckmanuals.com, n.d.

3. Giraldo, Elias A., MD, MS. "Subarachnoid Hemorrhage," Merckmanuals.com, n.d.

4. "Hemorrhagic Stroke," National Stroke Association, n.d.

5. "Hemorrhagic Strokes (Bleeds)," American Stroke Association, November 9, 2016.

6. "Stroke," Mayo Clinic, February 21, 2017.

7. "What is a Hemorrhagic Stroke?" Joe Niekro Foundation, n.d.

Section 12.2

Cerebral Aneurysm

This section contains text excerpted from the following sources: Text
in this section begins with the excerpts from "Cerebral Aneurysms
Information Page," National Institute of Neurological Disorders
and Stroke (NINDS), December 19, 2016; Text beginning with the
heading "What Causes a Cerebral Aneurysm?" is excerpted from
"Cerebral Aneurysms Fact Sheet," National Institute of Neurological
Disorders and Stroke (NINDS), July 2013. Reviewed April 2017.

A cerebral aneurysm is a weak or thin spot on a blood vessel in the
brain that balloons out and fills with blood. An aneurysm can press
on a nerve or surrounding tissue, and also leak or burst, which lets
blood spill into surrounding tissues (called a hemorrhage). Cerebral
aneurysms can occur at any age, although they are more common in
adults than in children and are slightly more common in women than
in men. The signs and symptoms of an unruptured cerebral aneurysm
will partly depend on its size and rate of growth. For example, a small,
unchanging aneurysm will generally produce no symptoms, whereas a
larger aneurysm that is steadily growing may produce symptoms such
as headache, numbness, loss of feeling in the face or problems with
the eyes. Immediately after an aneurysm ruptures, an individual may
experience such symptoms as a sudden and unusually severe headache, nausea, vision impairment, vomiting, and loss of consciousness.

What Causes a Cerebral Aneurysm?

Cerebral aneurysms can be congenital, resulting from an inborn
abnormality in an artery wall. Cerebral aneurysms are also more
common in people with certain genetic diseases, such as connective
tissue disorders and polycystic kidney disease, and certain circulatory
disorders, such as arteriovenous malformations (snarled tangles of
arteries and veins in the brain that disrupt blood flow).

Other causes include trauma or injury to the head, high blood
pressure, infection, tumors, atherosclerosis (a blood vessel disease
in which fats build up on the inside of artery walls) and other diseases of the vascular system, cigarette smoking, and drug abuse. Some

investigators have speculated that oral contraceptives may increase the risk of developing aneurysms.

Aneurysms that result from an infection in the arterial wall are called mycotic aneurysms. Cancer-related aneurysms are often associated with tumors of the head and neck. Drug abuse, particularly the habitual use of cocaine, can inflame blood vessels and lead to the development of brain aneurysms.

What Are the Symptoms?

Most cerebral aneurysms do not show symptoms until they either become very large or burst. Small, unchanging aneurysms generally will not produce symptoms, whereas a larger aneurysm that is steadily growing may press on tissues and nerves. Symptoms may include pain above and behind the eye; numbness, weakness, or paralysis on one side of the face; dilated pupils; and vision changes. When an aneurysm hemorrhages, an individual may experience a sudden and extremely severe headache, double vision, nausea, vomiting, stiff neck, and/or loss of consciousness. Individuals usually describe the headache as "the worst headache of my life" and it is generally different in severity and intensity from other headaches people may experience. "Sentinel" or warning headaches may result from an aneurysm that leaks for days to weeks prior to rupture. Only a minority of individuals have a sentinel headache prior to aneurysm rupture.

Other signs that a cerebral aneurysm has burst include nausea and vomiting associated with a severe headache, a drooping eyelid, sensitivity to light, and change in mental status or level of awareness. Some individuals may have seizures. Individuals may lose consciousness briefly or go into prolonged coma. People experiencing this "worst headache," especially when it is combined with any other symptoms, should seek immediate medical attention.

How Are Aneurysms Classified?

There are three types of cerebral aneurysm. A saccular aneurysm is a rounded or pouch-like sac of blood that is attached by a neck or stem to an artery or a branch of a blood vessel. Also known as a berry aneurysm (because it resembles a berry hanging from a vine), this most common form of cerebral aneurysm is typically found on arteries at the base of the brain. Saccular aneurysms occur most often in adults. A lateral aneurysm appears as a bulge on one wall of the blood vessel, while a fusiform aneurysm is formed by the widening along all walls of the vessel.

Aneurysms are also classified by size. Small aneurysms are less than 11 millimeters in diameter (about the size of a large pencil eraser), larger aneurysms are 11–25 millimeters (about the width of a dime), and giant aneurysms are greater than 25 millimeters in diameter (more than the width of a quarter).

Who Is at Risk?

Brain aneurysms can occur in anyone, at any age. They are more common in adults than in children and slightly more common in women than in men. People with certain inherited disorders are also at higher risk.

All cerebral aneurysms have the potential to rupture and cause bleeding within the brain. The incidence of reported ruptured aneurysm is about 10 in every 100,000 persons per year (about 30,000 individuals per year in the United States), most commonly in people between ages 30 and 60 years. Possible risk factors for rupture include hypertension, alcohol abuse, drug abuse (particularly cocaine), and smoking. In addition, the condition and size of the aneurysm affects the risk of rupture.

What Are the Dangers?

Aneurysms may burst and bleed into the brain, causing serious complications, including hemorrhagic stroke, permanent nerve damage, or death. Once it has burst, the aneurysm may burst again and bleed into the brain, and additional aneurysms may also occur. More commonly, rupture may cause a subarachnoid hemorrhage—bleeding into the space between the skull bone and the brain. A delayed but serious complication of subarachnoid hemorrhage is hydrocephalus, in which the excessive buildup of cerebrospinal fluid in the skull dilates fluid pathways called ventricles that can swell and press on the brain tissue. Another delayed postrupture complication is vasospasm, in which other blood vessels in the brain contract and limit blood flow to vital areas of the brain. This reduced blood flow can cause stroke or tissue damage.

How Are Cerebral Aneurysms Diagnosed?

Most cerebral aneurysms go unnoticed until they rupture or are detected by brain imaging that may have been obtained for another condition. Several diagnostic methods are available to provide information about the aneurysm and the best form of treatment. The tests are usually obtained after a subarachnoid hemorrhage, to confirm the diagnosis of an aneurysm.

Angiography

Angiography is a dye test used to analyze the arteries or veins. An intracerebral angiogram can detect the degree of narrowing or obstruction of an artery or blood vessel in the brain, head, or neck, and can identify changes in an artery or vein such as a weak spot like an aneurysm. It is used to diagnose stroke and to precisely determine the location, size, and shape of a brain tumor, aneurysm, or blood vessel that has bled. This test is usually performed in a hospital angiography suite. Following the injection of a local anesthetic, a flexible catheter is inserted into an artery and threaded through the body to the affected artery. A small amount of contrast dye (one that is highlighted on X-rays) is released into the bloodstream and allowed to travel into the head and neck. A series of X-rays is taken and changes, if present, are noted.

Computed Tomography (CT)

Computed tomography (CT) of the head is a fast, painless, non-invasive diagnostic tool that can reveal the presence of a cerebral aneurysm and determine, for those aneurysms that have burst, if blood has leaked into the brain. This is often the first diagnostic procedure ordered by a physician following suspected rupture. X-rays of the head are processed by a computer as two-dimensional cross-sectional images, or "slices," of the brain and skull. Occasionally a contrast dye is injected into the bloodstream prior to scanning. This process, called CT angiography, produces sharper, more detailed images of blood flow in the brain arteries. CT is usually conducted at a testing facility or hospital outpatient setting.

Magnetic Resonance Imaging (MRI)

Magnetic resonance imaging (MRI) uses computer-generated radio waves and a powerful magnetic field to produce detailed images of the brain and other body structures. Magnetic resonance angiography (MRA) produces more detailed images of blood vessels. The images may be seen as either three-dimensional pictures or two-dimensional cross-slices of the brain and vessels. These painless, noninvasive procedures can show the size and shape of an unruptured aneurysm and can detect bleeding in the brain.

Cerebrospinal Fluid (CSF) Analysis

Cerebrospinal fluid analysis may be ordered if a ruptured aneurysm is suspected. Following application of a local anesthetic, a small amount of this fluid (which protects the brain and spinal cord) is removed from the subarachnoid space—located between the spinal cord and the membranes that surround it—by a spinal needle and tested to detect any bleeding or brain hemorrhage. In individuals with suspected subarachnoid hemorrhage, this procedure is usually done in a hospital.

How Are Cerebral Aneurysms Treated?

Not all cerebral aneurysms burst. Some people with very small aneurysms may be monitored to detect any growth or onset of symptoms and to ensure aggressive treatment of coexisting medical problems and risk factors. Each case is unique, and considerations for treating an unruptured aneurysm include the type, size, and location of the aneurysm; risk of rupture; the individual's age, health, and personal and family medical history; and risk of treatment.

Two surgical options are available for treating cerebral aneurysms, both of which carry some risk to the individual (such as possible damage to other blood vessels, the potential for aneurysm recurrence and rebleeding, and the risk of postoperative stroke).

Microvascular clipping involves cutting off the flow of blood to the aneurysm. Under anesthesia, a section of the skull is removed and the aneurysm is located. The neurosurgeon uses a microscope to isolate the blood vessel that feeds the aneurysm and places a small, metal, clothespin-like clip on the aneurysm's neck, halting its blood supply. The clip remains in the person and prevents the risk of future bleeding. The piece of the skull is then replaced and the scalp is closed. Clipping has been shown to be highly effective, depending on the location, shape, and size of the aneurysm. In general, aneurysms that are completely clipped surgically do not return.

A related procedure is an occlusion, in which the surgeon clamps off (occludes) the entire artery that leads to the aneurysm. This procedure is often performed when the aneurysm has damaged the artery. An occlusion is sometimes accompanied by a bypass, in which a small blood vessel is surgically grafted to the brain artery, rerouting the flow of blood away from the section of the damaged artery.

Endovascular embolization is an alternative to surgery. Once the individual has been anesthetized, the doctor inserts a hollow plastic tube (a catheter) into an artery (usually in the groin) and threads it, using angiography, through the body to the site of the aneurysm. Using a guide wire, detachable coils (spirals of platinum wire) are passed through the catheter and released into the aneurysm. The coils fill the aneurysm, block it from circulation, and cause the blood to clot, which effectively destroys the aneurysm. The procedure may need to be performed more than once during the person's lifetime.

People who receive treatment for an aneurysm must remain in bed until the bleeding stops. Underlying conditions, such as high blood pressure, should be treated. Other treatment for cerebral aneurysm is symptomatic and may include anticonvulsants to prevent seizures and analgesics to treat headache. Vasospasm can be treated with calcium channel-blocking drugs and sedatives may be ordered if the person is restless. A shunt may be surgically inserted into a ventricle several months following rupture if the buildup of cerebrospinal fluid is causing harmful pressure on surrounding tissue. Individuals who have suffered a subarachnoid hemorrhage often need rehabilitative, speech, and occupational therapy to regain lost function and learn to cope with any permanent disability.

Can Cerebral Aneurysms Be Prevented?

There are no known ways to prevent a cerebral aneurysm from forming. People with a diagnosed brain aneurysm should carefully control high blood pressure, stop smoking, and avoid cocaine use or other stimulant drugs. They should also consult with a doctor about the benefits and risks of taking aspirin or other drugs that thin the blood. Women should check with their doctors about the use of oral contraceptives.

What Is the Prognosis?

An unruptured aneurysm may go unnoticed throughout a person's lifetime. A burst aneurysm, however, may be fatal or could lead to hemorrhagic stroke, vasospasm (the leading cause of disability or death following a burst aneurysm), hydrocephalus, coma, or short-term and/or permanent brain damage.

113

The prognosis for persons whose aneurysm has burst is largely dependent on the age and general health of the individual, other pre-existing neurological conditions, location of the aneurysm, extent of bleeding (and rebleeding), and time between rupture and medical attention. It is estimated that about 40 percent of individuals whose aneurysm has ruptured do not survive the first 24 hours; up to another 25 percent die from complications within 6 months. People who experience subarachnoid hemorrhage may have permanent neurological damage. Other individuals may recover with little or no neurological deficit. Delayed complications from a burst aneurysm may include hydrocephalus and vasospasm. Early diagnosis and treatment are important.

Individuals who receive treatment for an unruptured aneurysm generally require less rehabilitative therapy and recover more quickly than persons whose aneurysm has burst. Recovery from treatment or rupture may take weeks to months.

Clinical studies suggest that in the first six months after treatment patients treated with endovascular coiling have less disability than those with surgical clipping, but that beyond six months after treatment the amount of disability is about the same. Long-term results of coiling procedures are uncertain and investigators need to conduct more research on this topic, since some aneurysms can recur after coiling. Individuals may want to consult a specialist in both endovascular and surgical repair of aneurysms, to help provide greater understanding of treatment options.

Chapter 13

Mini-Stroke: Transient Ischemic Attack (TIA)

What Is a Transient Ischemic Attack?[1]

A transient ischemic attack (TIA) is a transient stroke that lasts only a few minutes. It occurs when the blood supply to part of the brain is briefly interrupted. TIA symptoms, which usually occur suddenly, are similar to those of stroke but do not last as long. Most symptoms of a TIA disappear within an hour, although they may persist for up to 24 hours. Symptoms can include:

- numbness or weakness in the face, arm, or leg, especially on one side of the body;

- confusion or difficulty in talking or understanding speech;

- trouble seeing in one or both eyes; and

- difficulty with walking, dizziness, or loss of balance and coordination.

This chapter includes text excerpted from documents published by two public domain sources. Text under headings marked 1 are excerpted from "Transient Ischemic Attack Information Page," National Institute of Neurological Disorders and Stroke (NINDS), April 4, 2017; Text under heading marked 2 is excerpted from "Stroke—How Is a Stroke Treated?" National Heart, Lung, and Blood Institute (NHLBI), January 27, 2017.

Treating an Ischemic Stroke[2]

A TIA occurs if an artery that supplies oxygen-rich blood to the brain becomes blocked. Often, blood clots cause the blockages that lead to TIA. Treatment for a TIA may include medicines and medical procedures.

Medicines

If you have a stroke caused by a blood clot, you may be given a clot-dissolving, or clot-busting, medication called tissue plasminogen activator (tPA). A doctor will inject tPA into a vein in your arm. This type of medication must be given within 4 hours of symptom onset. Ideally, it should be given as soon as possible. The sooner treatment begins, the better your chances of recovery. Thus, it's important to know the signs and symptoms of a stroke and to call 9-1-1 right away for emergency care.

If you can't have tPA for medical reasons, your doctor may give you antiplatelet medicine that helps stop platelets from clumping together to form blood clots or anticoagulant medicine (blood thinner) that keeps existing blood clots from getting larger. Two common medicines are aspirin and clopidogrel.

Medical Procedures

If you have carotid artery disease, your doctor may recommend a carotid endarterectomy or carotid artery angioplasty. Both procedures open blocked carotid arteries.

Researchers are testing other treatments for ischemic stroke, such as intra-arterial thrombolysis and mechanical clot removal in cerebral ischemia (MERCI). In intra-arterial thrombolysis, a long flexible tube called a catheter is put into your groin (upper thigh) and threaded to the tiny arteries of the brain. Your doctor can deliver medicine through this catheter to break up a blood clot in the brain. MERCI is a device that can remove blood clots from an artery. During the procedure, a catheter is threaded through a carotid artery to the affected artery in the brain. The device is then used to pull the blood clot out through the catheter.

Treating Stroke Risk Factors

After initial treatment for a TIA, your doctor will treat your risk factors. He or she may recommend heart-healthy lifestyle changes to help control your risk factors.

Heart-healthy lifestyle changes may include:

- Heart-healthy eating
- Aiming for a healthy weight
- Managing stress
- Physical activity
- Quitting smoking

If heart-healthy lifestyle changes aren't enough, you may need medicine to control your risk factors.

Prognosis of Transient Ischemic Attack[1]

TIAs are often warning signs that a person is at risk for a more serious and debilitating stroke. About one-third of those who have a TIA will have an acute stroke some time in the future. Many strokes can be prevented by heeding the warning signs of TIAs and treating underlying risk factors. The most important treatable factors linked to TIAs and stroke are high blood pressure, cigarette smoking, heart disease, carotid artery disease, diabetes, and heavy use of alcohol. Medical help is available to reduce and eliminate these factors. Lifestyle changes such as eating a balanced diet, maintaining healthy weight, exercising, and enrolling in smoking and alcohol cessation programs can also reduce these factors.

Chapter 14

Recurrent Stroke

As the name implies, a recurrent stroke is one that takes place after the original stroke has been stabilized. According to the National Stroke Association, of the more than 750,000 U.S. patients who experience a stroke each year, 5 to 14 percent will have a second occurrence within one year. And 42 percent of men and 24 percent of women will have a recurrence within five years. Additionally, recurrent strokes often result in higher fatality and disability rates because parts of the brain have already been damaged by the first stroke. So awareness and monitoring for recurrence is an important part of any stroke recovery plan.

Risk Factors for Recurrent Stroke

There a multiple risk factors that increase the chances of having a recurrent stroke. Among these are:

- age (being over 55)

- gender (men are more likely to experience recurrence)

- race (African-American patients are more at risk)

- family history of strokes

- hypertension (high blood pressure)

- atrial fibrillation (abnormal heart rhythm)

"What Is Recurrent Stroke?" © 2017 Omnigraphics. Reviewed April 2017.

- diabetes

- smoking

- excess alcohol consumption

- sedentary lifestyle

- obesity

- high cholesterol

Managing Risk Factors to Prevent Recurrent Stroke

Although some risk factors, such as age, gender, and race, are out of a patient's control, others can be managed to help reduce the chances of having a recurrent stroke. For example:

- **Hypertension.** Studies show that lowering blood pressure can reduce the risk of stroke by 30 to 40 percent. But it's also one of the most easily controlled risk factors through a variety of methods, including regular aerobic exercise, eating healthy foods, limiting salt and alcohol intake, losing weight, and medication.

- **Atrial fibrillation (AF).** An irregular heartbeat can cause blood to collect in the heart and possibly form clots, which can travel to the brain and cause a stroke. Treatment for AF can include electrical shocks or surgical procedures, but most often it is controlled through medication.

- **Diabetes.** Patients with diabetes (high glucose—or sugar—levels) are estimated to be four times as likely to have a recurrent stroke as other individuals, so it's important to keep the condition under control. Typically, this means maintaining a healthy diet, exercising, reducing blood pressure, losing weight, and taking insulin or oral hypoglycemic drugs to keep glucose levels in check.

- **Smoking.** Smokers are not only more at risk for a first stroke but are twice as likely to experience recurrent stroke than nonsmokers. Cigarette smoking causes atherosclerosis (buildup of plaque within the arteries) and other artery damage, constricting the blood vessels and reducing the flow of blood to the brain.

- **Alcohol consumption.** Very moderate alcohol use may actually help prevent ischemic stroke by increasing high-density lipoprotein ("good cholesterol") levels, but according to some studies, more than two drinks per day could increase stroke risk by 50 percent. Heavy drinking increases blood pressure, reduces blood flow to the brain, and can cause atrial fibrillation.

- **High cholesterol.** Elevated total cholesterol levels or low-density lipoprotein (LDL or "bad cholesterol") levels increase stroke risk by causing plaque to build up in the arteries and restrict blood flow to the brain. Medications called statins can help reduce cholesterol levels, as can lifestyle modifications, such as decreasing the intake of saturated fats, losing weight, and increasing physical activity.

- **Obesity.** There is still some debate about whether obesity directly increases the chances of having either an initial or recurrent stroke, but experts agree that obesity contributes to risk factors, such as hypertension and diabetes. Exercise and healthy eating habits are the best way to both lose weight and reduce stroke risk.

- **Sedentary lifestyle.** Studies show that patients who exercise five or more times per week are clearly less likely to have a recurrent stroke. Aerobic exercise improves cardiovascular fitness and reduces blood pressure, while strength training has the added benefit of improving balance and mobility after a stroke.

Other Ways to Prevent Recurrent Stroke

Although lifestyle changes and managing diseases to control risk factors are almost always suggested to help prevent recurrent stroke, doctors may recommend other methods, as well, depending on the details of the patient's original stroke, medical history, and overall physical condition. These might include:

- **Medication.** Drugs prescribed to help prevent recurrent stroke can include anticlotting medications, such as aspirin, dipyridamole, ticlopidine, and warfarin, as well as drugs to control hypertension, including diuretics, beta blockers, angiotensin II receptor blockers (ARBs), calcium channel blockers, and renin inhibitors.

- **Surgery.** Various surgical options are available to help prevent another stroke. Depending on the cause of the initial stroke, these can include carotid endarterectomy (removing a blockage in the carotid artery), extracranial or intracranial bypass (creating a new path around a damaged artery), and balloon angioplasty with stenting (expanding the artery and inserting a wire mesh tube to keep it open).

- **Physical therapy.** In patients for whom a sedentary lifestyle was a contributing factor to the original stroke and continues to put them at risk for a recurrent stroke, physical therapy might be recommended to help them make lifestyle changes. Many individuals find it easier to begin developing healthy habits by working with a trained professional, rather than trying to exercise on their own.

References

1. Dickerson, Lori M., PharmD, Peter J. Carek, MD, MS, and Robert Glen Quattlebaum, MD, MPH. "Prevention of Recurrent Ischemic Stroke," *American Family Physician*, April 1, 2007.

2. Jeffrey, Susan. "Risk for Recurrent Stroke, Death High in Hospitalized Stroke Patients," Medscape.com, February 25, 2010.

3. "New Guidelines for the Prevention of Recurrent Stroke," *Harvard Heart Letter*, July 2014.

4. "Preventing Another Stroke," National Stroke Association, n.d.5. "Recovery after Stroke: Recurrent Stroke," National Stroke Association, 2014.

Part Three

Stroke Risk Factors and Prevention

Chapter 15

Stroke Risks

Anyone can have a stroke at any age. But certain things can increase your chances of having a stroke. The best way to protect yourself and your loved ones from a stroke is to understand your risk and how to control it. While you can't control your age or family history, you can take steps to lower your chances of having a stroke.

Conditions That Increase Risk for Stroke

Many common medical conditions can increase your chances of having a stroke. Work with your healthcare team to control your risk.

Previous Stroke or Transient Ischemic Attack

If you have already had a stroke or a transient ischemic attack (TIA), also known as a "mini-stroke," your chances of having another stroke are higher.

High Blood Pressure

High blood pressure is a leading cause of stroke. It occurs when the pressure of the blood in your arteries and other blood vessels is too high. There are often no symptoms of high blood pressure. Get your blood pressure checked often. If you have high blood pressure,

This chapter includes text excerpted from "Stroke Risk," Centers for Disease Control and Prevention (CDC), January 17, 2017.

lowering your blood pressure through lifestyle changes or medicine can also lower your risk for stroke.

High Cholesterol

Cholesterol is a waxy, fat-like substance made by the liver or found in certain foods. Your liver makes enough for your body's needs, but we often get more cholesterol from the foods we eat. If we take in more cholesterol than the body can use, the extra cholesterol can build up in the arteries, including those of the brain. This can lead to stroke, narrowing of the arteries, and other problems. A blood test can tell your doctor if you have high levels of cholesterol and triglycerides (a related kind of fat) in your blood.

Heart Disease

Common heart disorders can increase your risk for stroke. For example, coronary artery disease increases your risk for stroke, because plaque builds up in the arteries and blocks the flow of oxygen-rich blood to the brain. Other heart conditions, such as heart valve defects, irregular heartbeat (including atrial fibrillation), and enlarged heart chambers, can cause blood clots that may break loose and cause a stroke.

Diabetes

Diabetes increases your risk for stroke. Your body needs glucose (sugar) for energy. Insulin is a hormone made in the pancreas that helps move glucose from the food you eat to your body's cells. If you have diabetes, your body doesn't make enough insulin, can't use its own insulin as well as it should, or both.

Diabetes causes sugars to build up in the blood and prevent oxygen and nutrients from getting to the various parts of your body, including your brain. High blood pressure is also common in people with diabetes. High blood pressure is the leading cause of stroke and is the main cause for increased risk of stroke among people with diabetes.

Talk to your doctor about ways to keep diabetes under control.

Sickle Cell Disease

Sickle cell disease is a blood disorder linked to ischemic stroke that affects mainly black and Hispanic children. The disease causes some red blood cells to form an abnormal sickle shape. A stroke can happen if sickle cells get stuck in a blood vessel and block the flow of blood to the brain.

Behaviors That Increase Risk for Stroke

Your lifestyle choices can affect your chances of having a stroke. To lower your risk, your doctor may suggest changes to your lifestyle.

The good news is that healthy behaviors can lower your risk for stroke.

Unhealthy Diet

Diets high in saturated fats, trans fat, and cholesterol have been linked to stroke and related conditions, such as heart disease. Also, getting too much salt (sodium) in the diet can raise blood pressure levels.

Physical Inactivity

Not getting enough physical activity can lead to other health conditions that can raise the risk for stroke. These health conditions include obesity, high blood pressure, high cholesterol, and diabetes. Regular physical activity can lower your chances for stroke.

Obesity

Obesity is excess body fat. Obesity is linked to higher "bad" cholesterol and triglyceride levels and to lower "good" cholesterol levels. Obesity can also lead to high blood pressure and diabetes.

Too Much Alcohol

Drinking too much alcohol can raise blood pressure levels and the risk for stroke. It also increases levels of triglycerides, a form of fat in your blood that can harden your arteries.

- Women should have no more than one drink a day.
- Men should have no more than two drinks a day.

Tobacco Use

Tobacco use increases the risk for stroke. Cigarette smoking can damage the heart and blood vessels, increasing your risk for stroke. The nicotine in cigarettes raises blood pressure, and the carbon monoxide from cigarette smoke reduces the amount of oxygen that your blood can carry. Even if you don't smoke, breathing in other people's secondhand smoke can make you more likely to have a stroke.

Family History and Other Characteristics That Increase Risk for Stroke

Family health history is a record of the diseases and health conditions that happen in your family. Family health history is a useful tool for understanding health risks and preventing health problems. Family members share genes, behaviors, lifestyles, and environments that can influence their health and their risk for disease. Stroke risk can be higher in some families than in others, and your chances of having a stroke can go up or down depending on your age, sex, and race or ethnicity.

You can't change your family history, but knowing your family's health history can help you know your risk for stroke and take steps to prevent stroke. The good news is you can take steps to prevent stroke. Work with your healthcare team to lower your risk for stroke.

Genetics and Family History

When members of a family pass traits from one generation to another through genes, that process is called heredity.

Genetic factors likely play some role in stroke, high blood pressure, and other related conditions. Several genetic disorders can cause a stroke, including sickle cell disease. People with a family history of stroke are also likely to share common environments and other potential factors that increase their risk.

The chances for stroke can increase even more when heredity combines with unhealthy lifestyle choices, such as smoking cigarettes and eating an unhealthy diet.

Age

The older you are, the more likely you are to have a stroke. The chance of having a stroke about doubles every 10 years after age 55. Although stroke is common among older adults, many people younger than 65 years also have strokes.

In fact, about one in seven strokes occur in adolescents and young adults ages 15 to 49.Experts think younger people are having more strokes because more young people are obese and have high blood pressure and diabetes.

Sex

Stroke is more common in women than men, and women of all ages are more likely than men to die from stroke. Pregnancy and use of birth control pills pose special stroke risks for women.

Race or Ethnicity

Blacks, Hispanics, American Indians, and Alaska Natives may be more likely to have a stroke than non-Hispanic whites or Asians. The risk of having a first stroke is nearly twice as high for blacks as for whites. Blacks are also more likely to die from stroke than whites are.

Chapter 16

Atherosclerosis and Carotid Artery Disease

Chapter Contents

Section 16.1—Atherosclerosis 132

Section 16.2—Carotid Artery Disease 144

Section 16.1

Atherosclerosis

This section includes text excerpted from "Atherosclerosis," National
Heart, Lung, and Blood Institute (NHLBI), June 22, 2016.

Atherosclerosis is a disease in which plaque builds up inside your
arteries. Arteries are blood vessels that carry oxygen-rich blood to
your heart and other parts of your body. Plaque is made up of fat,
cholesterol, calcium, and other substances found in the blood. Over
time, plaque hardens and narrows your arteries. This limits the flow of
oxygen-rich blood to your organs and other parts of your body. Atherosclerosis can lead to serious problems, including stroke, heart attack,
or even death.

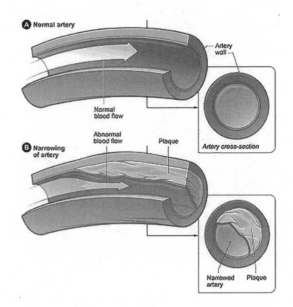

Figure 16.1. *Atherosclerosis*

*Figure section A shows a normal artery with normal blood flow. The inset image shows
a cross-section of a normal artery. Figure section B shows an artery with plaque buildup. The inset image shows a cross-section of an artery with plaque buildup.*

Atherosclerosis-Related Diseases

Atherosclerosis can affect any artery in the body, including arteries in the heart, brain, arms, legs, pelvis, and kidneys. As a result, different diseases may develop based on which arteries are affected.

Coronary Heart Disease

Coronary heart disease (CHD), also called coronary artery disease, occurs when plaque builds up in the coronary arteries. These arteries supply oxygen-rich blood to your heart. Plaque narrows the coronary arteries and reduces blood flow to your heart muscle. Plaque buildup also makes it more likely that blood clots will form in your arteries. Blood clots can partially or completely block blood flow.

If blood flow to your heart muscle is reduced or blocked, you may have angina (chest pain or discomfort) or a heart attack. Plaque also can form in the heart's smallest arteries. This disease is called coronary microvascular disease (MVD). In coronary MVD, plaque doesn't cause blockages in the arteries as it does in CHD.

Carotid Artery Disease

Carotid artery disease occurs if plaque builds up in the arteries on each side of your neck (the carotid arteries). These arteries supply oxygen-rich blood to your brain. If blood flow to your brain is reduced or blocked, you may have a stroke.

Peripheral Artery Disease

Peripheral artery disease (PAD) occurs if plaque builds up in the major arteries that supply oxygen-rich blood to your legs, arms, and pelvis. If blood flow to these parts of your body is reduced or blocked, you may have numbness, pain, and, sometimes, dangerous infections.

Chronic Kidney Disease

Chronic kidney disease can occur if plaque builds up in the renal arteries. These arteries supply oxygen-rich blood to your kidneys. Over time, chronic kidney disease causes a slow loss of kidney function. The main function of the kidneys is to remove waste and extra water from the body.

Causes of Atherosclerosis

The exact cause of atherosclerosis isn't known. However, studies show that atherosclerosis is a slow, complex disease that may start in childhood. It develops faster as you age.

Atherosclerosis may start when certain factors damage the inner layers of the arteries. These factors include:

- Smoking

- High amounts of certain fats and cholesterol in the blood

- High blood pressure

- High amounts of sugar in the blood due to insulin resistance or diabetes

Plaque may begin to build up where the arteries are damaged. Over time, plaque hardens and narrows the arteries. Eventually, an area of plaque can rupture (break open).

When this happens, blood cell fragments called platelets stick to the site of the injury. They may clump together to form blood clots. Clots narrow the arteries even more, limiting the flow of oxygen-rich blood to your body. Depending on which arteries are affected, blood clots can worsen angina (chest pain) or cause a stroke or heart attack.

Risk Factors for Atherosclerosis

The exact cause of atherosclerosis isn't known. However, certain traits, conditions, or habits may raise your risk for the disease. These conditions are known as risk factors. The more risk factors you have, the more likely it is that you'll develop atherosclerosis.

You can control most risk factors and help prevent or delay atherosclerosis. Other risk factors can't be controlled.

Major Risk Factors

- **Unhealthy blood cholesterol levels.** This includes high low-density lipoprotein (LDL) cholesterol (sometimes called "bad" cholesterol) and low high-density lipoprotein (HDL) cholesterol (sometimes called "good" cholesterol).

- **High blood pressure.** Blood pressure is considered high if it stays at or above 140/90 mmHg over time. If you have diabetes or chronic kidney disease, high blood pressure is defined as

130/80 mmHg or higher. (The mmHg is millimeters of mercury—the units used to measure blood pressure.)

- **Smoking.** Smoking can damage and tighten blood vessels, raise cholesterol levels, and raise blood pressure. Smoking also doesn't allow enough oxygen to reach the body's tissues.

- **Insulin resistance.** This condition occurs if the body can't use its insulin properly. Insulin is a hormone that helps move blood sugar into cells where it's used as an energy source. Insulin resistance may lead to diabetes.

- **Diabetes.** With this disease, the body's blood sugar level is too high because the body doesn't make enough insulin or doesn't use its insulin properly.

- **Overweight or obesity.** The terms "overweight" and "obesity" refer to body weight that's greater than what is considered healthy for a certain height.

- **Lack of physical activity.** A lack of physical activity can worsen other risk factors for atherosclerosis, such as unhealthy blood cholesterol levels, high blood pressure, diabetes, and over-weight and obesity.

- **Unhealthy diet.** An unhealthy diet can raise your risk for atherosclerosis. Foods that are high in saturated and trans fats, cholesterol, sodium (salt), and sugar, can worsen other atherosclerosis risk factors.

- **Older age.** As you get older, your risk for atherosclerosis increases. Genetic or lifestyle factors cause plaque to build up in your arteries as you age. By the time you're middle-aged or older, enough plaque has built up to cause signs or symptoms. In men, the risk increases after age 45. In women, the risk increases after age 55.

- **Family history of early heart disease.** Your risk for atherosclerosis increases if your father or a brother was diagnosed with heart disease before 55 years of age, or if your mother or a sister was diagnosed with heart disease before 65 years of age.

Although age and a family history of early heart disease are risk factors, it doesn't mean that you'll develop atherosclerosis if you have one or both. Controlling other risk factors often can lessen genetic influences and prevent atherosclerosis, even in older adults.

Studies show that an increasing number of children and youth are at risk for atherosclerosis. This is due to a number of causes, including rising childhood obesity rates.

Other Factors

Other factors also may raise your risk for atherosclerosis, such as:

- **Sleep apnea.** Sleep apnea is a disorder that causes one or more pauses in breathing or shallow breaths while you sleep. Untreated sleep apnea can raise your risk for high blood pressure, diabetes, and even a stroke or heart attack.

- **Stress.** Research shows that the most commonly reported "trigger" for a heart attack is an emotionally upsetting event, especially one involving anger.

- **Alcohol.** Heavy drinking can damage the heart muscle and worsen other risk factors for atherosclerosis. Men should have no more than two drinks containing alcohol a day. Women should have no more than one drink containing alcohol a day.

Signs and Symptoms of Atherosclerosis

Atherosclerosis usually doesn't cause signs and symptoms until it severely narrows or totally blocks an artery. Many people don't know they have the disease until they have a medical emergency, such as a stroke or heart attack. Some people may have signs and symptoms of the disease. Signs and symptoms will depend on which arteries are affected.

Coronary Arteries

The coronary arteries supply oxygen-rich blood to your heart. If plaque narrows or blocks these arteries (a disease called coronary heart disease, or CHD), a common symptom is angina. Angina is chest pain or discomfort that occurs when your heart muscle doesn't get enough oxygen-rich blood.

Angina may feel like pressure or squeezing in your chest. You also may feel it in your shoulders, arms, neck, jaw, or back. Angina pain may even feel like indigestion. The pain tends to get worse with activity and go away with rest. Emotional stress also can trigger the pain.

Other symptoms of CHD are shortness of breath and arrhythmias. Arrhythmias are problems with the rate or rhythm of the heartbeat.

Plaque also can form in the heart's smallest arteries. This disease is called coronary microvascular disease (MVD). Symptoms of coronary MVD include angina, shortness of breath, sleep problems, fatigue (tiredness), and lack of energy.

Carotid Arteries

The carotid arteries supply oxygen-rich blood to your brain. If plaque narrows or blocks these arteries (a disease called carotid artery disease), you may have symptoms of a stroke. These symptoms may include:

- Sudden weakness
- Paralysis (an inability to move) or numbness of the face, arms, or legs, especially on one side of the body
- Confusion
- Trouble speaking or understanding speech
- Trouble seeing in one or both eyes
- Problems breathing
- Dizziness, trouble walking, loss of balance or coordination, and unexplained falls
- Loss of consciousness
- Sudden and severe headache

Peripheral Arteries

Plaque also can build up in the major arteries that supply oxygen-rich blood to the legs, arms, and pelvis (a disease called peripheral artery disease). If these major arteries are narrowed or blocked, you may have numbness, pain, and, sometimes, dangerous infections.

Renal Arteries

The renal arteries supply oxygen-rich blood to your kidneys. If plaque builds up in these arteries, you may develop chronic kidney disease. Over time, chronic kidney disease causes a slow loss of kidney function.

Early kidney disease often has no signs or symptoms. As the disease gets worse it can cause tiredness, changes in how you urinate (more often or less often), loss of appetite, nausea (feeling sick to the stomach), swelling in the hands or feet, itchiness or numbness, and trouble concentrating.

Diagnosis of Atherosclerosis

Your doctor will diagnose atherosclerosis-based on your medical and family histories, a physical exam, and test results.

Specialists Involved

If you have atherosclerosis, a primary care doctor, such as an internist or family practitioner, may handle your care. Your doctor may recommend other healthcare specialists if you need expert care, such as:

- A **cardiologist.** This is a doctor who specializes in diagnosing and treating heart diseases and conditions. You may go to a cardiologist if you have peripheral artery disease (P.A.D.) or coronary microvascular disease (MVD).

- A **vascular specialist.** This is a doctor who specializes in diagnosing and treating blood vessel problems. You may go to a vascular specialist if you have P.A.D.

- A **neurologist.** This is a doctor who specializes in diagnosing and treating nervous system disorders. You may see a neurologist if you've had a stroke due to carotid artery disease.

- A **nephrologist**. This is a doctor who specializes in diagnosing and treating kidney diseases and conditions. You may go to a nephrologist if you have chronic kidney disease.

Physical Exam

During the physical exam, your doctor may listen to your arteries for an abnormal whooshing sound called a bruit. Your doctor can hear a bruit when placing a stethoscope over an affected artery. A bruit may indicate poor blood flow due to plaque buildup.

Your doctor also may check to see whether any of your pulses (for example, in the leg or foot) are weak or absent. A weak or absent pulse can be a sign of a blocked artery.

Diagnostic Tests

Your doctor may recommend one or more tests to diagnose atherosclerosis. These tests also can help your doctor learn the extent of your disease and plan the best treatment.

Blood Tests

Blood tests check the levels of certain fats, cholesterol, sugar, and proteins in your blood. Abnormal levels may be a sign that you're at risk for atherosclerosis.

Electrocardiogram (EKG)

An EKG is a simple, painless test that detects and records the heart's electrical activity. The test shows how fast the heart is beating and its rhythm (steady or irregular). An EKG also records the strength and timing of electrical signals as they pass through the heart.

An EKG can show signs of heart damage caused by CHD. The test also can show signs of a previous or current heart attack.

Chest X-Ray

A chest X-ray takes pictures of the organs and structures inside your chest, such as your heart, lungs, and blood vessels. A chest X-ray can reveal signs of heart failure.

Ankle-Brachial Index

This test compares the blood pressure in your ankle with the blood pressure in your arm to see how well your blood is flowing. This test can help diagnose P.A.D.

Echocardiography

Echocardiography (echo) uses sound waves to create a moving picture of your heart. The test provides information about the size and shape of your heart and how well your heart chambers and valves are working. Echo also can identify areas of poor blood flow to the heart, areas of heart muscle that aren't contracting normally, and previous injury to the heart muscle caused by poor blood flow.

Computed Tomography Scan

A computed tomography (CT) scan creates computer-generated pictures of the heart, brain, or other areas of the body. The test can show hardening and narrowing of large arteries.

A cardiac CT scan also can show whether calcium has built up in the walls of the coronary (heart) arteries. This may be an early sign of CHD.

Stress Testing

During stress testing, you exercise to make your heart work hard and beat fast while heart tests are done. If you can't exercise, you may be given medicine to make your heart work hard and beat fast. When your heart is working hard, it needs more blood and oxygen. Plaque-narrowed arteries can't supply enough oxygen-rich blood to meet your heart's needs.

A stress test can show possible signs and symptoms of CHD, such as:

- Abnormal changes in your heart rate or blood pressure
- Shortness of breath or chest pain
- Abnormal changes in your heart rhythm or your heart's electrical activity

As part of some stress tests, pictures are taken of your heart while you exercise and while you rest. These imaging stress tests can show how well blood is flowing in various parts of your heart. They also can show how well your heart pumps blood when it beats.

Angiography

Angiography is a test that uses dye and special X-rays to show the inside of your arteries. This test can show whether plaque is blocking your arteries and how severe the blockage is.

A thin, flexible tube called a catheter is put into a blood vessel in your arm, groin (upper thigh), or neck. Dye that can be seen on an X-ray picture is injected through the catheter into the arteries. By looking at the X-ray picture, your doctor can see the flow of blood through your arteries.

Other Tests

Other tests are being studied to see whether they can give a better view of plaque buildup in the arteries. Examples of these tests include magnetic resonance imaging (MRI) and positron emission tomography (PET).

Treatment of Atherosclerosis

Treatments for atherosclerosis may include heart-healthy lifestyle changes, medicines, and medical procedures or surgery. The goals of treatment include:

- Lowering the risk of blood clots forming

- Preventing atherosclerosis-related diseases

- Reducing risk factors in an effort to slow or stop the buildup of plaque

- Relieving symptoms

- Widening or bypassing plaque-clogged arteries

Heart-Healthy Lifestyle Changes

Your doctor may recommend heart-healthy lifestyle changes if you have atherosclerosis. Heart-healthy lifestyle changes include heart-healthy eating, aiming for a healthy weight, managing stress, physical activity and quitting smoking.

Medicines

Sometimes lifestyle changes alone aren't enough to control your cholesterol levels. For example, you also may need statin medications to control or lower your cholesterol. By lowering your blood cholesterol level, you can decrease your chance of having a stroke or heart attack. Doctors usually prescribe statins for people who have:

- Coronary heart disease, peripheral artery disease, or had a prior stroke

- Diabetes

- High LDL cholesterol levels

- Doctors may discuss beginning statin treatment with people who have an elevated risk for developing heart disease or having a stroke.

- Your doctor also may prescribe other medications to:

- Lower your blood pressure

- Lower your blood sugar levels

- Prevent blood clots, which can lead to heart attack and stroke

- Prevent inflammation

Take all medicines regularly, as your doctor prescribes. Don't change the amount of your medicine or skip a dose unless your doctor tells you to. You should still follow a heart healthy lifestyle, even if you take medicines to treat your atherosclerosis.

Medical Procedures and Surgery

If you have severe atherosclerosis, your doctor may recommend a medical procedure or surgery.

Percutaneous coronary intervention (PCI), also known as coronary angioplasty, is a procedure that's used to open blocked or narrowed coronary (heart) arteries. PCI can improve blood flow to the heart and relieve chest pain. Sometimes a small mesh tube called a stent is placed in the artery to keep it open after the procedure.

Coronary artery bypass grafting (CABG) is a type of surgery. In CABG, arteries or veins from other areas in your body are used to bypass or go around your narrowed coronary arteries. CABG can improve blood flow to your heart, relieve chest pain, and possibly prevent a heart attack.

Bypass grafting also can be used for leg arteries. For this surgery, a healthy blood vessel is used to bypass a narrowed or blocked artery in one of the legs. The healthy blood vessel redirects blood around the blocked artery, improving blood flow to the leg.

Carotid endarterectomy is a type of surgery to remove plaque buildup from the carotid arteries in the neck. This procedure restores blood flow to the brain, which can help prevent a stroke.

Prevention of Atherosclerosis

Taking action to control your risk factors can help prevent or delay atherosclerosis and its related diseases. Your risk for atherosclerosis increases with the number of risk factors you have.

One step you can take is to adopt a healthy lifestyle, which can include:

- **Heart-Healthy Eating.** Adopt heart-healthy eating habits, which include eating different fruits and vegetables (including beans and peas), whole grains, lean meats, poultry without skin, seafood, and fat-free or low-fat milk and dairy products. A heart-healthy diet is low in sodium, added sugar, solid fats, and refined grains. Following a heart-healthy diet is an important part of a healthy lifestyle.

- **Physical Activity.** Be as physically active as you can. Physical activity can improve your fitness level and your health. Ask your doctor what types and amounts of activity are safe for you.

- **Quit Smoking.** If you smoke, quit. Smoking can damage and tighten blood vessels and raise your risk for atherosclerosis. Talk with your doctor about programs and products that can help you quit. Also, try to avoid secondhand smoke.

- **Weight Control.** If you're overweight or obese, work with your doctor to create a reasonable weight-loss plan. Controlling your weight helps you control risk factors for atherosclerosis.

Other steps that can prevent or delay atherosclerosis include knowing your family history of atherosclerosis. If you or someone in your family has an atherosclerosis-related disease, be sure to tell your doctor.

If lifestyle changes aren't enough, your doctor may prescribe medicines to control your atherosclerosis risk factors. Take all of your medicines as your doctor advises.

Living with Atherosclerosis

Improved treatments have reduced the number of deaths from atherosclerosis-related diseases. These treatments also have improved the quality of life for people who have these diseases.

Adopting a healthy lifestyle may help you prevent or delay atherosclerosis and the problems it can cause. This, along with ongoing medical care, can help you avoid the problems of atherosclerosis and live a long, healthy life.

Researchers continue to look for ways to improve the health of people who have atherosclerosis or may develop it.

Ongoing Care

If you have atherosclerosis, work closely with your doctor and other healthcare providers to avoid serious problems, such as stroke and heart attack.

Follow your treatment plan and take all of your medicines as your doctor prescribes. Your doctor will let you know how often you should schedule office visits or blood tests. Be sure to let your doctor know if you have new or worsening symptoms.

Emotional Issues and Support

Having an atherosclerosis-related disease may cause fear, anxiety, depression, and stress. Talk about how you feel with your doctor.

Talking to a professional counselor also can help. If you're very depressed, your doctor may recommend medicines or other treatments that can improve your quality of life.

Community resources are available to help you learn more about atherosclerosis. Contact your local public health departments, hospitals, and local chapters of national health organizations to learn more about available resources in your area.

Talk about your lifestyle changes with your family and friends— whoever can provide support or needs to understand why you're changing your habits.

Family and friends may be able to help you make lifestyle changes. For example, they can help you plan healthier meals. Because atherosclerosis tends to run in families, your lifestyle changes may help many of your family members too.

Section 16.2

Carotid Artery Disease

This section includes text excerpted from "Carotid Artery Disease," National Heart, Lung, and Blood Institute (NHLBI), June 22, 2016.

Carotid artery disease is a disease in which a waxy substance called plaque builds up inside the carotid arteries. You have two common carotid arteries, one on each side of your neck. They each divide into internal and external carotid arteries. The internal carotid arteries supply oxygen-rich blood to your brain. The external carotid arteries supply oxygen-rich blood to your face, scalp, and neck.

Carotid artery disease is serious because it can cause a stroke, also called a "brain attack." A stroke occurs if blood flow to your brain is cut off. If blood flow is cut off for more than a few minutes, the cells in your brain start to die. This impairs the parts of the body that the brain cells control. A stroke can cause lasting brain damage; long-term disability, such as vision or speech problems or paralysis (an inability to move); or death.

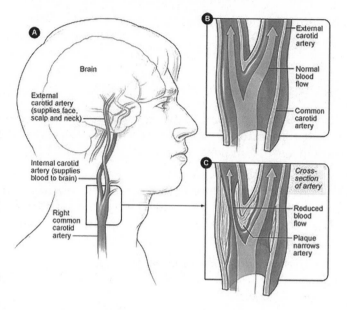

Figure 16.2. *Carotid Arteries*

Figure section A shows the location of the right carotid artery in the head and neck. Figure section B shows the inside of a normal carotid artery that has normal blood flow. Figure section C show the inside of a carotid artery that has plaque buildup and reduced blood flow.

Causes of Carotid Artery Disease

Carotid artery disease seems to start when damage occurs to the inner layers of the carotid arteries. Major factors that contribute to damage include:

- Smoking
- High levels of certain fats and cholesterol in the blood
- High blood pressure
- High levels of sugar in the blood due to insulin resistance or diabetes

When damage occurs, your body starts a healing process. The healing may cause plaque to build up where the arteries are damaged. The plaque in an artery can crack or rupture. If this happens, blood cell fragments called platelets will stick to the site of the injury and may clump together to form blood clots.

The buildup of plaque or blood clots can severely narrow or block the carotid arteries. This limits the flow of oxygen-rich blood to your brain, which can cause a stroke.

Risk Factors for Carotid Artery Disease

The major risk factors for carotid artery disease, listed below, also are the major risk factors for coronary heart disease (also called coronary artery disease) and peripheral artery disease.

- **Diabetes.** With this disease, the body's blood sugar level is too high because the body doesn't make enough insulin or doesn't use its insulin properly. People who have diabetes are four times more likely to have carotid artery disease than are people who don't have diabetes.

- **Family history of atherosclerosis.** People who have a family history of atherosclerosis are more likely to develop carotid artery disease.

- **High blood pressure (Hypertension).** Blood pressure is considered high if it stays at or above 140/90 mmHg over time. If you have diabetes or chronic kidney disease, high blood pressure is defined as 130/80 mmHg or higher. (The mmHg is millimeters of mercury—the units used to measure blood pressure.)

- **Lack of physical activity.** Too much sitting (sedentary lifestyle) and a lack of aerobic activity can worsen other risk factors for carotid artery disease, such as unhealthy blood cholesterol levels, high blood pressure, diabetes, and overweight or obesity.

- **Metabolic syndrome.** Metabolic syndrome is the name for a group of risk factors that raise your risk for stroke and other health problems, such as diabetes and heart disease. The five metabolic risk factors are a large waistline (abdominal obesity), a high triglyceride level (a type of fat found in the blood), a low HDL cholesterol level, high blood pressure, and high blood sugar. Metabolic syndrome is diagnosed if you have at least three of these metabolic risk factors.

- **Older age.** As you age, your risk for atherosclerosis increases. The process of atherosclerosis begins in youth and typically progresses over many decades before diseases develop.

- **Overweight or obesity.** The terms "overweight" and "obesity" refer to body weight that's greater than what is considered healthy for a certain height.

- **Smoking.** Smoking can damage and tighten blood vessels, lead to unhealthy cholesterol levels, and raise blood pressure. Smoking also can limit how much oxygen reaches the body's tissues.

- **Unhealthy blood cholesterol levels.** This includes high low-density lipoprotein (LDL) ("bad") cholesterol) and low high-density lipoprotein (HDL) ("good") cholesterol.

- **Unhealthy diet.** An unhealthy diet can raise your risk for carotid artery disease. Foods that are high in saturated and trans fats, cholesterol, sodium, and sugar can worsen other risk factors for carotid artery disease.

Having any of these risk factors does not guarantee that you'll develop carotid artery disease. However, if you know that you have one or more risk factors, you can take steps to help prevent or delay the disease.

If you have plaque buildup in your carotid arteries, you also may have plaque buildup in other arteries. People who have carotid artery disease also are at increased risk for coronary heart disease.

Signs and Symptoms of Carotid Artery Disease

Carotid artery disease may not cause signs or symptoms until it severely narrows or blocks a carotid artery. Signs and symptoms may include a bruit, a transient ischemic attack (TIA), or a stroke.

Bruit

During a physical exam, your doctor may listen to your carotid arteries with a stethoscope. He or she may hear a whooshing sound called a bruit. This sound may suggest changed or reduced blood flow due to plaque buildup. To find out more, your doctor may recommend tests.

Not all people who have carotid artery disease have bruits.

Transient Ischemic Attack (Mini-Stroke)

For some people, having a transient ischemic attack (TIA), or "mini-stroke," is the first sign of carotid artery disease. During a mini-stroke, you may have some or all of the symptoms of a stroke. However, the symptoms usually go away on their own within 24 hours.

Stroke and mini-stroke symptoms may include:

- A sudden, severe headache with no known cause

- Dizziness or loss of balance

- Inability to move one or more of your limbs

- Sudden trouble seeing in one or both eyes

- Sudden weakness or numbness in the face or limbs, often on just one side of the body

- Trouble speaking or understanding speech

A mini-stroke is a warning sign that you're at high risk of having a stroke. You shouldn't ignore these symptoms. Getting medical care can help find possible causes of a mini-stroke and help you manage risk factors. These actions might prevent a future stroke.

Although a mini-stroke may warn of a stroke, it doesn't predict when a stroke will happen. A stroke may occur days, weeks, or even months after a mini-stroke.

Stroke

The symptoms of a stroke are the same as those of a mini-stroke, but the results are not. A stroke can cause lasting brain damage; long-term disability, such as vision or speech problems or paralysis (an inability to move); or death. Most people who have strokes have not previously had warning mini-strokes.

Getting treatment for a stroke right away is very important. You have the best chance for full recovery if treatment to open a blocked artery is given within 4 hours of symptom onset. The sooner treatment occurs, the better your chances of recovery.

Make those close to you aware of stroke symptoms and the need for urgent action. Learning the signs and symptoms of a stroke will allow you to help yourself or someone close to you lower the risk of brain damage or death due to a stroke.

Diagnosis of Carotid Artery Disease

Your doctor will diagnose carotid artery disease based on your medical history, a physical exam, and test results.

Medical History

Your doctor will find out whether you have any of the major risk factors for carotid artery disease. He or she also will ask whether you've had any signs or symptoms of a mini-stroke or stroke.

Physical Exam

To check your carotid arteries, your doctor will listen to them with a stethoscope. He or she will listen for a whooshing sound called a bruit. This sound may indicate changed or reduced blood flow due to plaque buildup. To find out more, your doctor may recommend tests.

Diagnostic Tests

The following tests are common for diagnosing carotid artery disease. If you have symptoms of a mini-stroke or stroke, your doctor may use other tests as well.

Carotid Ultrasound. Carotid ultrasound (also called sonography) is the most common test for diagnosing carotid artery disease. It's a painless, harmless test that uses sound waves to create pictures of the insides of your carotid arteries. This test can show whether plaque has narrowed your carotid arteries and how narrow they are.

A standard carotid ultrasound shows the structure of your carotid arteries. A Doppler carotid ultrasound shows how blood moves through your carotid arteries.

Carotid Angiography. Carotid angiography is a special type of X-ray. This test may be used if the ultrasound results are unclear or don't give your doctor enough information.

For this test, your doctor will inject a substance (called contrast dye) into a vein, most often in your leg. The dye travels to your carotid arteries and highlights them on X-ray pictures.

Magnetic Resonance Angiography. Magnetic resonance angiography (MRA) uses a large magnet and radio waves to take pictures of your carotid arteries. Your doctor can see these pictures on a computer screen.

For this test, your doctor may give you contrast dye to highlight your carotid arteries on the pictures.

Computed Tomography Angiography. Computed tomography angiography, or CT angiography, takes X-ray pictures of the body from many angles. A computer combines the pictures into two- and three-dimensional images.

For this test, your doctor may give you contrast dye to highlight your carotid arteries on the pictures.

Treatment of Carotid Artery Disease

Treatments for carotid artery disease may include heart-healthy lifestyle changes, medicines, and medical procedures. The goals of treatment are to stop the disease from getting worse and to prevent a stroke. Your treatment will depend on your symptoms, how severe the disease is, and your age and overall health.

Heart-Healthy Lifestyle Changes

Your doctor may recommend heart-healthy lifestyle changes if you have carotid artery disease. Heart-healthy lifestyle changes include:

- Heart-healthy eating

- Aiming for a healthy weight

- Managing stress

- Physical activity

- Quitting smoking

- Medicines

If you have a stroke caused by a blood clot, you may be given a clot-dissolving, or clot-busting, medication. This type of medication must be given within 4 hours of symptom onset. The sooner treatment occurs, the better your chances of recovery.

Medicines to prevent blood clots are the mainstay treatment for people who have carotid artery disease. They prevent platelets from clumping together and forming blood clots in your carotid arteries, which can lead to a stroke. Two common medications are:

- Aspirin

- Clopidogrel

Sometimes lifestyle changes alone aren't enough to control your cholesterol levels. For example, you also may need statin medications to control or lower your cholesterol. By lowering your blood cholesterol level, you can decrease your chance of having a stroke or heart attack. Doctors usually prescribe statins for people who have:

- Diabetes

- Heart disease or have had a stroke

- High LDL cholesterol levels

Doctors may discuss beginning statin treatment with those who have an elevated risk for developing heart disease or having a stroke.

You may need other medications to treat diseases and conditions that damage the carotid arteries. Your doctor also may prescribe medications to:

- Lower your blood pressure.

- Lower your blood sugar level.

- Prevent blood clots from forming, which can lead to stroke.

- Prevent or reduce inflammation.

Take all medicines regularly, as your doctor prescribes. Don't change the amount of your medicine or skip a dose unless your doctor tells you to. Your healthcare team will help find a treatment plan that's right for you.

Medical Procedures

You may need a medical procedure if you have symptoms caused by the narrowing of the carotid artery. Doctors use one of two methods to open narrowed or blocked carotid arteries: carotid endarterectomy and carotid artery angioplasty and stenting.

Carotid Endarterectomy. Carotid endarterectomy is mainly for people whose carotid arteries are blocked 50 percent or more.

For the procedure, a surgeon will make a cut in your neck to reach the narrowed or blocked carotid artery. Next, he or she will make a cut in the blocked part of the artery and remove the artery's inner lining that is blocking the blood flow.

Finally, your surgeon will close the artery with stitches and stop any bleeding. He or she will then close the cut in your neck.

Carotid Artery Angioplasty and Stenting. Doctors use a procedure called angioplasty to widen the carotid arteries and restore blood flow to the brain.

A thin tube with a deflated balloon on the end is threaded through a blood vessel in your neck to the narrowed or blocked carotid artery. Once in place, the balloon is inflated to push the plaque outward against the wall of the artery.

A stent (a small mesh tube) is then put in the artery to support the inner artery wall. The stent also helps prevent the artery from becoming narrowed or blocked again.

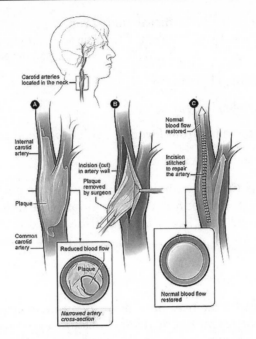

Figure 16.3. *Carotid Endarterectomy*

The illustration shows the process of carotid endarterectomy. Figure A shows a carotid artery with plaque buildup. The inset image shows a cross-section of the narrowed carotid artery. Figure B shows how the carotid artery is cut and how the plaque is removed. Figure C shows the artery stitched up and normal blood flow restored. The inset image shows a cross-section of the artery with plaque removed and normal blood flow restored.

Prevention of Carotid Artery Disease

Taking action to control your risk factors can help prevent or delay carotid artery disease and stroke. Your risk for carotid artery disease increases with the number of risk factors you have.

One step you can take is to make heart-healthy lifestyle changes, which can include:

- **Heart-Healthy Eating.** Following heart-healthy eating is an important part of a healthy lifestyle. Dietary Approaches to Stop Hypertension (DASH) is a program that promotes heart-healthy eating.

- **Aiming for a Healthy Weight.** If you're overweight or obese, work with your doctor to create a reasonable plan for weight

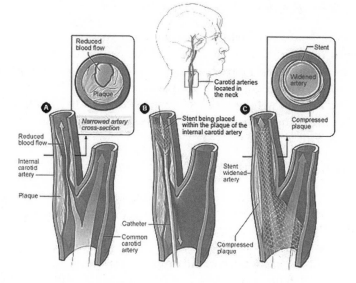

Figure 16.4. *Carotid Artery Stenting*

The illustration shows the process of carotid artery stenting. Figure A shows an internal carotid artery that has plaque buildup and reduced blood flow. The inset image shows a cross-section of the narrowed carotid artery. Figure B shows a stent being placed in the carotid artery to support the inner artery wall and keep the artery open. Figure C shows normal blood flow restored in the stent-widened artery. The inset image shows a cross-section of the stent-widened artery.

loss. Controlling your weight helps you control risk factors for carotid artery disease.

• **Physical Activity.** Be as physically active as you can. Physical activity can improve your fitness level and your health. Ask your doctor what types and amounts of activity are safe for you.

• **Quit Smoking.** If you smoke, quit. Talk with your doctor about programs and products that can help you quit.

Other steps that can prevent or delay carotid artery disease include knowing your family history of carotid artery disease. If you or someone in your family has carotid artery disease, be sure to tell your doctor.

If lifestyle changes aren't enough, your doctor may prescribe medicines to control your carotid artery disease risk factors. Take all of your medicines as your doctor advises.

Living with Carotid Artery Disease

If you have carotid artery disease, you can take steps to manage the condition, reduce risk factors, and prevent complications. These steps include making heart-healthy lifestyle changes, following your treatment plan, and getting ongoing care.

Having carotid artery disease raises your risk of having a stroke. Know the warning signs of a stroke—such as weakness and trouble speaking—and what to do if they occur.

Treatment Plan

Following your treatment plan may help prevent your carotid artery disease from getting worse. It also can lower your risk for stroke and other health problems.

You may need to take medicines to control certain risk factors and to prevent blood clots that could cause a stroke. Taking prescribed medicines and following a healthy lifestyle can help control carotid artery disease. However, they don't cure the disease. You'll likely have to stick with your treatment plan for life.

Ongoing Care

If you have carotid artery disease, having ongoing medical care is important. Most people who have the disease will need to have their blood pressure checked regularly and their blood sugar and blood cholesterol levels tested one or more times a year. If you have diabetes, you'll need routine blood sugar tests and other tests. Testing shows whether these conditions are under control, or whether your doctor needs to adjust your treatment for better results.

If you've had a stroke or procedures to restore blood flow in your carotid arteries, you'll likely need a yearly carotid Doppler ultrasound test. This test shows how well blood flows through your carotid arteries. Repeating this test over time will show whether the narrowing in your carotid arteries is getting worse. Results also can show how well procedures to treat your arteries have worked.

Follow up with your doctor regularly. The sooner your doctor spots problems, the sooner he or she can prescribe treatment.

Stroke Warning Signs

The signs and symptoms of stroke may include:

- Sudden weakness or numbness in the face or limbs, often on only one side of the body

- The inability to move one or more of your limbs
- Trouble speaking or understanding speech
- Sudden trouble seeing in one or both eyes
- Dizziness or loss of balance
- A sudden, severe headache with no known cause

If you're a candidate for clot-busting therapy, you have the best chance for full recovery if treatment to open a blocked artery is given within 4 hours of symptom onset. The sooner treatment occurs, the better your chances of recovery.

Chapter 17

Atrial Fibrillation and Stroke

Atrial fibrillation, or AF, is the most common type of arrhythmia. An arrhythmia is a problem with the rate or rhythm of the heartbeat. During an arrhythmia, the heart can beat too fast, too slow, or with an irregular rhythm. AF occurs if rapid, disorganized electrical signals cause the heart's two upper chambers—called the atria—to fibrillate. The term "fibrillate" means to contract very fast and irregularly.

In AF, blood pools in the atria. It isn't pumped completely into the heart's two lower chambers, called the ventricles. As a result, the heart's upper and lower chambers don't work together as they should. People who have AF may not feel symptoms. However, even when AF isn't noticed, it can increase the risk of stroke. In some people, AF can cause chest pain or heart failure, especially if the heart rhythm is very rapid. AF may happen rarely or every now and then, or it may become an ongoing or long-term heart problem that lasts for years.

Types of Atrial Fibrillation

Paroxysmal Atrial Fibrillation. In paroxysmal atrial fibrillation (AF), the faulty electrical signals and rapid heart rate begin suddenly and then stop on their own. Symptoms can be mild or severe. They stop within about a week, but usually in less than 24 hours.

This chapter includes text excerpted from "Atrial Fibrillation," National Heart, Lung, and Blood Institute (NHLBI), September 18, 2014.

Persistent Atrial Fibrillation. Persistent AF is a condition in which the abnormal heart rhythm continues for more than a week. It may stop on its own, or it can be stopped with treatment.

Permanent Atrial Fibrillation. Permanent AF is a condition in which a normal heart rhythm can't be restored with treatment. Both paroxysmal and persistent AF may become more frequent and, over time, result in permanent AF.

Causes of Atrial Fibrillation

Atrial fibrillation (AF) occurs if the heart's electrical signals don't travel through the heart in a normal way. Instead, they become very rapid and disorganized. Damage to the heart's electrical system causes AF. The damage most often is the result of other conditions that affect the health of the heart, such as high blood pressure and coronary heart disease. The risk of AF increases as you age. Inflammation also is thought to play a role in causing AF.

Sometimes, the cause of AF is unknown.

Risk Factors for Atrial Fibrillation

Atrial fibrillation (AF) affects millions of people, and the number is rising. Men are more likely than women to have the condition. In the United States, AF is more common among Whites than African Americans or Hispanic Americans.

The risk of AF increases as you age. This is mostly because your risk for heart disease and other conditions that can cause AF also increases as you age. However, about half of the people who have AF are younger than 75.

AF is uncommon in children.

Major Risk Factors

AF is more common in people who have:

- High blood pressure
- Coronary heart disease (CHD)
- Heart failure
- Rheumatic heart disease
- Structural heart defects, such as mitral valve prolapse

- Pericarditis (a condition in which the membrane, or sac, around your heart is inflamed)

- Congenital heart defects

- Sick sinus syndrome (a condition in which the heart's electrical signals don't fire properly and the heart rate slows down; sometimes the heart will switch back and forth between a slow rate and a fast rate).

AF also is more common in people who are having heart attacks or who have just had surgery.

Other Risk Factors

Other conditions that raise your risk for AF include hyperthyroidism (too much thyroid hormone), obesity, diabetes, and lung disease. Certain factors also can raise your risk for AF. For example, drinking large amounts of alcohol, especially binge drinking, raises your risk. Even modest amounts of alcohol can trigger AF in some people. Caffeine or psychological stress also may trigger AF in some people.

Some data suggest that people who have sleep apnea are at greater risk for AF. Sleep apnea is a common disorder that causes one or more pauses in breathing or shallow breaths while you sleep. Metabolic syndrome also raises your risk for AF. Metabolic syndrome is the name for a group of risk factors that raises your risk for CHD and other health problems, such as diabetes and stroke.

Research suggests that people who receive high-dose steroid therapy are at increased risk for AF. This therapy is used for asthma and some inflammatory conditions. It may act as a trigger in people who have other AF risk factors.

Genetic factors also may play a role in causing AF. However, their role isn't fully known.

Signs and Symptoms of Atrial Fibrillation

Atrial fibrillation (AF) usually causes the heart's lower chambers, the ventricles, to contract faster than normal.

When this happens, the ventricles can't completely fill with blood. Thus, they may not be able to pump enough blood to the lungs and body. This can lead to signs and symptoms, such as:

- Palpitations (feelings that your heart is skipping a beat, fluttering, or beating too hard or fast)

159

- Shortness of breath

- Weakness or problems exercising

- Chest pain

- Dizziness or fainting

- Fatigue (tiredness)

- Confusion

Atrial Fibrillation Complications

AF has two major complications—stroke and heart failure.

Stroke

During AF, the heart's upper chambers, the atria, don't pump all of their blood to the ventricles. Some blood pools in the atria. When this happens, a blood clot (also called a thrombus) can form.

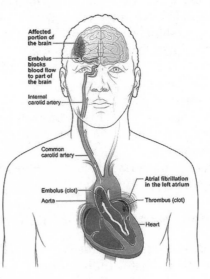

Figure 17.1. *Atrial Fibrillation and Stroke*

The illustration shows how a stroke can occur during atrial fibrillation. A blood clot (thrombus) can form in the left atrium of the heart. If a piece of the clot breaks off and travels to an artery in the brain, it can block blood flow through the artery. The lack of blood flow to the portion of the brain fed by the artery causes a stroke.

If the clot breaks off and travels to the brain, it can cause a stroke. (A clot that forms in one part of the body and travels in the bloodstream to another part of the body is called an embolus.)

Blood-thinning medicines that reduce the risk of stroke are an important part of treatment for people who have AF.

Heart Failure

Heart failure occurs if the heart can't pump enough blood to meet the body's needs. AF can lead to heart failure because the ventricles are beating very fast and can't completely fill with blood. Thus, they may not be able to pump enough blood to the lungs and body.

Fatigue and shortness of breath are common symptoms of heart failure. A buildup of fluid in the lungs causes these symptoms. Fluid also can build up in the feet, ankles, and legs, causing weight gain.

Lifestyle changes, medicines, and procedures or surgery (rarely, a mechanical heart pump or heart transplant) are the main treatments for heart failure.

Diagnosis of Atrial Fibrillation

Atrial fibrillation (AF) is diagnosed based on your medical and family histories, a physical exam, and the results from tests and procedures. Sometimes AF doesn't cause signs or symptoms. Thus, it may be found during a physical exam or EKG (electrocardiogram) test done for another purpose.

If you have AF, your doctor will want to find out what is causing it. This will help him or her plan the best way to treat the condition.

Specialists Involved

Primary care doctors often are involved in the diagnosis and treatment of AF. These doctors include family practitioners and internists.

Doctors who specialize in the diagnosis and treatment of heart disease also may be involved, such as:

- **Cardiologists.** These are doctors who diagnose and treat heart diseases and conditions.

- **Electrophysiologists.** These are cardiologists who specialize in arrhythmias.

161

Medical and Family Histories

Your doctor will likely ask questions about your:

- **Signs and symptoms.** What symptoms are you having? Have you had palpitations? Are you dizzy or short of breath? Are your feet or ankles swollen (a possible sign of heart failure)? Do you have any chest pain?

- **Medical history.** Do you have other health problems, such as a history of heart disease, high blood pressure, lung disease, diabetes, or thyroid problems?

- **Family's medical history.** Does anyone in your family have a history of AF? Has anyone in your family ever had heart disease or high blood pressure? Has anyone had thyroid problems? Does your family have a history of other illnesses or health problems?

- **Health habits.** Do you smoke or use alcohol or caffeine?

Physical Exam

Your doctor will do a complete cardiac exam. He or she will listen to the rate and rhythm of your heartbeat and take your pulse and blood pressure reading. Your doctor will likely check for any signs of heart muscle or heart valve problems. He or she will listen to your lungs to check for signs of heart failure.

Your doctor also will check for swelling in your legs or feet and look for an enlarged thyroid gland or other signs of hyperthyroidism (too much thyroid hormone).

Diagnostic Tests and Procedures

Electrocardiogram (EKG)

An EKG is a simple, painless test that records the heart's electrical activity. It's the most useful test for diagnosing AF. An EKG shows how fast your heart is beating and its rhythm (steady or irregular). It also records the strength and timing of electrical signals as they pass through your heart.

A standard EKG only records the heartbeat for a few seconds. It won't detect AF that doesn't happen during the test.

Holter and Event Monitors

The two most common types of portable EKGs are Holter and event monitors.

- A Holter monitor records the heart's electrical activity for a full 24-or 48-hour period. You wear small patches called electrodes on your chest. Wires connect these patches to a small, portable recorder. The recorder can be clipped to a belt, kept in a pocket, or hung around your neck. You wear the Holter monitor while you do your normal daily activities. This allows the monitor to record your heart for a longer time than a standard EKG.

- An event monitor is similar to a Holter monitor. You wear an event monitor while doing your normal activities. However, an event monitor only records your heart's electrical activity at certain times while you're wearing it.

Stress Test

Some heart problems are easier to diagnose when your heart is working hard and beating fast. During stress testing, you exercise to make your heart work hard and beat fast while heart tests are done. If you can't exercise, you may be given medicine to make your heart work hard and beat fast.

Echocardiography

Echocardiography (echo) uses sound waves to create a moving picture of your heart. The test shows the size and shape of your heart and how well your heart chambers and valves are working. Echo also can identify areas of poor blood flow to the heart, areas of heart muscle that aren't contracting normally, and previous injury to the heart muscle caused by poor blood flow.

This test sometimes is called transthoracic echocardiography. It's painless and noninvasive (no instruments are inserted into the body).

Transesophageal Echocardiography

Transesophageal echo, or TEE, uses sound waves to take pictures of your heart through the esophagus. Your heart's upper chambers, the atria, are deep in your chest. They often can't be seen very well using transthoracic echo. Your doctor can see the atria much better using TEE. During this test, the transducer is attached to the end of a flexible tube. The tube is guided down your throat and into your esophagus. TEE is used to detect blood clots that may be forming in the atria because of AF.

Chest X-Ray

A chest X-ray is a painless test that creates pictures of the structures in your chest, such as your heart and lungs. This test can show fluid buildup in the lungs and signs of other AF complications.

Blood Tests

Blood tests check the level of thyroid hormone in your body and the balance of your body's electrolytes. Electrolytes are minerals that help maintain fluid levels and acid-base balance in the body. They're essential for normal health and functioning of your body's cells and organs.

Treatment of Atrial Fibrillation

Treatment for atrial fibrillation (AF) depends on how often you have symptoms, how severe they are, and whether you already have heart disease. General treatment options include medicines, medical procedures, and lifestyle changes.

Goals of Treatment

The goals of treating AF include:

• Preventing blood clots from forming, thus lowering the risk of stroke.

• Controlling how many times a minute the ventricles contract. This is called rate control. Rate control is important because it allows the ventricles enough time to completely fill with blood. With this approach, the abnormal heart rhythm continues, but you feel better and have fewer symptoms.

• Restoring a normal heart rhythm. This is called rhythm control. Rhythm control allows the atria and ventricles to work together to efficiently pump blood to the body.

• Treating any underlying disorder that's causing or raising the risk of AF—for example, hyperthyroidism (too much thyroid hormone).

Who Needs Treatment for Atrial Fibrillation?

People who have AF but don't have symptoms or related heart problems may not need treatment. AF may even go back to a normal heart rhythm on its own. (This also can occur in people who have AF with symptoms.)

In some people who have AF for the first time, doctors may choose to use an electrical procedure or medicine to restore a normal heart rhythm.

Repeat episodes of AF tend to cause changes to the heart's electrical system, leading to persistent or permanent AF. Most people who have persistent or permanent AF need treatment to control their heart rate and prevent complications.

Prevention of Atrial Fibrillation

Following a healthy lifestyle and taking steps to lower your risk for heart disease may help you prevent atrial fibrillation (AF). These steps include:

- Following a heart healthy diet that's low in saturated fat, trans fat, and cholesterol. A healthy diet includes a variety of whole grains, fruits, and vegetables daily.

- Not smoking.

- Being physically active.

- Maintaining a healthy weight.

If you already have heart disease or other AF risk factors, work with your doctor to manage your condition. In addition to adopting the healthy habits above, which can help control heart disease, your doctor may advise you to:

- Follow the Dietary Approaches to Stop Hypertension (DASH) eating plan to help lower your blood pressure.

- Keep your cholesterol and triglycerides at healthy levels with dietary changes and medicines (if prescribed).

- Limit or avoid alcohol.

- Control your blood sugar level if you have diabetes.

- Get ongoing medical care and take your medicines as prescribed.

Living with Atrial Fibrillation

People who have atrial fibrillation (AF)—even permanent AF— can live normal, active lives. If you have AF, ongoing medical care is important.

Keep all your medical appointments. Bring a list of all the medicines you're taking to every doctor and emergency room visit. This will help your doctor know exactly what medicines you're taking.

Follow your doctor's instructions for taking medicines. Be careful about taking over-the-counter medicines, nutritional supplements, and cold and allergy medicines. Some of these products contain stimulants that can trigger rapid heart rhythms. Also, some over-the-counter medicines can have harmful interactions with heart rhythm medicines.

Tell your doctor if your medicines are causing side effects, if your symptoms are getting worse, or if you have new symptoms.

If you're taking blood-thinning medicines, you'll need to be carefully monitored. For example, you may need routine blood tests to check how the medicines are working. Also, talk with your doctor about your diet. Some foods, such as leafy green vegetables, may interfere with warfarin, a blood-thinning medicine.

Ask your doctor about physical activity, weight control, and alcohol use. Find out what steps you can take to manage your condition.

Chapter 18

Blood Clotting Disorders and Stroke

What Is a Hypercoagulable State?

When a person has an abnormally strong tendency for the blood to thicken and clot, it is called a hypercoagulable state. It can be the result of environmental factors (such as the effects of hormones, surgery, or cancer), or it can be caused by an inherited defect in one of the molecules involved in blood clotting. Blood clotting problems like these are more likely to increase your risk of developing harmful blood clots in the deep veins of the legs (deep vein thrombosis or DVT) than blood clots in the arteries that can result in a stroke or heart attack. A blood clot or thrombus in the veins of the legs can break off and travel through the bloodstream to block an artery in the lungs, causing the life-threatening condition, pulmonary embolism.

What Causes Blood Clotting Problems?

There are several causes for blood clotting problems. You are more prone to developing blood clots after surgery (especially hip or knee), or when you are immobilized for more than 4 days, or as a result of

This chapter includes text excerpted from "Blood Clotting Problems and Stroke Risk," Office on Women's Health (OWH), U.S. Department of Health and Human Services (HHS), February 6, 2017.

injuries from a severe accident. Cancer can also lead to a hypercoagulable state: 1 percent to 15 percent of cancer patients develop blood clots in their veins.

Some people have a higher risk of blood clotting problems because they inherit mutations (variations) in the genes for blood clotting proteins.

Hormones, including estrogen found in hormone therapy and birth control pills, can increase your risk of developing blood clots, especially if you have an inherited blood clotting disorder or have a history of unexplained blood clots.

Can Inherited Blood Clotting Problems Increase My Risk of Having a Stroke?

Blood clotting disorders may be to blame for 5 percent to 10 percent of blocked-vessel (ischemic) strokes—possibly more in younger, otherwise healthy people. Typical clotting disorders result in a greater likelihood of clots forming inside of blood vessels, which can cause a blocked-vessel stroke. Clotting disorders that predispose to the formation of blood clots are not risk factors for bleeding (hemorrhagic) stroke. There are some rare inherited disorders that make the blood unable to clot, which does increase the chances of a bleeding stroke.

What Is Factor V Leiden?

The most commonly inherited blood clotting problem is called Factor V Leiden (FVL), so-called because it affects the Factor V (5) clotting protein. FVL occurs in about 5 percent of white women and men; rates are lower for Hispanics and it is rare in people of Asian or African descent.

Does FVL Increase My Risk of Stroke?

Inheriting the FVL mutation may increase your risk of stroke in the presence of other risk factors, such as birth control pills. The mutation by itself accounts for an increase in stroke risk less than that associated with the birth control pill alone. However, women with a single defective FVL gene have a 30-fold higher risk of developing blood clots while using birth control pills, a 15-fold higher risk with postmenopausal hormone therapy, and a 7-fold higher risk during pregnancy compared with women without this mutation. Women who carry two abnormal FVL genes have an even greater risk of developing blood clots. It is likely that these women will experience at least one blood clotting event during their lifetime. Whether the FVL mutation increases stroke risk in younger people without other risk factors is controversial.

A recent European study of 240 stroke patients found that FVL together with another genetic clotting condition (prothrombin, discussed below) accounted for an overall 4-fold increased risk of stroke compared with patients with similar risk factors but no genetic clotting condition. Compared with men, women in this study had a greater stroke risk (5-fold) associated with these disorders.

What Other Inherited Blood Clotting Problems May Be Linked to Stroke?

A common genetic risk factor for blood clots is a mutation in the gene encoding the clotting factor 'prothrombin'. The mutation is found in about 1 in 50 persons in the United States. It raises the risk of blood clots for both women and men of all ages, but appears to increase stroke risk only if you have other risk factors such as a congenital heart defect (especially Patent Foramen Ovale), other clotting problems, or are taking birth control pills. If you know you have an inherited blood clotting disorder, or have had a blood clot before, it is very important you address your other risk factors for stroke such as quitting smoking, managing high blood pressure and talking to your doctor about birth control pills.

Results from the Framingham Heart Study showed that one particular blood marker was an independent risk factor for blocked-vessel stroke and transient ischemic attack (TIA) in women but not in men. The blood marker in question is called an anticardiolipin antibody (aCL). aCL is a protein found in the blood that, if present in excessive amounts, is associated with clotting abnormalities as well as multiple pregnancy miscarriages. The study in question found that women with a high level of aCL in their blood were almost 3 times as likely to suffer a blocked-vessel stroke as women with normal aCL levels. No association between stroke and aCL was found for men.

Chapter 19

Peripheral Artery Disease

Peripheral artery disease (PAD) is a disease in which plaque builds up in the arteries that carry blood to your head, organs, and limbs. Plaque is made up of fat, cholesterol, calcium, fibrous tissue, and other substances in the blood.

When plaque builds up in the body's arteries, the condition is called atherosclerosis. Over time, plaque can harden and narrow the arteries. This limits the flow of oxygen-rich blood to your organs and other parts of your body.

PAD usually affects the arteries in the legs, but it also can affect the arteries that carry blood from your heart to your head, arms, kidneys, and stomach. This chapter focuses on PAD that affects blood flow to the legs.

Causes of Peripheral Artery Disease

The most common cause of peripheral artery disease (PAD) is atherosclerosis. Atherosclerosis is a disease in which plaque builds up in your arteries. The exact cause of atherosclerosis isn't known.

The disease may start if certain factors damage the inner layers of the arteries. These factors include:

- Smoking

- High amounts of certain fats and cholesterol in the blood

This chapter includes text excerpted from "Peripheral Artery Disease," National Heart, Lung, and Blood Institute (NHLBI), June 22, 2016.

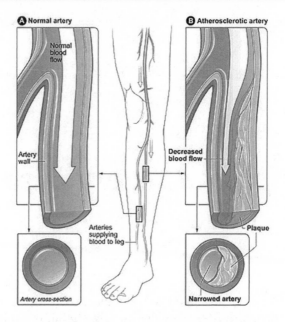

Figure 19.1. *Normal Artery and Artery with Plaque Buildup*

The illustration shows how PAD can affect arteries in the legs. Figure A shows a normal artery with normal blood flow. The inset image shows a cross-section of the normal artery. Figure B shows an artery with plaque buildup that's partially blocking blood flow. The inset image shows a cross-section of the narrowed artery.

- High blood pressure
- High amounts of sugar in the blood due to insulin resistance or
- Diabetes

When damage occurs, your body starts a healing process. The healing may cause plaque to build up where the arteries are damaged.

Eventually, a section of plaque can rupture (break open), causing a blood clot to form at the site. The buildup of plaque or blood clots can severely narrow or block the arteries and limit the flow of oxygen-rich blood to your body.

Risk Factors for Peripheral Artery Disease

Peripheral artery disease (PAD) affects millions of people in the United States. The disease is more common in blacks than any other racial or ethnic group. The major risk factors for PAD are smoking, older age, and having certain diseases or conditions.

Smoking

Smoking is the main risk factor for PAD and your risk increases if you smoke or have a history of smoking. Quitting smoking slows the progress of PAD. People who smoke and people who have diabetes are at highest risk for PAD complications, such as gangrene (tissue death) in the leg from decreased blood flow.

Older Age

Older age also is a risk factor for PAD Plaque builds up in your arteries as you age. Older age combined with other risk factors, such as smoking or diabetes, also puts you at higher risk for PAD

Diseases and Conditions

Many diseases and conditions can raise your risk of PAD, including:

- Stroke
- Diabetes
- High blood pressure
- High blood cholesterol
- Coronary heart disease
- Metabolic syndrome

Signs and Symptoms of Peripheral Artery Disease

Many people who have PAD don't have any signs or symptoms. Even if you don't have signs or symptoms, ask your doctor whether you should get checked for PAD if you're:

- Aged 70 or older
- Aged 50 or older and have a history of smoking or diabetes
- Younger than 50 and have diabetes and one or more risk factors for atherosclerosis

Intermittent Claudication

People who have PAD may have symptoms when walking or climbing stairs, which may include pain, numbness, aching, or heaviness in the leg muscles. Symptoms also may include cramping in the affected leg(s) and in the buttocks, thighs, calves, and feet. Symptoms may ease after resting. These symptoms are called intermittent claudication.

During physical activity, your muscles need increased blood flow. If your blood vessels are narrowed or blocked, your muscles won't get enough blood, which will lead to symptoms. When resting, the muscles need less blood flow, so the symptoms will go away.

Other Signs and Symptoms

Other signs and symptoms of PAD include:

- Weak or absent pulses in the legs or feet
- Sores or wounds on the toes, feet, or legs that heal slowly, poorly, or not at all
- A pale or bluish color to the skin
- A lower temperature in one leg compared to the other leg
- Poor nail growth on the toes and decreased hair growth on the legs
- Erectile dysfunction, especially among men who have diabetes

Diagnosis of Peripheral Artery Disease

PAD is diagnosed based on your medical and family histories, a physical exam, and test results.

PAD often is diagnosed after symptoms are reported. A correct diagnosis is important because people who have PAD are at higher risk for stroke and transient ischemic attack ("mini-stroke"), coronary heart disease (CHD), and heart attack. If you have PAD, your doctor also may want to check for signs of these diseases and conditions.

Specialists Involved

Primary care doctors, such as internists and family doctors, may treat people who have mild PAD For more advanced PAD, a vascular specialist may be involved. This is a doctor who specializes in treating blood vessel diseases and conditions.

A cardiologist also may be involved in treating people who have PAD Cardiologists treat heart problems, such as CHD and heart attack, which often affect people who have PAD

Medical and Family Histories

Your doctor may ask:

- Whether you have any risk factors for PAD. For example, he or she may ask whether you smoke or have diabetes.

- About your symptoms, including any symptoms that occur when walking, exercising, sitting, standing, or climbing.

- About your diet.

- About any medicines you take, including prescription and over-the-counter medicines.

- Whether anyone in your family has a history of heart or blood vessel diseases.

Physical Exam

During the physical exam, your doctor will look for signs of PAD He or she may check the blood flow in your legs or feet to see whether you have weak or absent pulses.

Your doctor also may check the pulses in your leg arteries for an abnormal whooshing sound called a bruit. He or she can hear this sound with a stethoscope. A bruit may be a warning sign of a narrowed or blocked artery.

Your doctor may compare blood pressure between your limbs to see whether the pressure is lower in the affected limb. He or she also may check for poor wound healing or any changes in your hair, skin, or nails that may be signs of PAD

Diagnostic Tests

Ankle-Brachial Index

- A simple test called an ankle-brachial index (ABI) often is used to diagnose PAD The ABI compares blood pressure in your ankle to blood pressure in your arm. This test shows how well blood is flowing in your limbs.

- ABI can show whether PAD is affecting your limbs, but it won't show which blood vessels are narrowed or blocked.

- A normal ABI result is 1.0 or greater (with a range of 0.90 to 1.30). The test takes about 10 to 15 minutes to measure both arms and both ankles. This test may be done yearly to see whether PAD is getting worse.

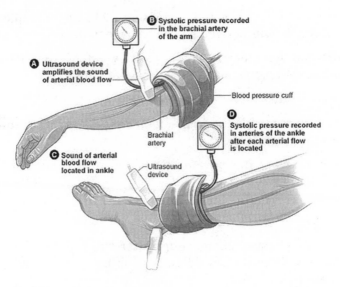

Figure 19.2. *Ankle-Brachial Index*

The illustration shows the ankle-brachial index test. The test compares blood pressure in the ankle to blood pressure in the arm. As the blood pressure cuff deflates, the blood pressure in the arteries is recorded.

Doppler Ultrasound

A Doppler ultrasound looks at blood flow in the major arteries and veins in the limbs. During this test, a handheld device is placed on your body and passed back and forth over the affected area. A computer converts sound waves into a picture of blood flow in the arteries and veins.

The results of this test can show whether a blood vessel is blocked. The results also can help show the severity of PAD.

Treadmill Test

A treadmill test can show the severity of symptoms and the level of exercise that brings them on. You'll walk on a treadmill for this test. This shows whether you have any problems during normal walking.

You may have an ABI test before and after the treadmill test. This will help compare blood flow in your arms and legs before and after exercise.

Magnetic Resonance Angiogram

A magnetic resonance angiogram (MRA) uses magnetic and radio wave energy to take pictures of your blood vessels. This test is a type of magnetic resonance imaging (MRI).

An MRA can show the location and severity of a blocked blood vessel. If you have a pacemaker, man-made joint, stent, surgical clips, mechanical heart valve, or other metallic devices in your body, you might not be able to have an MRA. Ask your doctor whether an MRA is an option for you.

Arteriogram

An arteriogram provides a "road map" of the arteries. Doctors use this test to find the exact location of a blocked artery.

For this test, dye is injected through a needle or catheter (tube) into one of your arteries. This may make you feel mildly flushed. After the dye is injected, an X-ray is taken. The X-ray can show the location, type, and extent of the blockage in the artery.

Some doctors use a newer method of arteriogram that uses tiny ultrasound cameras. These cameras take pictures of the insides of the blood vessels. This method is called intravascular ultrasound.

Blood Tests

Your doctor may recommend blood tests to check for PAD risk factors. For example, blood tests can help diagnose conditions such as diabetes and high blood cholesterol.

Treatment of Peripheral Artery Disease

Treatments for PAD include heart-healthy lifestyle changes, medicines, and surgery or procedures.

The overall goals of treating PAD include reducing risk of stroke and heart attack; reducing symptoms of claudication; improving mobility and overall quality of life; and preventing complications. Treatment is based on your signs and symptoms, risk factors, and the results of physical exams and tests.

Treatment may slow or stop the progression of the disease and reduce the risk of complications. Without treatment, PAD may progress, resulting in serious tissue damage in the form of sores or gangrene (tissue death) due to inadequate blood flow. In extreme cases of

PAD, also referred to as critical limb ischemia (CLI), removal (amputation) of part of the leg or foot may be necessary.

Heart-Healthy Lifestyle Changes

Treatment often includes making life-long heart-healthy lifestyle changes such as:

- Physical activity

- Quitting smoking

- Heart-healthy eating

Surgery or Procedures

Bypass Grafting

Your doctor may recommend bypass grafting surgery if blood flow in your limb is blocked or nearly blocked. For this surgery, your doctor uses a blood vessel from another part of your body or a synthetic tube to make a graft.

This graft bypasses (that is, goes around) the blocked part of the artery. The bypass allows blood to flow around the blockage. This surgery doesn't cure PAD, but it may increase blood flow to the affected limb.

Angioplasty and Stent Placement

Your doctor may recommend angioplasty to restore blood flow through a narrowed or blocked artery.

During this procedure, a catheter (thin tube) with a balloon at the tip is inserted into a blocked artery. The balloon is then inflated, which pushes plaque outward against the artery wall. This widens the artery and restores blood flow.

A stent (a small mesh tube) may be placed in the artery during angioplasty. A stent helps keep the artery open after angioplasty is done. Some stents are coated with medicine to help prevent blockages in the artery.

Atherectomy

Atherectomy is a procedure that removes plaque buildup from an artery. During the procedure, a catheter is used to insert a small cutting device into the blocked artery. The device is used to shave or cut off plaque.

The bits of plaque are removed from the body through the catheter or washed away in the bloodstream (if they're small enough).

Doctors also can perform atherectomy using a special laser that dissolves the blockage.

Other Types of Treatment

Researchers are studying cell and gene therapies to treat PAD However, these treatments aren't yet available outside of clinical trials.

Prevention of Peripheral Artery Disease

Taking action to control your risk factors can help prevent or delay peripheral artery disease (PAD) and its complications. Know your family history of health problems related to PAD If you or someone in your family has the disease, be sure to tell your doctor. Controlling risk factors includes the following.

- Be physically active.

- Be screened for PAD A simple office test, called an ankle-brachial index or ABI, can help determine whether you have PAD

- Follow heart-healthy eating.

- If you smoke, quit. Talk with your doctor about programs and products that can help you quit smoking.

- If you're overweight or obese, work with your doctor to create a reasonable weight-loss plan.

The lifestyle changes described above can reduce your risk of developing PAD. These changes also can help prevent and control conditions that can be associated with PAD, such as stroke, coronary heart disease, diabetes, high blood pressure, and high blood cholesterol.

Living with Peripheral Artery Disease

If you have peripheral artery disease (PAD), you're more likely to also have stroke, transient ischemic attack ("mini-stroke"), coronary heart disease, and heart attack. However, you can take steps to treat and control PAD and lower your risk for these other conditions.

Living with Peripheral Artery Disease Symptoms

If you have PAD, you may feel pain in your calf or thigh muscles after walking. Try to take a break and allow the pain to ease before walking again. Over time, this may increase the distance that you can walk without pain.

Talk with your doctor about taking part in a supervised exercise program. This type of program has been shown to reduce PAD symptoms.

Check your feet and toes regularly for sores or possible infections. Wear comfortable shoes that fit well. Maintain good foot hygiene and have professional medical treatment for corns, bunions, or calluses.

Ongoing Healthcare Needs and Lifestyle Changes

See your doctor for checkups as he or she advises. If you have PAD without symptoms, you still should see your doctor regularly. Take all medicines as your doctor prescribes.

Heart-healthy lifestyle changes can help prevent or delay PAD and other related problems, such as stroke, transient ischemic attack (TIA), coronary heart disease, and heart attack. Heart-healthy lifestyle changes include physical activity, quitting smoking, and heart-healthy eating.

Chapter 20

Diabetes and Stroke Risk

Having diabetes means that you are more likely to develop heart disease and have a greater chance of a stroke or a heart attack. People with diabetes are also more likely to have certain conditions, or risk factors, that increase the chances of having heart disease or stroke, such as high blood pressure or high cholesterol. If you have diabetes, you can protect your heart and health by managing your blood glucose, also called blood sugar, as well as your blood pressure and cholesterol. If you smoke, get help to stop.

Link among Diabetes, Heart Disease, and Stroke

Over time, high blood glucose from diabetes can damage your blood vessels and the nerves that control your heart and blood vessels. The longer you have diabetes, the higher the chances that you will develop heart disease.

People with diabetes tend to develop heart disease at a younger age than people without diabetes. In adults with diabetes, the most common causes of death are heart disease and stroke. Adults with diabetes are nearly twice as likely to die from heart disease or stroke as people without diabetes.

The good news is that the steps you take to manage your diabetes also help to lower your chances of having heart disease or stroke.

This chapter includes text excerpted from "Diabetes, Heart Disease, and Stroke," National Institute of Diabetes and Digestive and Kidney Diseases (NIDDK), February 2017.

Risk Factors for Diabetes

If you have diabetes, other factors add to your chances of developing heart disease or having a stroke.

Smoking

Smoking raises your risk of developing heart disease. If you have diabetes, it is important to stop smoking because both smoking and diabetes narrow blood vessels. Smoking also increases your chances of developing other long-term problems such as lung disease. Smoking also can damage the blood vessels in your legs and increase the risk of lower leg infections, ulcers, and amputation.

High Blood Pressure

If you have high blood pressure, your heart must work harder to pump blood. High blood pressure can strain your heart, damage blood vessels, and increase your risk of stroke, heart attack, eye problems, and kidney problems.

Abnormal Cholesterol Levels

Cholesterol is a type of fat produced by your liver and found in your blood. You have two kinds of cholesterol in your blood: Low-Density Lipoprotein (LDL) and High-Density Lipoprotein (HDL).

LDL, often called "bad" cholesterol, can build up and clog your blood vessels. High levels of LDL cholesterol raise your risk of developing heart disease.

Another type of blood fat, triglycerides, also can raise your risk of heart disease when the levels are higher than recommended by your healthcare team.

Obesity and Belly Fat

Being overweight or obese can affect your ability to manage your diabetes and increase your risk for many health problems, including heart disease and high blood pressure. If you are overweight, a healthy eating plan with reduced calories often will lower your glucose levels and reduce your need for medications.

Excess belly fat around your waist, even if you are not overweight, can raise your chances of developing heart disease.

You have excess belly fat if your waist measures:

- more than 40 inches and you are a man
- more than 35 inches and you are a woman

Family History of Heart Disease

A family history of heart disease may also add to your chances of developing heart disease. If one or more of your family members had a heart attack before age 50, you may have an even higher chance of developing heart disease.

You can't change whether heart disease runs in your family, but if you have diabetes, it's even more important to take steps to protect yourself from heart disease and decrease your chances of having a stroke.

Prevention of Diabetes

Taking care of your diabetes is important to help you take care of your heart. You can lower your chances of having a stroke or heart attack or by taking the following steps to manage your diabetes to keep your heart and blood vessels healthy.

Manage Your Diabetes ABCs

Knowing your diabetes ABCs will help you manage your blood glucose, blood pressure, and cholesterol. Stopping smoking if you have diabetes is also important to lower your chances for heart disease.

A is for the A1C test. The A1C test shows your average blood glucose level over the past 3 months. This is different from the blood glucose checks that you do every day. The higher your A1C number, the higher your blood glucose levels have been during the past 3 months. High levels of blood glucose can harm your heart, blood vessels, kidneys, feet, and eyes.

The A1C goal for many people with diabetes is below 7 percent. Some people may do better with a slightly higher A1C goal. Ask your healthcare team what your goal should be.

B is for blood pressure. Blood pressure is the force of your blood against the wall of your blood vessels. If your blood pressure gets too high, it makes your heart work too hard. High blood pressure can cause a stroke or heart attack and damage your kidneys and eyes.

The blood pressure goal for most people with diabetes is below 140/90 mm Hg. Ask what your goal should be.

C is for cholesterol. You have two kinds of cholesterol in your blood: LDL and HDL. LDL or "bad" cholesterol can build up and clog your blood vessels. Too much bad cholesterol can cause a stroke or heart attack. HDL or "good" cholesterol helps remove the "bad" cholesterol from your blood vessels.

Ask your healthcare team what your cholesterol numbers should be. If you are over 40 years of age, you may need to take medicine such as a statin to lower your cholesterol and protect your heart. Some people with very high LDL ("bad") cholesterol may need to take medicine at a younger age.

S is for stop smoking. Not smoking is especially important for people with diabetes because both smoking and diabetes narrow blood vessels, so your heart has to work harder.

If you quit smoking:

- you will lower your risk for stroke, heart attack, nerve disease, kidney disease, eye disease, and amputation

- your blood glucose, blood pressure, and cholesterol levels may improve

- your blood circulation will improve

- you may have an easier time being physically active

If you smoke or use other tobacco products, stop. Ask for help so you don't have to do it alone. You can start by calling the national quitline at 1-800-QUITNOW or 1-800-784-8669. Smokefree.gov provides tips on quitting.

Ask your healthcare team about your goals for A1C, blood pressure, and cholesterol, and what you can do to reach these goals.

Develop or Maintain Healthy Lifestyle Habits

Developing or maintaining healthy lifestyle habits can help you manage your diabetes and prevent heart disease.

- Follow your healthy eating plan.

- Make physical activity part of your routine.

- Stay at or get to a healthy weight.

- Get enough sleep.

Learn to Manage Stress

Managing diabetes is not always easy. Feeling stressed, sad, or angry is common when you are living with diabetes. You may know what to do to stay healthy but may have trouble sticking with your plan over time. Long-term stress can raise your blood glucose and blood pressure, but you can learn ways to lower your stress. Try deep breathing, gardening, taking a walk, doing yoga, meditating, doing a hobby, or listening to your favorite music.

Take Medicine to Protect Your Heart

Medicines may be an important part of your treatment plan. Your doctor will prescribe medicine based on your specific needs. Medicine may help you:

- Meet your A1C (blood glucose), blood pressure, and cholesterol goals.

- Reduce your risk of blood clots, heart attack, or stroke.

- Treat angina, or chest pain that is often a symptom of heart disease. (Angina can also be an early symptom of a heart attack.)

Ask your doctor whether you should take aspirin. Aspirin is not safe for everyone. Your doctor can tell you whether taking aspirin is right for you and exactly how much to take.

Statins can reduce the risk of having a stroke or heart attack in some people with diabetes. Statins are a type of medicine often used to help people meet their cholesterol goals. Talk with your doctor to find out whether taking a statin is right for you.

Talk with your doctor if you have questions about your medicines. Before you start a new medicine, ask your doctor about possible side effects and how you can avoid them. If the side effects of your medicine bother you, tell your doctor. Don't stop taking your medicines without checking with your doctor first.

Diagnosing Heart Disease in Diabetes

Doctors diagnose heart disease in diabetes based on:

- your symptoms

- your medical and family history

- how likely you are to have heart disease

- a physical exam

- results from tests and procedures

Tests used to monitor your diabetes—A1C, blood pressure, and cholesterol—help your doctor decide whether it is important to do other tests to check your heart health.

Warning Signs of Heart Attack and Stroke

Warning signs of a heart attack includes:

- pain or pressure in your chest that lasts longer than a few minutes or goes away and comes back

- pain or discomfort in one or both of your arms or shoulders; or your back, neck, or jaw

- shortness of breath

- sweating or light-headedness

- indigestion or nausea (feeling sick to your stomach)

- feeling very tired

Treatment works best when it is given right away. Warning signs can be different in different people. You may not have all of these symptoms.

If you have angina, it's important to know how and when to seek medical treatment.

Women sometimes have nausea and vomiting, feel very tired (sometimes for days), and have pain in the back, shoulders, or jaw without any chest pain.

People with diabetes-related nerve damage may not notice any chest pain.

Warning signs of a stroke, includes sudden:

- weakness or numbness of your face, arm, or leg on one side of your body

- confusion, or trouble talking or understanding

- dizziness, loss of balance, or trouble walking

- trouble seeing out of one or both eyes

- sudden severe headache

If you have any one of these warning signs, call 9-1-1. You can help prevent permanent damage by getting to a hospital within an hour of a stroke.

Chapter 21

High Blood Pressure and High Cholesterol

Chapter Contents

Section 21.1—High Blood Pressure 190

Section 21.2—High Blood Cholesterol 202

Section 21.1

High Blood Pressure

This section includes text excerpted from "High Blood Pressure," National Heart, Lung, and Blood Institute (NHLBI), September 10, 2015.

What Is High Blood Pressure?

High blood pressure is a common disease in which blood flows through blood vessels (arteries) at higher than normal pressures.

Blood pressure is the force of blood pushing against the walls of the arteries as the heart pumps blood. High blood pressure, sometimes called hypertension, happens when this force is too high. Healthcare workers check blood pressure readings the same way for children, teens, and adults. They use a gauge, stethoscope or electronic sensor, and a blood pressure cuff. With this equipment, they measure:

- **Systolic Pressure:** blood pressure when the heart beats while pumping blood

- **Diastolic Pressure:** blood pressure when the heart is at rest between beats

- Healthcare workers write blood pressure numbers with the systolic number above the diastolic number. For example: 118/76 mmHg (People read "118 over 76"millimeters of mercury.)

Normal Blood Pressure

Normal blood pressure for adults is defined as a systolic pressure below 120 mmHg and a diastolic pressure below 80 mmHg. It is normal for blood pressures to change when you sleep, wake up, or are excited or nervous. When you are active, it is normal for your blood pressure to increase. However, once the activity stops, your blood pressure returns to your normal baseline range.

Blood pressure normally rises with age and body size. Newborn babies often have very low blood pressure numbers that are considered normal for babies, while older teens have numbers similar to adults.

Abnormal Blood Pressure

Abnormal increases in blood pressure are defined as having blood pressures higher than 120/80 mmHg. The following table outlines and defines high blood pressure severity levels.

Stages of High Blood Pressure in Adults

Table 21.1. Stages of High Blood Pressure in Adults

Stages	Systolic (Top Number)		Diastolic (Bottom Number)
Prehypertension	120–139	OR	80–89
High blood pressure Stage 1	140–159	OR	90–99
High blood pressure Stage 2	160 or higher	OR	100 or higher

The ranges in the table are blood pressure guides for adults who do not have any short-term serious illnesses. People with diabetes or chronic kidney disease should keep their blood pressure below 130/80 mmHg.

Although blood pressure increases seen in prehypertension are less than those used to diagnose high blood pressure, prehypertension can progress to high blood pressure and should be taken seriously. Over time, consistently high blood pressure weakens and damages your blood vessels, which can lead to complications.

Types of High Blood Pressure

There are two main types of high blood pressure: primary and secondary high blood pressure.

Primary High Blood Pressure

Primary, or essential, high blood pressure is the most common type of high blood pressure. This type of high blood pressure tends to develop over years as a person ages.

Secondary High Blood Pressure

Secondary high blood pressure is caused by another medical condition or use of certain medicines. This type usually resolves after the cause is treated or removed.

Causes of High Blood Pressure

Changes, either from genes or the environment, in the body's normal functions may cause high blood pressure, including changes to kidney fluid and salt balances, the renin-angiotensin-aldosterone system, sympathetic nervous system activity, and blood vessel structure and function.

Biology and High Blood Pressure

Researchers continue to study how various changes in normal body functions cause high blood pressure. The key functions affected in high blood pressure include:

Kidney Fluid and Salt Balances

The kidneys normally regulate the body's salt balance by retaining sodium and water and excreting potassium. Imbalances in this kidney function can expand blood volumes, which can cause high blood pressure.

Renin-Angiotensin-Aldosterone System

The renin-angiotensin-aldosterone system makes angiotensin and aldosterone hormones. Angiotensin narrows or constricts blood vessels, which can lead to an increase in blood pressure. Aldosterone controls how the kidneys balance fluid and salt levels. Increased aldosterone levels or activity may change this kidney function, leading to increased blood volumes and high blood pressure.

Sympathetic Nervous System Activity

The sympathetic nervous system has important functions in blood pressure regulation, including heart rate, blood pressure, and breathing rate. Researchers are investigating whether imbalances in this system cause high blood pressure.

Blood Vessel Structure and Function

Changes in the structure and function of small and large arteries may contribute to high blood pressure. The angiotensin pathway and the immune system may stiffen small and large arteries, which can affect blood pressure.

Genetic Causes of High Blood Pressure

Much of the understanding of the body systems involved in high blood pressure has come from genetic studies. High blood pressure often runs in families. Years of research have identified many genes and other mutations associated with high blood pressure, some in the renal salt regulatory and renin-angiotensin-aldosterone pathways. However, these known genetic factors only account for 2 to 3 percent of all cases. Emerging research suggests that certain DNA changes during fetal development also may cause the development of high blood pressure later in life.

Environmental Causes of High Blood Pressure

Environmental causes of high blood pressure include unhealthy lifestyle habits, being overweight or obese, and medicines.

Unhealthy Lifestyle Habits

Unhealthy lifestyle habits can cause high blood pressure, including:

- High dietary sodium intake and sodium sensitivity
- Drinking excess amounts of alcohol
- Lack of physical activity

Overweight and Obesity

Research studies show that being overweight or obese can increase the resistance in the blood vessels, causing the heart to work harder and leading to high blood pressure.

Medicines

Prescription medicines such as asthma or hormone therapies, including birth control pills and estrogen, and over-the-counter medicines such as cold relief medicines may cause this form of high blood pressure. This happens because medicines can change the way your body controls fluid and salt balances, cause your blood vessels to constrict, or impact the renin-angiotensin-aldosterone system leading to high blood pressure.

Other Medical Causes of High Blood Pressure

Other medical causes of high blood pressure include other medical conditions such as chronic kidney disease, sleep apnea, thyroid problems, or certain tumors. This happens because these other conditions change the way your body controls fluids, sodium, and hormones in your blood, which leads to secondary high blood pressure.

Risk Factors of High Blood Pressure

Anyone can develop high blood pressure; however, age, race or ethnicity, being overweight, gender, lifestyle habits, and a family history of high blood pressure can increase your risk for developing high blood pressure.

Age

Blood pressure tends to rise with age. About 65 percent of Americans age 60 or older have high blood pressure. However, the risk for prehypertension and high blood pressure is increasing for children and teens, possibly due to the rise in the number of overweight children and teens.

Race/Ethnicity

High blood pressure is more common in African-American adults than in Caucasian or Hispanic-American adults. Compared with these ethnic groups, African Americans:

- Tend to get high blood pressure earlier in life.

- Often, on average, have higher blood pressure numbers.

- Are less likely to achieve target blood pressure goals with treatment.

Overweight

You are more likely to develop prehypertension or high blood pressure if you're overweight or obese. The terms "overweight" and "obese" refer to body weight that's greater than what is considered healthy for a certain height.

Gender

Before age 55, men are more likely than women to develop high blood pressure. After age 55, women are more likely than men to develop high blood pressure.

Lifestyle Habits

Unhealthy lifestyle habits can raise your risk for high blood pressure, and they include:

- Eating too much sodium or too little potassium
- Lack of physical activity
- Drinking too much alcohol
- Stress

Family History

A family history of high blood pressure raises the risk of developing prehypertension or high blood pressure. Some people have a high sensitivity to sodium and salt, which may increase their risk for high blood pressure and may run in families. Genetic causes of this condition are why family history is a risk factor for this condition.

Signs, Symptoms and Complications of High Blood Pressure

Because diagnosis is based on blood pressure readings, this condition can go undetected for years, as symptoms do not usually appear until the body is damaged from chronic high blood pressure.

Complications of High Blood Pressure

When blood pressure stays high over time, it can damage the body and cause complications. Some common complications and their signs and symptoms include:

- **Stroke:** When the flow of oxygen-rich blood to a portion of the brain is blocked. The symptoms of a stroke include sudden onset of weakness; paralysis or numbness of the face, arms, or legs; trouble speaking or understanding speech; and trouble seeing.

- **Aneurysms:** When an abnormal bulge forms in the wall of an artery. Aneurysms develop and grow for years without causing signs or symptoms until they rupture, grow large enough to press on nearby body parts, or block blood flow. The signs and symptoms that develop depend on the location of the aneurysm.

- **Chronic Kidney Disease:** When blood vessels narrow in the kidneys, possibly causing kidney failure.

- **Cognitive Changes:** Research shows that over time, higher blood pressure numbers can lead to cognitive changes. Signs and symptoms include memory loss, difficulty finding words, and losing focus during conversations.

- **Eye Damage:** When blood vessels in the eyes burst or bleed. Signs and symptoms include vision changes or blindness.

- **Heart Attack:** When the flow of oxygen-rich blood to a section of heart muscle suddenly becomes blocked and the heart doesn't get oxygen. The most common warning symptoms of a heart attack are chest pain or discomfort, upper body discomfort, and shortness of breath.

- **Heart Failure:** When the heart can't pump enough blood to meet the body's needs. Common signs and symptoms of heart failure include shortness of breath or trouble breathing; feeling tired; and swelling in the ankles, feet, legs, abdomen, and veins in the neck.

- **Peripheral Artery Disease:** A disease in which plaque builds up in leg arteries and affects blood flow in the legs. When people have symptoms, the most common are pain, cramping, numbness, aching, or heaviness in the legs, feet, and buttocks after walking or climbing stairs.

Diagnosing High Blood Pressure

For most patients, healthcare providers diagnose high blood pressure when blood pressure readings are consistently 140/90 mmHg or above.

Confirming High Blood Pressure

A blood pressure test is easy and painless and can be done in a healthcare provider's office or clinic. To prepare for the test:

- Don't drink coffee or smoke cigarettes for 30 minutes prior to the test.

- Go to the bathroom before the test.

- Sit for 5 minutes before the test.

To track blood pressure readings over a period of time, the health-care provider may ask you to come into the office on different days and at different times to take your blood pressure. The healthcare provider also may ask you to check readings at home or at other locations that have blood pressure equipment and to keep a written log of all your results.

Whenever you have an appointment with the healthcare provider, be sure to bring your log of blood pressure readings. Every time you visit the healthcare provider, he or she should tell you what your blood pressure numbers are; if he or she does not, you should ask for your readings.

Blood Pressure Severity and Type

Your healthcare provider usually takes 2–3 readings at several medical appointments to diagnose high blood pressure. Using the results of your blood pressure test, your healthcare provider will diag-nose prehypertension or high blood pressure if:

- Your systolic or diastolic readings are consistently higher than 120/80 mmHg.

- Your child's blood pressure numbers are outside average num-bers for children of the same age, gender, and height.

Once your healthcare provider determines the severity of your blood pressure, he or she can order additional tests to determine if your blood pressure is due to other conditions or medicines or if you have primary high blood pressure. Healthcare providers can use this information to develop your treatment plan.

Some people have "white coat hypertension." This happens when blood pressure readings are only high when taken in a healthcare provider's office compared with readings taken in any other location. Healthcare providers diagnose this type of high blood pressure by reviewing readings in the office and readings taken anywhere else. Researchers believe stress, which can occur during the medical appointment, causes white coat hypertension.

Treatment of High Blood Pressure

Based on your diagnosis, healthcare providers develop treatment plans for high blood pressure that include lifelong lifestyle changes and medicines to control high blood pressure; lifestyle changes such as weight loss can be highly effective in treating high blood pressure.

Treatment Plans

Healthcare providers work with you to develop a treatment plan based on whether you were diagnosed with primary or secondary high blood pressure and if there is a suspected or known cause. Treatment plans may evolve until blood pressure control is achieved.

If your healthcare provider diagnoses you with secondary high blood pressure, he or she will work to treat the other condition or change the medicine suspected of causing your high blood pressure. If high blood pressure persists or is first diagnosed as primary high blood pressure, your treatment plan will include lifestyle changes. When lifestyle changes alone do not control or lower blood pressure, your healthcare provider may change or update your treatment plan by prescribing medicines to treat the disease. Healthcare providers prescribe children and teens medicines at special doses that are safe and effective in children.

If your healthcare provider prescribes medicines as a part of your treatment plan, keep up your healthy lifestyle habits. The combination of the medicines and the healthy lifestyle habits helps control and lower your high blood pressure.

Some people develop "resistant" or uncontrolled high blood pressure. This can happen when the medications they are taking do not work well for them or another medical condition is leading to uncontrolled blood pressure. Healthcare providers treat resistant or uncontrolled high blood pressure with an intensive treatment plan that can include a different set of blood pressure medications or other special treatments.

To achieve the best control of your blood pressure, follow your treatment plan and take all medications as prescribed. Following your prescribed treatment plan is important because it can prevent or delay complications that high blood pressure can cause and can lower your risk for other related problems.

Healthy Lifestyle Changes

Healthy lifestyle habits can help you control high blood pressure. These habits include:

- Healthy eating
- Being physically active
- Maintaining a healthy weight
- Limiting alcohol intake
- Managing and coping with stress

To help make lifelong lifestyle changes, try making one healthy lifestyle change at a time and add another change when you feel that you have successfully adopted the earlier changes. When you practice several healthy lifestyle habits, you are more likely to lower your blood pressure and maintain normal blood pressure readings.

Medicines

Blood pressure medicines work in different ways to stop or slow some of the body's functions that cause high blood pressure. Medicines to lower blood pressure include:

- Diuretics (water or fluid pills)
- Beta blockers
- Angiotensin-converting enzyme (ACE) inhibitors
- Angiotensin II receptor blockers (ARBs)
- Calcium channel blockers
- Alpha blockers
- Alpha-beta blockers
- Central acting agents
- Vasodilators

To lower and control blood pressure, many people take two or more medicines. If you have side effects from your medicines, don't stop taking your medicines. Instead, talk with your healthcare provider about the side effects to see if the dose can be changed or a new medicine prescribed.

Future Treatments

Scientists, doctors, and researchers continue to study the changes that cause high blood pressure, to develop new medicines and treatments to control high blood pressure. Possible future treatments under investigation include new combination medicines, vaccines, and interventions aimed at the sympathetic nervous system, such as kidney nerve ablation.

Prevention of High Blood Pressure

Healthy lifestyle habits, proper use of medicines, and regular medical care can prevent high blood pressure or its complications.

Preventing High Blood Pressure Onset

Healthy lifestyle habits can help prevent high blood pressure from developing. It is important to check your blood pressure regularly. Children should have their blood pressure checked starting at 3 years of age. If prehypertension is detected, it should be taken seriously to avoid progressing to high blood pressure.

Preventing Worsening High Blood Pressure or Complications

If you have been diagnosed with high blood pressure, it is important to obtain regular medical care and to follow your prescribed treatment plan, which will include healthy lifestyle habit recommendations and possibly medicines. Not only can healthy lifestyle habits prevent high blood pressure from occurring, but they can reverse prehypertension and help control existing high blood pressure or prevent complications and long-term problems associated with this condition, such as coronary heart disease, stroke, or kidney disease.

Living with High Blood Pressure

If you have high blood pressure, the best thing to do is to talk with your healthcare provider and take steps to control your blood pressure by making healthy lifestyle changes and taking medications, if any have been prescribed for you.

For a healthy future, follow your treatment plan closely and work with your healthcare team.

Healthy Lifestyle Changes

You can help control your blood pressure by making these healthy lifestyle changes:

- Follow a healthy diet.
- Be physically active.
- Maintain a healthy weight.
- Limit alcohol intake.

Other lifestyle changes can improve your overall health, such as:

- If you smoke, quit.

- Get plenty of sleep.

- Drink more water.

Medicines

Take all blood pressure medicines that your healthcare provider prescribes. Know the names and doses of your medicines and how to take them. If you have questions about your medicines, talk with your healthcare provider or pharmacist. Make sure you refill your medicines before they run out. Take your medicines exactly as your healthcare provider directs, and never skip days or cut pills in half.

Ongoing Care

Keeping track of your blood pressure is important. Check your blood pressure and have regular medical checkups or tests as your healthcare provider advises. You may want to learn how to check your blood pressure at home. Your healthcare provider can help you learn how to do this. Each time you check your own blood pressure, you should write down your numbers and the date. Take the log of your blood pressure readings with you to appointments with your healthcare provider.

During checkups, talk to your healthcare provider about:

- Blood pressure readings

- Your overall health

- Your treatment plan

- Your healthcare provider may need to change or add medicines to your treatment plan over time.

Pregnancy Planning

High blood pressure can cause problems for mother and baby. High blood pressure can harm the mother's kidneys and other organs and can cause early birth and low birth weight. If you're thinking about having a baby and have high blood pressure, talk with your healthcare team so you can take steps to control your blood pressure before and during the pregnancy.

Some women develop high blood pressure during pregnancy. When this happens, your healthcare provider will closely monitor you and your baby and provide special care to lower the chance of complications. With such care, most women and babies have good outcomes.

Section 21.2

High Blood Cholesterol

This section includes text excerpted from "High Blood Cholesterol," National Heart, Lung, and Blood Institute (NHLBI), April 8, 2016.

To understand high blood cholesterol, it helps to learn about cholesterol. Cholesterol is a waxy, fat-like substance that's found in all cells of the body. Your body needs some cholesterol to make hormones, vitamin D, and substances that help you digest foods. Your body makes all the cholesterol it needs. However, cholesterol also is found in some of the foods you eat.

Cholesterol travels through your bloodstream in small packages called lipoproteins. These packages are made of fat (lipid) on the inside and proteins on the outside. Two kinds of lipoproteins carry cholesterol throughout your body: low-density lipoproteins (LDL) and high-density lipoproteins (HDL). Having healthy levels of both types of lipoproteins is important.

LDL cholesterol sometimes is called "bad" cholesterol. A high LDL level leads to a buildup of cholesterol in your arteries. (Arteries are blood vessels that carry blood from your heart to your body.)

HDL cholesterol sometimes is called "good" cholesterol. This is because it carries cholesterol from other parts of your body back to your liver. Your liver removes the cholesterol from your body.

What Is High Blood Cholesterol?

High blood cholesterol is a condition in which you have too much cholesterol in your blood. By itself, the condition usually has no signs or symptoms. Thus, many people don't know that their cholesterol levels are too high.

People who have high blood cholesterol have a greater chance of getting coronary heart disease, also called coronary artery disease. (In this section, the term "heart disease" refers to coronary heart disease.)

The higher the level of LDL cholesterol in your blood, the GREATER your chance is of getting heart disease. The higher the level of HDL cholesterol in your blood, the LOWER your chance is of getting heart disease.

Coronary heart disease is a condition in which plaque builds up inside the coronary (heart) arteries. Plaque is made up of cholesterol, fat, calcium, and other substances found in the blood. When plaque builds up in the arteries, the condition is called atherosclerosis.

Over time, plaque hardens and narrows your coronary arteries. This limits the flow of oxygen-rich blood to the heart.

Eventually, an area of plaque can rupture (break open). This causes a blood clot to form on the surface of the plaque. If the clot becomes large enough, it can mostly or completely block blood flow through a coronary artery.

If the flow of oxygen-rich blood to your heart muscle is reduced or blocked, angina or a heart attack may occur.

Angina is chest pain or discomfort. It may feel like pressure or squeezing in your chest. The pain also may occur in your shoulders, arms, neck, jaw, or back. Angina pain may even feel like indigestion.

A heart attack occurs if the flow of oxygen-rich blood to a section of heart muscle is cut off. If blood flow isn't restored quickly, the section of heart muscle begins to die. Without quick treatment, a heart attack can lead to serious problems or death.

Plaque also can build up in other arteries in your body, such as the arteries that bring oxygen-rich blood to your brain and limbs. This can lead to problems such as carotid artery disease, stroke, and peripheral artery disease.

Causes of High Blood Cholesterol

Many factors can affect the cholesterol levels in your blood. You can control some factors, but not others.

Factors You Can Control

Diet

Cholesterol is found in foods that come from animal sources, such as egg yolks, meat, and cheese. Some foods have fats that raise your cholesterol level.

For example, saturated fat raises your low-density lipoprotein (LDL) cholesterol level more than anything else in your diet. Saturated fat is found in some meats, dairy products, chocolate, baked goods, and deep-fried and processed foods.

Trans fatty acids (*trans* fats) raise your LDL cholesterol and lower your high-density lipoprotein (HDL) cholesterol. Trans fats are made when hydrogen is added to vegetable oil to harden it. Trans fats are found in some fried and processed foods.

Limiting foods with cholesterol, saturated fat, and trans fats can help you control your cholesterol levels.

Physical Activity and Weight

Lack of physical activity can lead to weight gain. Being overweight tends to raise your LDL level, lower your HDL level, and increase your total cholesterol level. (Total cholesterol is a measure of the total amount of cholesterol in your blood, including LDL and HDL.)

Routine physical activity can help you lose weight and lower your LDL cholesterol. Being physically active also can help you raise your HDL cholesterol level.

Factors You Can't Control

Heredity

High blood cholesterol can run in families. An inherited condition called familial hypercholesterolemia causes very high LDL cholesterol. ("Inherited" means the condition is passed from parents to children through genes.) This condition begins at birth, and it may cause a heart attack at an early age.

Age and Sex

Starting at puberty, men often have lower levels of HDL cholesterol than women. As women and men age, their LDL cholesterol levels often rise. Before age 55, women usually have lower LDL cholesterol levels than men. However, after age 55, women can have higher LDL levels than men.

Signs and Symptoms of High Blood Cholesterol

High blood cholesterol usually has no signs or symptoms. Thus, many people don't know that their cholesterol levels are too high.

If you're 20 years old or older, have your cholesterol levels checked at least once every 5 years. Talk with your doctor about how often you should be tested.

Diagnosis of High Blood Cholesterol

Your doctor will diagnose high blood cholesterol by checking the cholesterol levels in your blood. A blood test called a lipoprotein panel can measure your cholesterol levels. Before the test, you'll need to fast (not eat or drink anything but water) for 9 to 12 hours.

The lipoprotein panel will give your doctor information about your:

- **Total cholesterol.** Total cholesterol is a measure of the total amount of cholesterol in your blood, including low-density lipoprotein (LDL) cholesterol and high-density lipoprotein (HDL) cholesterol.

- **LDL cholesterol.** LDL, or "bad," cholesterol is the main source of cholesterol buildup and blockages in the arteries.

- **HDL cholesterol.** HDL, or "good," cholesterol helps remove cholesterol from your arteries.

- **Triglycerides.** Triglycerides are a type of fat found in your blood. Some studies suggest that a high level of triglycerides in the blood may raise the risk of coronary heart disease, especially in women.

If it's not possible to have a lipoprotein panel, knowing your total cholesterol and HDL cholesterol can give you a general idea about your cholesterol levels.

Testing for total and HDL cholesterol does not require fasting. If your total cholesterol is 200 mg/dL or more, or if your HDL cholesterol is less than 40 mg/dL, your doctor will likely recommend that you have a lipoprotein panel. (Cholesterol is measured as milligrams (mg) of cholesterol per deciliter (dL) of blood.)

The tables below show total, LDL, and HDL cholesterol levels and their corresponding categories. See how your cholesterol numbers compare to the numbers in the tables below.

Table 21.2. Total Cholesterol Level

Total Cholesterol Level	Total Cholesterol Category
Less than 200 mg/dL	Desirable
200–239 mg/dL	Borderline high
240 mg/dL and higher	High

Table 21.3. LDL Cholesterol Level

LDL Cholesterol Level	LDL Cholesterol Category
Less than 100 mg/dL	Optimal
100–129 mg/dL	Near optimal/above optimal
130–159 mg/dL	Borderline high
160–189 mg/dL	High
190 mg/dL and higher	Very high

Table 21.4. HDL Cholesterol Level

HDL Cholesterol Level	HDL Cholesterol Category
Less than 40 mg/dL	A major risk factor for heart disease
40–59 mg/dL	The higher, the better
60 mg/dL and higher	Considered protective against heart disease

Triglycerides also can raise your risk for heart disease. If your triglyceride level is borderline high (150–199 mg/dL) or high (200 mg/dL or higher), you may need treatment.

Factors that can raise your triglyceride level include:

- Overweight and obesity

- Lack of physical activity

- Cigarette smoking

- Excessive alcohol use

- A very high carbohydrate diet

- Certain diseases and medicines

- Some genetic disorders

Treatment of High Blood Cholesterol

High blood cholesterol is treated with lifestyle changes and medicines. The main goal of treatment is to lower your low-density lipoprotein (LDL) cholesterol level enough to reduce your risk for coronary heart disease, heart attack, and other related health problems.

Your risk for heart disease and heart attack goes up as your LDL cholesterol level rises and your number of heart disease risk factors increases.

Some people are at high risk for heart attacks because they already have heart disease. Other people are at high risk for heart disease because they have diabetes or more than one heart disease risk factor.

Talk with your doctor about lowering your cholesterol and your risk for heart disease. Also, check the list to find out whether you have risk factors that affect your LDL cholesterol goal:

- Cigarette smoking

- High blood pressure (140/90 mmHg or higher), or you're on medicine to treat high blood pressure

- Low high-density lipoprotein (HDL) cholesterol (less than 40 mg/dL)

- Family history of early heart disease (heart disease in father or brother before age 55; heart disease in mother or sister before age 65)

- Age (men 45 years or older; women 55 years or older)

You can use the NHLBI 10-Year Risk Calculator (cvdrisk.nhlbi.nih. gov/calculator.asp) to find your risk score. The score, given as a percentage, refers to your chance of having a heart attack in the next 10 years.

Based on your medical history, number of risk factors, and risk score, figure out your risk of getting heart disease or having a heart attack using the table below.

Table 21.5. NHLBI 10-Year Risk Calculator

If You Have	You Are in Category	Your LDL Goal Is
Heart disease, diabetes, or a risk score higher than 20%	I. High risk*	Less than 100 mg/dL
Two or more risk factors and a risk score of 10–20%	II. Moderately high risk	Less than 130 mg/dL
Two or more risk factors and a risk score lower than 10%	III. Moderate risk	Less than 130 mg/dL
One or no risk factors	IV. Low to moderate risk	Less than 160 mg/dL

*Some people in this category are at very high risk because they've just had a heart attack or they have diabetes and heart disease, severe risk factors, or metabolic syndrome. If you're at very high risk, your doctor may set your LDL goal even lower, to less than 70 mg/dL. Your doctor also may set your LDL goal at this lower level if you have heart disease alone.

After following the above steps, you should have an idea about your risk for heart disease and heart attack.

The two main ways to lower your cholesterol (and, thus, your heart disease risk) include:

- **Therapeutic Lifestyle Changes (TLC).** TLC is a three-part program that includes a healthy diet, weight management, and physical activity. TLC is for anyone whose LDL cholesterol level is above goal.

- **Medicines.** If cholesterol-lowering medicines are needed, they're used with the TLC program to help lower your LDL cholesterol level.

Your doctor will set your LDL goal. The higher your risk for heart disease, the lower he or she will set your LDL goal. Using the following guide, you and your doctor can create a plan for treating your high blood cholesterol.

Category I, high risk, your LDL goal is less than 100 mg/dL.*

Table 21.6. Treatment Plan for High LDL

Your LDL Level	Treatment
If your LDL level is 100 or higher	You will need to begin the TLC diet and take medicines as prescribed.
Even if your LDL level is below 100	You should follow the TLC diet to keep your LDL level as low as possible.

* Your LDL goal may be set even lower, to less than 70 mg/dL, if you're at very high risk or if you have heart disease. If you have this lower goal and your LDL is 70 mg/dL or higher, you'll need to begin the TLC diet and take medicines as prescribed.

Category II, moderately high risk, your LDL goal is less than 130 mg/dL

Table 21.7. Treatment Plan for High LDL

Your LDL Level	Treatment
If your LDL level is 130 mg/dL or higher	You will need to begin the TLC diet.
If your LDL level is 130 mg/dL or higher after 3 months on the TLC diet	You may need medicines along with the TLC diet.
If your LDL level is less than 130 mg/dL	You will need to follow a heart healthy diet.

Category III, moderate risk, your LDL goal is less than 130 mg/dL.

Table 21.8. Treatment Plan for High LDL

Your LDL Level	Treatment
If your LDL level is 130 mg/dL or higher	You will need to begin the TLC diet.
If your LDL level is 160 mg/dL or higher after 3 months on the TLC diet	You may need medicines along with the TLC diet.
If your LDL level is less than 130 mg/dL	You will need to follow a heart healthy diet.

Category IV, low to moderate risk, your LDL goal is less than 160 mg/dL.

Table 21.9. Treatment Plan for High LDL

Your LDL Level	Treatment
If your LDL level is 160 mg/dL or higher	You will need to begin the TLC diet.
If your LDL level is 160 mg/dL or higher after 3 months on the TLC diet	You may need medicines along with the TLC diet.
If your LDL level is less than 160 mg/dL	You will need to follow a heart healthy diet.

Lowering Cholesterol Using Therapeutic Lifestyle Changes

TLC is a set of lifestyle changes that can help you lower your LDL cholesterol. The main parts of the TLC program are a healthy diet, weight management, and physical activity.

The TLC Diet

With the TLC diet, less than 7 percent of your daily calories should come from saturated fat. This kind of fat is found in some meats, dairy products, chocolate, baked goods, and deep-fried and processed foods.

No more than 25 to 35 percent of your daily calories should come from all fats, including saturated, trans, monounsaturated, and poly-unsaturated fats.

You also should have less than 200 mg a day of cholesterol. The amounts of cholesterol and the types of fat in prepared foods can be found on the foods' Nutrition Facts labels.

Foods high in soluble fiber also are part of the TLC diet. They help prevent the digestive tract from absorbing cholesterol. These foods include:

- Whole-grain cereals such as oatmeal and oat bran

- Fruits such as apples, bananas, oranges, pears, and prunes

- Legumes such as kidney beans, lentils, chickpeas, black-eyed peas, and lima beans

A diet rich in fruits and vegetables can increase important cholesterol-lowering compounds in your diet. These compounds, called plant stanols or sterols, work like soluble fiber.

A healthy diet also includes some types of fish, such as salmon, tuna (canned or fresh), and mackerel. These fish are a good source of omega-3 fatty acids. These acids may help protect the heart from blood clots and inflammation and reduce the risk of heart attack. Try to have about two fish meals every week.

You also should try to limit the amount of sodium (salt) that you eat. This means choosing low-salt and "no added salt" foods and seasonings at the table or while cooking. The Nutrition Facts label on food packaging shows the amount of sodium in the item.

Weight Management

If you're overweight or obese, losing weight can help lower LDL cholesterol. Maintaining a healthy weight is especially important if you have a condition called metabolic syndrome.

Metabolic syndrome is the name for a group of risk factors that raise your risk for heart disease and other health problems, such as diabetes and stroke.

The five metabolic risk factors are a large waistline (abdominal obesity), a high triglyceride level, a low HDL cholesterol level, high blood pressure, and high blood sugar. Metabolic syndrome is diagnosed if you have at least three of these metabolic risk factors.

Try to limit drinks with alcohol. Too much alcohol will raise your blood pressure and triglyceride level. (Triglycerides are a type of fat found in the blood.) Alcohol also adds extra calories, which will cause weight gain.

Men should have no more than two drinks containing alcohol a day. Women should have no more than one drink containing alcohol a day. One drink is a glass of wine, beer, or a small amount of hard liquor.

Physical Activity

Routine physical activity can lower LDL cholesterol and triglycerides and raise your HDL cholesterol level.

People gain health benefits from as little as 60 minutes of moderate-intensity aerobic activity per week. The more active you are, the more you will benefit.

Cholesterol-Lowering Medicines

In addition to lifestyle changes, your doctor may prescribe medicines to help lower your cholesterol. Even with medicines, you should continue the TLC program.

Medicines can help control high blood cholesterol, but they don't cure it. Thus, you must continue taking your medicine to keep your cholesterol level in the recommended range.

The five major types of cholesterol-lowering medicines are statins, bile acid sequestrants, nicotinic acid, fibrates, and ezetimibe.

- **Statins** work well at lowering LDL cholesterol. These medicines are safe for most people. Rare side effects include muscle and liver problems.

- **Bile acid sequestrants** also help lower LDL cholesterol. These medicines usually aren't prescribed as the only medicine to lower cholesterol. Sometimes they're prescribed with statins.

- **Nicotinic acid** lowers LDL cholesterol and triglycerides and raises HDL cholesterol. You should only use this type of medicine with a doctor's supervision.

- **Fibrates** lower triglycerides, and they may raise HDL cholesterol. When used with statins, fibrates may increase the risk of muscle problems.

- **Ezetimibe** lowers LDL cholesterol. This medicine works by blocking the intestine from absorbing cholesterol.

While you're being treated for high blood cholesterol, you'll need ongoing care. Your doctor will want to make sure your cholesterol levels are controlled. He or she also will want to check for other health problems.

If needed, your doctor may prescribe medicines for other health problems. Take all medicines exactly as your doctor prescribes. The combination of medicines may lower your risk for heart disease and heart attack.

While trying to manage your cholesterol, take steps to manage other heart disease risk factors too. For example, if you have high blood pressure, work with your doctor to lower it.

If you smoke, quit. Talk with your doctor about programs and products that can help you quit smoking. Also, try to avoid secondhand smoke. If you're overweight or obese, try to lose weight. Your doctor can help you create a reasonable weight-loss plan.

Chapter 22

Overweight, Obesity, and Stroke Risk

Overweight and obesity are increasingly common conditions in the United States. They are caused by the increase in the size and the amount of fat cells in the body. Doctors measure body mass index (BMI) and waist circumference to screen and diagnose overweight and obesity. Obesity is a serious medical condition that can cause complications such as metabolic syndrome, high blood pressure, atherosclerosis, heart disease, diabetes, high blood cholesterol, cancers, and sleep disorders. Treatment depends on the cause and severity of your condition and whether you have complications. Treatments include lifestyle changes, such as heart-healthy eating and increased physical activity, and U.S. Food and Drug Administration (FDA)-approved weight-loss medicines. For some people, surgery may be a treatment option.

Causes of Overweight and Obesity

Energy imbalances, some genetic or endocrine medical conditions, and certain medicines are known to cause overweight or obesity.

Energy Imbalances Cause the Body to Store Fat

Energy imbalances can cause overweight and obesity. An energy imbalance means that your energy in does not equal your energy out.

This chapter includes text excerpted from "Overweight and Obesity," National Heart, Lung, and Blood Institute (NHLBI), February 23, 2017.

This energy is measured in calories. Energy in is the amount of calories you get from food and drinks. Energy out is the amount of calories that your body uses for things such as breathing, digesting, being physically active, and regulating body temperature.

Overweight and obesity develop over time when you take in more calories than you use, or when energy in is more than your energy out. This type of energy imbalance causes your body to store fat.

Your body uses certain nutrients such as carbohydrates or sugars, proteins, and fats from the foods you eat to:

- Make energy for immediate use to power routine daily body functions and physical activity.

- Store energy for future use by your body. Sugars are stored as glycogen in the liver and muscles. Fats are stored mainly as triglycerides in fat tissue.

The amount of energy that your body gets from the food you eat depends on the type of foods you eat, how the food is prepared, and how long it has been since you last ate.

The body has three types of fat tissue—white, brown, and beige—that it uses to fuel itself, regulate its temperature in response to cold, and store energy for future use. Learn about the role of each fat type in maintaining energy balance in the body.

- **White fat tissue** can be found around the kidneys and under the skin in the buttocks, thighs, and abdomen. This fat type stores energy, makes hormones that control the way the body regulates urges to eat or stop eating, and makes inflammatory substances that can lead to complications.

- **Brown fat tissue** is located in the upper back area of human infants. This fat type releases stored energy as heat energy when a baby is cold. It also can make inflammatory substances. Brown fat can be seen in children and adults.

- **Beige fat tissue** is seen in the neck, shoulders, back, chest and abdomen of adults and resembles brown fat tissue. This fat type, which uses carbohydrates and fats to produce heat, increases when children and adults are exposed to cold.

Medical Conditions

Some genetic syndromes and endocrine disorders can cause overweight or obesity.

Genetic Syndromes

Several genetic syndromes are associated with overweight and obesity, including the following:

- Prader-Willi syndrome
- Bardet-Biedl syndrome
- Alström syndrome
- Cohen syndrome

The study of these genetic syndromes has helped researchers understand obesity.

Endocrine Disorders

Because the endocrine system produces hormones that help maintain energy balances in the body, the following endocrine disorders or tumors affecting the endocrine system can cause overweight and obesity.

- **Hypothyroidism.** People with this condition have low levels of thyroid hormones. These low levels are associated with decreased metabolism and weight gain, even when food intake is reduced. People with hypothyroidism also produce less body heat, have a lower body temperature, and do not efficiently use stored fat for energy.

- **Cushing syndrome.** People with this condition have high levels of glucocorticoids, such as cortisol, in the blood. High cortisol levels make the body feel like it is under chronic stress. As a result, people have an increase in appetite and the body will store more fat. Cushing syndrome may develop after taking certain medicines or because the body naturally makes too much cortisol.

- **Tumors.** Some tumors, such as craneopharingioma, can cause severe obesity because the tumors develop near parts of the brain that control hunger.

Medicines

Medicines such as antipsychotics, antidepressants, antiepileptics, and antihyperglycemics can cause weight gain and lead to overweight and obesity.

215

Talk to your doctor if you notice weight gain while you are using one of these medicines. Ask if there are other forms of the same medicine or other medicines that can treat your medical condition, but have less of an effect on your weight. Do not stop taking the medicine without talking to your doctor.

Several parts of your body, such as your stomach, intestines, pancreas, and fat tissue, use hormones to control how your brain decides if you are hungry or full. Some of these hormones are insulin, leptin, glucagon-like peptide (GLP-1), peptide YY, and ghrelin.

Risk Factors for Overweight and Obesity

There are many risk factors for overweight and obesity. Some risk factors can be changed, such as unhealthy lifestyle habits and environments. Other risk factors, such as age, family history and genetics, race and ethnicity, and sex, cannot be changed. Healthy lifestyle changes can decrease your risk for developing overweight and obesity.

Lack of Physical Activity

Lack of physical activity due to high amounts of TV, computer, video game or other screen usage has been associated with a high body mass index (BMI). Healthy lifestyle changes, such as being physically active and reducing screen time, can help you aim for a healthy weight.

Unhealthy Eating Behaviors

Some unhealthy eating behaviors can increase your risk for overweight and obesity.

- **Eating more calories than you use.** The amount of calories you need will vary based on your sex, age, and physical activity level. Find out your daily calorie needs or goals with the Body Weight Planner (www.supertracker.usda.gov/bwp/index.html).

- **Eating too much saturated and *trans* fats.**

- **Eating foods high in added sugars.**

Not Enough Sleep

Many studies have seen a high BMI in people who do not get enough sleep. Some studies have seen a relationship between sleep and the way our bodies use nutrients for energy and how lack of sleep can affect hormones that control hunger urges.

High Amounts of Stress

Acute stress and chronic stress affect the brain and trigger the production of hormones, such as cortisol, that control our energy balances and hunger urges. Acute stress can trigger hormone changes that make you not want to eat. If the stress becomes chronic, hormone changes can make you eat more and store more fat.

Age

Childhood obesity remains a serious problem in the United States, and some populations are more at risk for childhood obesity than others. The risk of unhealthy weight gain increases as you age. Adults who have a healthy BMI often start to gain weight in young adulthood and continue to gain weight until 60 to 65 years old, when they tend to start losing weight.

Unhealthy Environments

Many environmental factors can increase your risk for overweight and obesity:

- **Social factors** such as having a low socioeconomic status or an unhealthy social or unsafe environment in the neighborhood

- **Built environment factors** such as easy access to unhealthy fast foods, limited access to recreational facilities or parks, and few safe or easy ways to walk in your neighborhood

- **Exposure to chemicals** known as obesogens that can change hormones and increase fatty tissue in our bodies

Family History and Genetics

Genetic studies have found that overweight and obesity can run in families, so it is possible that our genes or deoxyribonucleic acid (DNA) can cause these conditions. Research studies have found that certain DNA elements are associated with obesity.

Eating too much or eating too little during your pregnancy can change your baby's DNA and can affect how your child stores and uses fat later in life. Also, studies have shown that obese fathers have DNA changes in their sperm that can be passed on to their children.

217

Race or Ethnicity

Overweight and obesity is highly prevalent in some racial and ethnic minority groups. Rates of obesity in American adults are highest in blacks, followed by Hispanics, then whites. This is true for men or women. While Asian men and women have the lowest rates of unhealthy BMIs, they may have high amounts of unhealthy fat in the abdomen. Samoans may be at risk for overweight and obesity because they may carry a DNA variant that is associated with increased BMI but not with common obesity-related complications.

Sex

In the United States, obesity is more common in black or Hispanic women than in black or Hispanic men. A person's sex may also affect the way the body stores fat. For example, women tend to store less unhealthy fat in the abdomen than men do.

Overweight and obesity is also common in women with polycystic ovary syndrome (PCOS). This is an endocrine condition that causes large ovaries and prevents proper ovulation, which can reduce fertility.

Screening and Prevention of Obesity

Children and adults should be screened at least annually to see if they have a high or increasing body mass index (BMI), which allows doctors to recommend healthy lifestyle changes to prevent overweight and obesity.

Screening for a High or Increasing Body Mass Index (BMI)

To screen for overweight and obesity, doctors measure BMI using calculations that depend on whether you are a child or an adult. After reading the information below, talk to your doctor or your child's doctor to determine if you or your child has a high or increasing BMI.

- **Children:** A healthy weight is usually when your child's BMI is at the 5th percentile up to the 85th percentile, based on growth charts for children who are the same age and sex. To figure out your child's BMI, use the Center for Disease Control and Prevention (CDC) BMI Percentile Calculator for Child and Teen (nccd.cdc.gov/dnpabmi/calculator.aspx) and compare the BMI with Table 22.1.

- **Adults:** A healthy weight for adults is usually when your BMI is 18.5 to less than 25. To figure out your BMI, use the National

Heart, Lung, and Blood Institute's online BMI calculator (www. nhlbi.nih.gov/health/educational/lose_wt/BMI/bmicalc.htm) and compare it with the Table 22.1.

Healthy Lifestyle Changes to Prevent Overweight and Obesity

If your BMI indicates you are getting close to being overweight, or if you have certain risk factors, your doctor may recommend you adopt healthy lifestyle changes to prevent you from becoming overweight and obese. Changes include healthy eating, being physically active, aiming for a healthy weight, and getting healthy amounts of sleep.

Signs, Symptoms, and Complications of Overweight and Obesity

There are no specific symptoms of overweight and obesity. The signs of overweight and obesity include a high body mass index (BMI) and an unhealthy body fat distribution that can be estimated by measuring your waist circumference. Obesity can cause complications in many parts of your body.

High Body Mass Index (BMI)

A high BMI is the most common sign of overweight and obesity.

Table 22.1. Weight Category and BMI

Weight Category	Body Mass Index	
	Children	**Adult**
Underweight	Below 5th Percentile*	Below 18.5
Healthyweight	5th Percentile to less than 85th percentile	18.5 to 24.5
Overweight	85th Percentile to less than 85th percentile	25 to 29.9
Obese	95th Percentile or above	30 or above

*Body mass index (BMI) is used to determine if you or your child are underweight, healthy, or overweight or obese. Children are underweight if their BMI is below the 5th percentile, healthy weight if their BMI is between the 5th to less than the 85th percentile, overweight if their BMI is the 85th percentile to less than the 95th percentile, and obese if their BMI is the 95th percentile or above. Adults are underweight if their BMI is below 18.5, healthy weight if their BMI is 18.5 to 24.9, overweight if their BMI is 25 to 29.9, and obese if their BMI is 30 or above. *A child's BMI percentile is calculated by comparing your child's BMI to growth charts for children who are the same age and sex as your child.*

Unhealthy Body Fat Distribution

Another sign of overweight and obesity is having an unhealthy body fat distribution. Fatty tissue is found in different parts of your body and has many functions. Having an increased waist circumference suggests that you have increased amounts of fat in your abdomen. An increased waist circumference is a sign of obesity and can increase your risk for obesity-related complications.

Did you know that fatty tissue has different functions depending on its location in your body? Visceral fat is the fatty tissue inside of your abdomen and organs. While we do not know what causes the body to create and store visceral fat, it is known that this type of fat interferes with the body's endocrine and immune systems and promotes chronic inflammation and contributes to obesity-related complications.

Complications

- Diseases of the heart and blood vessels such as stroke, high blood pressure, atherosclerosis, and heart attacks

- Metabolic Syndrome

- Type 2 diabetes

- High blood cholesterol and high triglyceride levels in the blood

- Respiratory problems such as obstructive sleep apnea, asthma, and obesity hypoventilation syndrome

- Back pain

- Non-alcoholic fatty liver disease (NAFLD)

- Osteoarthritis, a chronic inflammation that damages the cartilage and bone in or around the affected joint. It can cause mild or severe pain and usually affects weight-bearing joints in people who are obese. It is a major cause of knee replacement surgery in patients who are obese for a long time.

- Urinary incontinence, the unintentional leakage of urine. Chronic obesity can weaken pelvic muscles, making it harder to maintain bladder control. While it can happen to both sexes, it usually affects women as they age.

- Gallbladder disease

- Emotional health issues such as low self-esteem or depression. This may commonly occur in children.

- Cancers of the esophagus, pancreas, colon, rectum, kidney, endometrium, ovaries, gallbladder, breast, or liver.

Did you know inflammation is thought to play a role in the onset of certain obesity-related complications?

Researchers now know more about visceral fat, which is deep in the abdomen of overweight and obese patients. Visceral fat releases factors that promote inflammation. Chronic obesity-related inflammation is thought to lead to insulin resistance and diabetes, changes in the liver or non-alcoholic fatty acid liver disease, and cancers. More research is needed to understand what triggers inflammation in some obese patients and to find new treatments.

Diagnosis of Overweight and Obesity

Your doctor may diagnose overweight and obesity based on your medical history, physical exams that confirm you have a high body mass index (BMI) and possibly a high waist circumference, and tests to rule out other medical conditions.

Confirming a High Body Mass Index

To diagnose overweight and obesity, doctors measure BMI using calculations that depend on whether you are a child or an adult.

- **Children:** A healthy weight is usually when your child's BMI is at the 5th percentile up to less than the 85th percentile based on growth charts for children who are the same age and sex. To figure out your child's BMI, use the Center for Disease Control and Prevention (CDC) BMI Percentile Calculator for Child and Teen and compare the BMI with the table below.

- **Adults:** A healthy weight for adults is usually when your BMI is 18.5 to less than 25. To figure out your BMI, use the National Heart, Lung, and Blood Institute's online BMI calculator (www.nhlbi.nih.gov/health/educational/lose_wt/BMI/bmicalc.htm) and compare it with the Table 22.1. Even if your BMI is in the healthy range, it is possible to be diagnosed as obese if you have a large waist circumference that suggests increased amounts of fat in your abdomen that can lead to complications.

Medical History

Your doctor will ask about your eating and physical activity habits, family history, and will see if you have other risk factors. Your doctor may ask if you have any other signs or symptoms. This information can help determine if you have other conditions that may be causing you to be overweight or obese or if you have complications from being overweight or obese.

Physical Exam

During your physical exam, your doctor will measure your weight and height to calculate your BMI. Your doctor may also measure your waist circumference to estimate the amount of unhealthy fat in your abdomen. In adults, a waist circumference over 35 inches for women who are not pregnant or 40 inches for men can help diagnose obesity and assess risk of future complications. If you are of South Asian or Central and South American descent, your doctor may use smaller waist circumference values to diagnose your obesity. People from these backgrounds often don't show signs of a large waist circumference even though they may have unhealthy amounts of fat deep in their abdomens and may be diagnosed with obesity.

Tests to Identify Other Medical Conditions

Your doctor may order some of the following tests to identify medical conditions that may be causing your overweight and obesity.

- **Blood tests.** Blood tests that check your thyroid hormone levels can help rule out hypothyroidism as a cause of your overweight or obesity. Cortisol and adrenocorticotropic hormone (ACTH) tests can rule out Cushing syndrome. Total testosterone and dehydroepiandrosterone sulphate (DHEAS) tests can help rule out polycystic ovary syndrome (PCOS).

- **Pelvic ultrasound** to examine the ovaries and detect cysts. This can rule out PCOS.

Treating Overweight and Obesity

Treatment for overweight and obesity depends on the cause and severity of your condition. Possible treatments include healthy lifestyle changes, behavioral weight-loss treatment programs, medicines, and possibly surgery. You may need treatments for any complications that you have.

Healthy Lifestyle Changes

To help you aim for and maintain a healthy weight, your doctor may recommend that you adopt lifelong healthy lifestyle changes.

- **Heart-healthy eating.** Learn about which foods and nutrients are part of a healthy eating pattern. It's important to eat the right amount of calories to maintain a healthy weight. If you need to lose weight, try to reduce your total daily calories gradually. Use the Body Weight Planner (www.supertracker.usda.gov/bwp/index.html) to find out your daily calorie needs and to set goals. Talk with your doctor before beginning any diet or eating plan.

- **Physical activity.** Many health benefits are associated with physical activity and getting the recommended amount of physical activity needed each week. Physical activity is an important factor in determining whether a person can maintain a healthy body weight, lose excess body weight, or maintain successful weight loss. Before starting any exercise program, ask your doctor about what level of physical activity is right for you.

- **Healthy Sleep.** Studies have shown some relationship between lack of sleep and obesity.

Making lifelong healthy lifestyle changes, such as heart-healthy eating and physical activity, can help you modify your energy balance to help you aim for and maintain a healthy weight. For example:

- To aim for a healthy weight, or lose weight, you want your energy OUT to be more than your energy IN.

- To maintain weight loss you want your energy IN and energy OUT to be the same.

Behavioral Weight-Loss Programs

Your doctor may recommend you enroll in individual or group behavioral weight-loss programs to treat your overweight and obesity. In these programs, a trained healthcare professional will customize a weight-loss plan for you. This plan will include a moderately-reduced calorie diet, physical activity goals, and behavioral strategies to help you make and maintain these lifestyle changes.

223

Did you know your brain's pleasure and reward centers can be stimulated by food and the act of eating, making it harder to change eating patterns and lose weight?

Researchers know that our brains can become patterned so that we feel pleasure or reward from eating. This can make us unconsciously crave food so our bodies feel that sense of pleasure. It can also make it hard to change our eating patterns, lose weight, or maintain a healthy weight. Researchers are studying whether cognitive behavioral therapies can be an effective treatment for overweight and obesity by retraining the brain to not associate pleasure with food and the act of eating.

Medicines

When healthy lifestyle changes are not enough, your doctor may treat your overweight and obesity with FDA-approved medicines. These medicines work in the following parts of your body.

- **Brain.** Several medicines change the way the brain regulates the urge to eat, which can help to decrease appetite. Some examples of these medicines are diethylpropion, phendimetrazine, lorcaserin, naltrexone/bupropion, and liraglutide.

- **Gastrointestinal tract.** Orlistat is the only available medicine. It blocks your intestines from absorbing fat from foods in your diet.

Weight-loss medicines are not recommended as a single treatment for weight loss. These medicines can help you lose weight but when combined with lifestyle changes may result in greater weight loss. Some of these medicines should not be used if you have certain conditions or are taking certain medicines. Also, these medicines have side effects. Talk to your doctor if you are pregnant, planning to get pregnant, breastfeeding, or have a family history of cardiovascular diseases such as stroke, high blood pressure, or heart attack.

Surgical Procedures

Some patients with obesity do not respond to healthy lifestyle changes and medicines. When these patients develop certain obesity-related complications, they may be eligible for the following surgeries.

- **Gastric bypass surgery.** A small part of the stomach is connected to the middle part of the intestine, bypassing the first part of intestine. This decreases the amount of food that you can eat and the amount of fat your body can take in and store.

- **Gastrectomy.** A big portion of the stomach is removed to decrease the amount of food that you can eat.

- **Gastric banding.** A hollow band is placed around the upper part of the stomach creating a smaller stomach. This decreases the amount of food you can eat.

Talk to your doctor to learn more about the benefits and risks of each type of surgery. Possible complications include bleeding, infection, internal rupture of sutures, or even death.

Interested in learning why these surgeries lead to weight loss in some patients?

First, these surgeries reduce the amount of food stored in the stomach and the amount of calories your body can take in. This can help your body restore energy balance. Second, these surgeries change the levels of certain hormones and the way the brain responds to these hormones to control hunger urges. After surgery, some people are less interested in eating or they prefer to eat healthier foods. In some cases, genetic differences may affect how much weight loss patients experience after bariatric surgery.

Living with Overweight and Obesity

If you have been diagnosed with overweight and obesity, it is important that you continue your treatment. Read about tips to help you aim for a healthy weight, the benefit of finding and continuing a behavioral weight-loss program, and ways your doctor may monitor if your condition is stable, worsening, or improving and assess your risk for complications.

Tips to Aim for a Healthy Weight

Changing lifestyle habits takes time and patience. Follow these tips to help you maintain the healthy lifestyle changes your doctor recommended to aim for a healthy weight.

- **Use daily food and activity diary.** You, your doctor, or healthcare provider can use Daily Food and Activity Diary to monitor your progress.

- **Set specific goals.** An example of a specific goal is to "walk 30 minutes, 5 days a week." Be realistic about your time and abilities.

- **Set doable goals** that don't change too much at once. Consecutive goals that can move you ahead in small steps, are the best way to reach a distant point. When starting a new lifestyle, try to avoid changing too much at once. Slow changes lead to success. Remember, quick weight-loss methods do not provide lasting results.

- **Learn from your slips.** Everyone slips, especially when learning something new. Don't worry if work, the weather, or your family causes you to have an occasional slip. Remember that changing your lifestyle is a long-term process. Find out what triggered the slip and restart your eating and physical activity plan.

- **Celebrate your success.** Reward yourself along the way as you meet your goals. Instead of eating out to celebrate your success, try a night at the movies, go shopping for workout clothes, visit the library or bookstore, or go on a hike.

- **Identify temptations.** Learn what environments or social activities, such as watching TV or going out with friends, may be keeping you from meeting your goals. Once you have identified them, use creative strategies to help keep you on track.

- **Plan regular physical activity with a friend.** Find a fun activity that you both enjoy, such as Zumba, jogging, biking or swimming. You are more likely to stick with that activity if you and a friend have committed to it.

Find and Continue a Behavioral Weight-Loss Program

Some people find it is easier to aim and maintain a healthy weight when they have support from a weight-loss specialist or other individuals who also are trying to lose weight. Behavioral weight-loss programs can provide this support, and they can help you set goals that are specific to your needs. Your weight-loss specialist usually reviews or modifies your goals every six months based on your progress and overall health.

When you are choosing a behavioral weight-loss program, you may want to consider whether the program should:

- **offer the service of multiple professionals**, such as registered dietitians, doctors, nurses, psychologists, and exercise physiologists.

- **provide goals that have been customized for you** that consider things such as the types of food you like, your schedule, your physical fitness, and your overall health.

- **provide individual or group counseling** to help you change your eating patterns and personal unhealthy habits.

- **teach long-term strategies** to deal with problems that can lead to future weight gain, such as stress or slipping back into unhealthy habits.

When selecting a program, you may want to ask about:

- the percentage of people who complete the program

- the average weight loss for people who finish the program

- possible side effects

- fees or costs for additional items such as dietary supplements

Monitoring Your Condition and Its Health Risks

You should visit your healthcare provider periodically to monitor for possible complications, which if left untreated can be life-threatening. Your doctor may do any of the following to monitor your condition.

- **Assess your weight loss since your last visit.** A weight loss of approximately five percent in an overweight patient may improve the function of the fat tissue and help lower bad cholesterol and other substances that can predispose to complications.

- **Measure your waist circumference if you are an adult.** If your waist circumference is greater than 35 inches for women or greater than 40 inches for men, you may be at risk for stroke, heart disease, or type 2 diabetes. South Asians and South and Central Americans have a higher risk of complications, so waist circumference should be smaller than 35 for man and 31 for women. To correctly measure your waist, stand and place a tape measure around your middle, just above your hip bones. Measure your waist just after you breathe out.

- **Order blood tests to screen for complications.** A lipid panel test can check if you have high cholesterol or triglyceride levels in your blood. A liver function test can determine if your liver is working properly. A fasting glucose test can find out if you have prediabetes or diabetes.

Chapter 23

Other Stroke Risk Factors

Chapter Contents

Section 23.1—Inactivity, Exercise, and Stroke 230

Section 23.2—Migraine and Stroke Risk................................. 235

Section 23.3—Sleep Apnea Increases Risk of Stroke............... 239

Section 23.4—Stress and Stroke Risk...................................... 244

Section 23.5—Stress at Work and Stroke Risk 246

Section 23.6—Alcohol and Stroke 248

Section 23.7—Smoking and Stroke.. 251

Section 23.8—Illegal Substance Use and Stroke 254

Section 23.9—Traumatic Brain Injury (TBI) and
Stroke.. 257

Section 23.1

Inactivity, Exercise, and Stroke

This section contains text excerpted from the following sources:
Text in this section begins with excerpts from "Working up a Sweat
May Help Reduce Stroke Risk," National Institutes of Health
(NIH), August 5, 2013. Reviewed April 2017; Text beginning with
the heading "The Benefits of Physical Activity" is excerpted from
"Physical Activity and Health," Centers for Disease Control and
Prevention (CDC), June 4, 2015.

Stroke occurs when blood vessels that supply the brain become
ruptured or blocked. As a result, brain cells die from lack of oxygen
and other nutrients. Even when a stroke isn't fatal, the damage to
brain cells can lead to permanent speech, movement or memory problems. It's still not known why most strokes occur, but various risk
factors have been identified, including high blood pressure, diabetes
and inactivity.

A Study on Physical Activity and Stroke

To investigate the relationship between physical activity and
stroke, a team led by Dr. Michelle N. McDonnell from the University of
South Australia and Dr. Virginia Howard of the University of Alabama
at Birmingham analyzed data from the Reasons for Geographic and
Racial Differences in Stroke (REGARDS) study. The dataset included
information on more than 27,000 black and white participants, both
men and women, from across the country. They were at least 45 years
old at the time of recruitment and had no prior history of stroke.

The participants were asked how many times per week they exercised to the point of sweating. They were then contacted every 6 months
to see if they had experienced a stroke or a mini-stroke known as a
transient ischemic attack (TIA). Participants were followed for an
average of 5.7 years. Medical records confirmed their responses. The
study was funded by National Institutes of Health's (NIH) National
Institute of Neurological Disorders and Stroke (NINDS).

Participants who were inactive (exercising less than once a week)
were 20 percent more likely to have a stroke or TIA than those who

exercised at least 4 times a week. After adjusting for traditional stroke risk factors (diabetes, hypertension, body mass index, alcohol use and smoking) exercise was not a significant independent predictor of stroke risk, suggesting that the effect of physical activity is mediated through its association with obesity, hypertension and diabetes.

"Physical inactivity is a major modifiable risk factor for stroke," Howard says. "This should be emphasized in routine physician checkups."

"Exercise reduces blood pressure, weight and diabetes. If exercise was a pill, you'd be taking one pill to treat 4 or 5 different conditions," McDonnell says.

One limitation of the study is that it included self-reported data on the frequency of exercise, but not on the duration of activity. Official guidelines recommend that healthy adults (ages 18 to 64) get at least 2.5 hours of moderate aerobic physical activity each week. Activity should be done for at least 10 minutes at a time.

The Benefits of Physical Activity

Regular physical activity is one of the most important things you can do for your health. It can help:

- Control your weight
- Reduce your risk of cardiovascular disease
- Reduce your risk for type 2 diabetes and metabolic syndrome
- Reduce your risk of some cancers
- Strengthen your bones and muscles
- Improve your mental health and mood
- Improve your ability to do daily activities and prevent falls, if you're an older adult
- Increase your chances of living longer

If you're not sure about becoming active or boosting your level of physical activity because you're afraid of getting hurt, the good news is that moderate-intensity aerobic activity, like brisk walking, is generally safe for most people.

Start slowly. Cardiac events, such as a heart attack, are rare during physical activity. But the risk does go up when you suddenly become much more active than usual. For example, you can put yourself at risk if you don't usually get much physical activity and then all of a sudden do vigorous-intensity aerobic activity, like shoveling snow. That's why it's important to start slowly and gradually increase your level of activity.

If you have a chronic health condition such as arthritis, diabetes, or heart disease, talk with your doctor to find out if your condition limits, in any way, your ability to be active. Then, work with your doctor to come up with a physical activity plan that matches your abilities. If your condition stops you from meeting the minimum Guidelines, try to do as much as you can. What's important is that you avoid being inactive. Even 60 minutes a week of moderate-intensity aerobic activity is good for you.

The bottom line is—the health benefits of physical activity far outweigh the risks of getting hurt.

Control Your Weight

Looking to get to or stay at a healthy weight? Both diet and physical activity play a critical role in controlling your weight. You gain weight when the calories you burn, including those burned during physical activity, are less than the calories you eat or drink. When it comes to weight management, people vary greatly in how much physical activity they need. You may need to be more active than others to achieve or maintain a healthy weight.

To maintain your weight: Work your way up to 150 minutes of moderate-intensity aerobic activity, 75 minutes of vigorous-intensity aerobic activity, or an equivalent mix of the two each week. Strong scientific evidence shows that physical activity can help you maintain your weight over time. However, the exact amount of physical activity needed to do this is not clear since it varies greatly from person to person. It's possible that you may need to do more than the equivalent of 150 minutes of moderate-intensity activity a week to maintain your weight.

To lose weight and keep it off: You will need a high amount of physical activity unless you also adjust your diet and reduce the amount of calories you're eating and drinking. Getting to and staying at a healthy weight requires both regular physical activity and a healthy eating plan.

Reduce Your Risk of Cardiovascular Disease

Stroke and heart disease are two of the leading causes of death in the United States. But following the Guidelines and getting at least

150 minutes a week (2 hours and 30 minutes) of moderate-intensity aerobic activity can put you at a lower risk for these diseases. You can reduce your risk even further with more physical activity. Regular physical activity can also lower your blood pressure and improve your cholesterol levels.

Reduce Your Risk for Type 2 Diabetes and Metabolic Syndrome

Regular physical activity can reduce your risk of developing type 2 diabetes and metabolic syndrome. Metabolic syndrome is a condition in which you have some combination of too much fat around the waist, high blood pressure, low high-density lipoproteins (HDL) cholesterol, high triglycerides, or high blood sugar. Research shows that lower rates of these conditions are seen with 120 to 150 minutes (2 hours to 2 hours and 30 minutes) a week of at least moderate-intensity aerobic activity. And the more physical activity you do, the lower your risk will be.

Reduce Your Risk of Some Cancers

Being physically active lowers your risk for two types of cancer: colon and breast. Research shows that:

- Physically active people have a lower risk of colon cancer than do people who are not active.

- Physically active women have a lower risk of breast cancer than do people who are not active.

Reduce your risk of endometrial and lung cancer. Although the research is not yet final, some findings suggest that your risk of endometrial cancer and lung cancer may be lower if you get regular physical activity compared to people who are not active.

Improve your quality of life. If you are a cancer survivor, research shows that getting regular physical activity not only helps give you a better quality of life, but also improves your physical fitness.

Strengthen Your Bones and Muscles

As you age, it's important to protect your bones, joints and muscles. Not only do they support your body and help you move, but keeping bones, joints and muscles healthy can help ensure that you're able to do your daily activities and be physically active. Research shows that doing aerobic, muscle-strengthening and bone-strengthening physical activity of at least a moderately-intense level can slow the loss of bone density that comes with age.

Hip fracture is a serious health condition that can have life-changing negative effects, especially if you're an older adult. But research shows that people who do 120 to 300 minutes of at least moderate-intensity aerobic activity each week have a lower risk of hip fracture.

Regular physical activity helps with arthritis and other conditions affecting the joints. If you have arthritis, research shows that doing 130 to 150 (2 hours and 10 minutes to 2 hours and 30 minutes) a week of moderate-intensity, low-impact aerobic activity can not only improve your ability to manage pain and do everyday tasks, but it can also make your quality of life better.

Build strong, healthy muscles. Muscle-strengthening activities can help you increase or maintain your muscle mass and strength. Slowly increasing the amount of weight and number of repetitions you do will give you even more benefits, no matter your age.

Improve Your Mental Health and Mood

Regular physical activity can help keep your thinking, learning, and judgment skills sharp as you age. It can also reduce your risk of depression and may help you sleep better. Research has shown that doing aerobics or a mix of aerobic and muscle-strengthening activities 3 to 5 times a week for 30 to 60 minutes can give you these mental health benefits. Some scientific evidence has also shown that even lower levels of physical activity can be beneficial.

Improve Your Ability to Do Daily Activities and Prevent Falls

A functional limitation is a loss of the ability to do everyday activities such as climbing stairs, grocery shopping, or playing with your grandchildren.

How does this relate to physical activity? If you're a physically active middle-aged or older adult, you have a lower risk of functional limitations than people who are inactive.

Already have trouble doing some of your everyday activities? Aerobic and muscle-strengthening activities can help improve your ability to do these types of tasks.

Are you an older adult who is at risk for falls? Research shows that doing balance and muscle-strengthening activities each week along with moderate-intensity aerobic activity, like brisk walking, can help reduce your risk of falling.

Increase Your Chances of Living Longer

Science shows that physical activity can reduce your risk of dying early from the leading causes of death, like heart disease and some cancers. This is remarkable in two ways:

1. Only a few lifestyle choices have as large an impact on your health as physical activity. People who are physically active for about 7 hours a week have a 40 percent lower risk of dying early than those who are active for less than 30 minutes a week.

2. You don't have to do high amounts of activity or vigorous-intensity activity to reduce your risk of premature death. You can put yourself at lower risk of dying early by doing at least 150 minutes a week of moderate-intensity aerobic activity.

Everyone can gain the health benefits of physical activity—age, ethnicity, shape or size do not matter.

Section 23.2

Migraine and Stroke Risk

Text in this section is from "Migraine, Stroke and Heart Disease," © 2017 American Migraine Foundation. Reprinted with permission.

Both migraine and stroke are common disorders, but they usually occur in quite different populations. Stroke most commonly affects elderly men, and migraine, young women, but over the past 40 years study after study has shown an independent link between migraine and stroke. Despite much exploration, the complex relationship of migraine and stroke is still unfolding. The following is list of ways in which the two conditions may be connected:

*   Migraine causes of stroke (migrainous infarction)—stroke occurs during the migraine attack.

*   Migraine is a risk factor for stroke—stroke occurs more frequently in person who have or have had migraine, but not during an attack.

- Migraine mimics stroke, and stroke mimics migraine.

- Migraine is caused by stroke (symptomatic migraine)—ischemia or hemorrhage trigger a migraine-like, or aura-like event.

- Migraine and stroke share a common cause—such as cardiac shunt (known as patent foramen ovale), or an abnormality of blood vessels (known as vasculopathy) due to a genetic condition, such as CADASIL (Cerebral Autosomal-Dominant Arteriopathy with Subcortical Infarcts and Leukoencephalopathy).

- Migraine is associated with silent stroke—stroke-like lesions seen on MRI without symptoms of stroke.

What Is the Risk of Stroke with Migraine?

Fortunately, the absolute risk of migraine-related stroke is low. In the U.S. the yearly number of strokes from all causes is about 800,000 (split fairly evenly between the sexes) in a population of over 322 million persons. The yearly risk of stroke in women with migraine is about 3 times what it is for women without migraine, with an estimated 13 strokes per 100,000 women that are tied to migraine rather than to another diagnosis. This means that out of 28 million women in the U.S. with migraine, the number of stroke per year related to that diagnosis is about 3600, which is less than 1 percent of the total strokes affecting women.

Who Is at Risk?

The main type of migraine associated with stroke is migraine with aura, a subtype affecting about 25 percent of persons with migraine. The main type of stroke associated with migraine is ischemic stroke (resulting from decreased blood flow to a portion of the brain) but persons with migraine also have an increased risk of hemorrhagic stroke (resulting from bleeding into or around the brain). Women with aura are 2 to 3 times more likely to have stroke than women without migraine, all other things being equal. Women with aura are also at higher risk of stroke than men with aura. Interestingly, young persons (below the age of 45 years old) are at greater risk for migraine-related stroke than are older individuals, and the strongest association of migraine and stroke is in persons without traditional stroke risk factors such as high blood pressure, diabetes mellitus and high cholesterol.

Migraine Aura or Transient Ischemic Attack?

Due to an overlap of clinical features it is sometimes difficult to tell a typical migraine aura from a TIA, an event often referred to as a "mini-stroke." Both aura and TIA involve brief (usually 60 minutes or less), focal neurological symptoms, which may or may not be followed by headache. Symptoms in aura are typically "positive" and expanding, such as a growing bright, crescent with jagged edges obscuring part of the vision, or a 5-minute long march of tingling from fingertips on one side up to the face.

Symptoms of TIA are, in contrast, often "negative" and of sudden onset, such one-sided visual loss (eye or field of vision), and numbness. Some aura symptoms, including visual loss in one eye (retinal migraine), one-sided weakness (hemiplegic migraine), vertigo (basilar migraine), and migraine with prolonged aura are difficult to clinically differentiate from TIA. In both conditions labs and MRI may be normal. An additional wrinkle in the complex relationship of migraine aura and brain ischemia is the fact that ischemia may trigger an electrical brain phenomenon known as cortical spreading depression, which manifests itself aura. This phenomenon is referred to as symptomatic migraine. This means that in some cases aura symptoms may be due to a TIA-like event.

The ABCs of Migraine-Stroke Linking Mechanisms

A is for Arteries. Atherosclerosis, the most common cause of stroke in the general population is not enhanced in persons with migraine. Stroke occurring during the migraine with aura attack may be due to vasospasm, which is a reversible constriction of one or more arteries. The rare condition is known as migrainous infarction. Cervical artery dissection, another vascular cause of stroke, refers to a tear within the inner lining of an artery carrying blood to the brain. This may be due to quick movement of the neck traumatizing the artery. Arterial dissection is more likely to occur in young persons with a history of migraine, and the most common presenting symptoms of head and neck pain may not be initially recognized as having another cause. The rare genetic condition, CADASIL, shows abnormalities of the small and medium sized arteries and clinical features of migraine with aura, TIAs, strokes, and eventually, vascular dementia. Even under normal circumstances, there is growing evidence that migraine attacks perturb or activate the inner cell lining (endothelium) of the arteries, leading to release of substances involved in inflammation, and coagulation, and decreasing the ability of the vessel to fully dilate.

B is for Blood. Blockage of an artery from a clot may cause stroke, but if the blockage is temporary the result may be a TIA or aura-like episode. When blood clots more than normal, this is referred to hypercoagulability. It may be caused by genetic, acquired, or lifestyle factors, such as cigarette smoking or use of estrogen containing contraceptives (risk varies with dose). One study of young persons with stroke showed that those with migraine with aura were over twice as likely to have at least one factor causing hypercoagulability as those with migraine without aura, or no migraine at all. For some persons use of daily aspirin prevents aura.

C is for Cardiac. About 15–25 percent of persons are born with a passageway between the right and left upper chambers (atria) of the heart, and this is known as a patent foramen ovale (PFO). Clots forming in or shunting through the PFO may be pumped to the brain and result in stroke, TIA, or aura-like episodes. Wide variation of results from studies investigating the frequency of PFO in persons with migraine (range: 15 to 90%), and of migraine in persons with PFO (range: 16 to 64%) have clouded the potential role of PFO as a link between migraine and stroke. Clinical trials of PFO closure have not proven that this is an effective way to prevent migraine.

Migraine and Heart Disease

Most of the studies examining migraine and vascular disease have naturally focused on stroke, another brain condition. There is, however, also strong evidence that migraine increases the risk of heart disease, such as myocardial infarction (heart attacks) and angina. The link between migraine and heart disease has been uncovered in men and women over a vast range of ages and across the globe. Most recently the large (23,000 women) Nurses' Health Study, which enrolled persons, ages 25 to 42 years old, about 20 years earlier, showed that migraine increases the risk of stroke, coronary events, and related death by about 50 percent. In several other study populations the risk of ischemic heart disease was doubled. The mechanisms are unknown but likely involve inflammation, coagulation, and dysfunction of endothelial lining of the arteries.

Tips for lowering risk of stroke and heart disease:

- Maintain a healthful diet, drink plenty of water, and get regular exercise and at least 8 hours of sleep

- Be evaluated and treated for conditions known to cause stroke and heart disease such as high blood pressure, high cholesterol and diabetes

- No cigarette smoking

- Use migraine preventive strategies. In addition to decreasing attacks of migraine aura and headache, this may also prevent stroke. In addition to the traditional migraine preventives, ask your doctor whether meds, which in addition to decreasing inflammation, decrease clotting (such as daily aspirin), or repair the endothelium (such as a statin with Vitamin D) are right for you

- Avoid use of estrogen containing contraceptives, especially if you smoke or have a personal or family history of blood clots. Progestogen-contraception has less risk.

- Avoid chiropractic manipulation of the neck, in order to decrease risk of cervical artery dissection

- Do not use triptans or other medications that constrict blood vessels if you have a history of heart disease or stroke, or if you have attacks weakness on one side (possible hemiplegic migraine) vertigo and gait imbalance (possible basilar migraine).

Section 23.3

Sleep Apnea Increases Risk of Stroke

This section contains text excerpted from the following sources: Text in this section begins with the excerpts from "Always Tired? You May Have Sleep Apnea," U.S. Food and Drug Administration (FDA), March 4, 2016; Text under the heading "Sleep Apnea Tied to Increased Risk of Stroke" is excerpted from "Sleep Apnea Tied to Increased Risk of Stroke," National Heart, Lung, and Blood Institute (NHLBI), April 7, 2010. Reviewed April 2017.

Your spouse says your snoring is driving her nuts.
You wake up feeling unrested and irritable.

These are common signs that you may have obstructive sleep apnea (OSA), a sleep disorder that—left untreated—can take its toll on the body and mind.

Untreated OSA has been linked to high blood pressure, heart attacks, strokes, car accidents, work-related accidents and depression. According to the American Sleep Association, OSA affects more than 12 million Americans.

The U.S. Food and Drug Administration (FDA) ensures the safety and effectiveness of medical devices, including the device most often used by those affected by OSA—the Continuous Positive Airway Pressure machine, commonly known as CPAP—and a new device, the Inspire Upper Airway Stimulation (UAS) System.

What Is Sleep Apnea?

The Greek word "apnea" literally means "without breath." With sleep apnea, your breathing pauses multiple times during sleep. The pauses can last from a few seconds to minutes and can occur more than five times per hour, to as high as 100 times per hour. (Fewer than five times per hour is normal). Sometimes when you start breathing again, you make a loud snort or choking sound.

Obstructive sleep apnea (OSA), the most common type, is caused by a blockage of the airway, usually when the soft tissue in the back of the throat collapses. The less common form, central sleep apnea, happens if the area of your brain that controls breathing doesn't send the correct signals to your breathing muscles.

According to Eric Mann, M.D., Ph.D., deputy director of FDA's Division of Ophthalmic, Neurological, and Ear, Nose and Throat Devices (DOED), you may be unaware of these events since they happen while you're sleeping. Because you partially wake up when your breathing pauses, your sleep is interrupted, and you often feel tired and irritable the next day.

Sleep apnea is almost twice as common in men as it is in women. Other risk factors include:

- being overweight, as extra fat tissue around the neck makes it harder to keep the airway open,
- being over age 40,
- smoking,
- having a family history of sleep apnea, and
- having a nasal obstruction due to a deviated septum, allergies or sinus problem.

Children also get sleep apnea, most commonly between ages 3 and 6. The most common cause is enlarged tonsils and adenoids in the upper airway.

"You should certainly tell your physician if you think you, or your child, is experiencing symptoms of sleep apnea," Mann says. "But the diagnosis of sleep disorders such as obstructive sleep apnea requires a formal sleep study."

Polysomnogram (PSG) is the most common sleep study for sleep apnea and often takes place in a sleep center or lab to record brain activity, eye movement, blood pressure and the amount of air that moves in and out of your lungs.

Sleep Apnea Tied to Increased Risk of Stroke

Obstructive sleep apnea is associated with an increased risk of stroke in middle-aged and older adults, especially men, according to results from a landmark study supported by the National Heart, Lung, and Blood Institute (NHLBI) of the National Institutes of Health (NIH). Overall, sleep apnea more than doubles the risk of stroke in men. Obstructive sleep apnea is a common disorder in which the upper airway is intermittently narrowed or blocked, disrupting sleep and breathing during sleep.

Researchers from the Sleep Heart Health Study (SHHS) report that the risk of stroke appears in men with mild sleep apnea and rises with the severity of sleep apnea. Men with moderate to severe sleep apnea were nearly three times more likely to have a stroke than men without sleep apnea or with mild sleep apnea. The risk from sleep apnea is independent of other risk factors such as weight, high blood pressure, race, smoking, and diabetes.

Link between Sleep Apnea and Increased Risk of Stroke

They also report for the first time a link between sleep apnea and increased risk of stroke in women. Obstructive Sleep Apnea Hypopnea and Incident Stroke: The Sleep Heart Health Study (SHHS), was published in the *American Journal of Respiratory and Critical Care Medicine (AJRCCM)*.

Stroke is the second leading cause of death worldwide. "Although scientists have uncovered several risk factors for stroke—such as age, high blood pressure and atrial fibrillation, and diabetes—there are still many cases in which the cause or contributing factors are unknown," noted NHLBI Acting Director Susan B. Shurin, M.D. "This is the largest study to date to link sleep apnea with an increased risk of stroke. The time is right for researchers to study whether treating sleep apnea could prevent or delay stroke in some individuals."

Conducted in nine medical centers across the United States, the SHHS is the largest and most comprehensive prospective, multi-center study on the risk of cardiovascular disease and other conditions related to sleep apnea. In a report, researchers studied stroke risk in 5,422 participants aged 40 years and older without a history of stroke. At the start of the study, participants performed a standard at-home sleep test, which determined whether they had sleep apnea and, if so, the severity of the sleep apnea.

Researchers followed the participants for an average of about nine years. They report that during the study, 193 participants had a stroke—85 men (of 2,462 men enrolled) and 108 women (out of 2,960 enrolled).

After adjusting for several cardiovascular risk factors, the researchers found that the effect of sleep apnea on stroke risk was stronger in men than in women. In men, a progressive increase in stroke risk was observed as sleep apnea severity increased from mild levels to moderate to severe levels. In women, however, the increased risk of stroke was significant only with severe levels of sleep apnea.

The researchers suggest that the differences between men and women might be because men are more likely to develop sleep apnea at younger ages. Therefore, they tend to have untreated sleep apnea for longer periods of time than women. "It's possible that the stroke risk is related to cumulative effects of sleep apnea adversely influencing health over many years," said Susan Redline, M.D., MPH, professor of medicine, pediatrics, and epidemiology and biostatistics, at Case Western Reserve University in Cleveland and lead author of the paper.

"Our findings provide compelling evidence that obstructive sleep apnea is a risk factor for stroke, especially in men," noted Redline. "Overall, the increased risk of stroke in men with sleep apnea is comparable to adding 10 years to a man's age. Importantly, we found that increased stroke risk in men occurs even with relatively mild levels of sleep apnea."

"Research on the effects of sleep apnea not only increases our understanding of how lapses of breathing during sleep affects our health and well being, but it can also provide important insight into how cardiovascular problems such as stroke and high blood pressure develop," noted Michael J. Twery, Ph.D., director of the NIH National Center on Sleep Disorders Research, an office administered by the NHLBI.

These results support earlier findings that have linked sleep apnea to stroke risk. SHHS researchers have also reported that untreated sleep apnea is associated with an increased risk of high blood pressure, heart attack, irregular heartbeats, heart failure, and death from any cause. Other studies have also linked untreated sleep apnea with overweight and obesity and diabetes. It is also linked to excessive daytime sleepiness, which lowers performance in the workplace and at school, and increases the risk of injuries and death from drowsy driving and other accidents.

More than 12 million American adults are believed to have sleep apnea, and most are not diagnosed or treated. Treatments to restore regular breathing during sleep include mouthpieces, surgery, and breathing devices, such as continuous positive airway pressure, or CPAP. In people who are overweight or obese, weight loss can also help.

These treatments can help improve breathing and reduce the severity of symptoms such as loud snoring and excessive daytime sleepiness, thereby improving sleep-related quality of life and performance at work or in school. Randomized clinical trials to test whether treating sleep apnea lowers the risk of stroke, other cardiovascular diseases, or death are needed.

"We now have abundant evidence that sleep apnea is associated with cardiovascular risk factors and diseases. The next logical step is to determine if treating sleep apnea can lower a person's risk of these leading killers," said Redline.

"With stimulus funds, our research group is now developing the additional research and resources to begin answering this important question."

Through funding from the American Recovery and Reinvestment Act (ARRA), the NHLBI is awarding approximately $4.4 million to Redline to conduct the first NIH-funded comparative effectiveness study of treatments for sleep apnea. In the two-year multi-center pilot study, SHHS researchers and others will compare the cardiovascular effects of adding either CPAP or supplemental oxygen during sleep to standard care in patients with moderate to severe sleep apnea who are at high risk for cardiovascular disease events such as stroke or heart attack.

Section 23.4

Stress and Stroke Risk

"Stress and Stroke Risk," © 2017 Omnigraphics.
Reviewed April 2017.

Stress and Health

Within the context of personal health, stress is defined as the mental or emotional pressure people experience when they are in very demanding circumstances. Examples of life events that often result in stress include job loss, death of a loved one, change in financial circumstances, change in housing, uncertainty about the future, and so on. Stress can also result from positive life events such as becoming a new parent or guardian of a child, starting a challenging new job, graduation from school, or getting married. Any significant life event can cause a person to experience high levels of stress.

When a person is experiencing stress, the brain releases a series of hormones intended to help the body react to the perceived threat to well-being. This is generally known as the "fight or flight" response. Stress hormones essentially provide a sudden burst of energy to the body in an effort to prepare or react in a stressful situation. These hormones affect involuntary body functions such as breathing, blood pressure, heart rate, and activity in key blood vessels and airways. People living with chronic stress experience elevated stress hormones much of the time, which is known to contribute to a greater risk of stroke.

Risk Factors

High stress can develop as a result of situations in which people feel they have little control over events. For example, people may experience high levels of stress at work when they have little control over the amount of work they have, the amount of time in which the work must be completed, and the number of tasks that must be coordinated at the same time. Men with high-stress jobs have a 22 percent higher risk of stroke than those with low-stress jobs, while the risk rises to 33 percent among women in high-stress jobs. Other examples of stressful life situations include job insecurity, poverty or financial crisis, health problems in loved ones, or experiencing a major life event during the past eight months (job loss, death of a loved one, change of housing, etc.).

Stress, particularly if it is chronic or experienced over a long period of time, often leads to unhealthy behaviors, such as being quick-tempered, aggressive, or impatient in daily life, excessive consumption of alcohol, excessive consumption of caffeine (coffee, energy drinks, sodas, etc.), smoking or other tobacco use.

Experiencing chronic or long-term stress can result in further health problems that are known risks for stroke, including:

- High blood pressure (hypertension)
- Heart disease or heart rhythm disorders
- Artery disease (atherosclerosis)
- Diabetes
- High cholesterol
- Sleep apnea
- Depression
- Obesity
- Posttraumatic stress disorder (PTSD)

Prevention

Stress management is the best way to prevent stress-related risk of stroke. Identifying the areas of life that produce the greatest amount of stress and working to remove or reduce some of that stress can produce health benefits. Even small, simple changes can be beneficial. Choosing healthy food and drinks, finding ways to include exercise or physical activity to daily routines, and ending unhealthy behaviors such as smoking can all be helpful in reducing the effect of stress on the body. Meditation, yoga, or other spiritual practice can also provide a respite from chronic stress.

References

1. Blaszczak-Boxe, Agata. "High-Stress Jobs May Raise Stroke Risk," Live Science, October 14, 2015.

2. Boyles, Salynn. "Stress Linked to Stroke," WebMD, August 30, 2012.

3. "Can Stress Cause a Stroke?" November 4, 2015.

4. "How Stress May Increase Risk of Heart Disease and Stroke," Science Daily, January 11, 2017.

Section 23.5

Stress at Work and Stroke Risk

Text in this section is from "Stressed at Work? You May Have a
Higher Risk of Stroke," © 1995-2017 Cleveland Clinic.
Reprinted with permission.

It's already known that stress from work can increase your risk for cardiovascular disease, particularly high blood pressure and heart disease. But a study now links work stress to an increased risk of stroke, especially for women.

Dimensions of Work

In the study, researchers in China compiled data from six studies with 138,782 participants. The researchers evaluated the link between job stress and future stroke risk. The researchers looked at two dimensions of work called psychological job demand and job control.

Psychological job demand means a worker's time pressure, mental load and level of responsibilities. Job control is your control over decisions. The researchers found that jobs with high demands and low control, such as waitress or nurses aide, were associated with a 22 percent increased risk of stroke compared with jobs with low demand and high control, such as architect or natural scientist.

The results were more pronounced for ischemic stroke, a type of stroke that is caused by a blood clot. Women were at greatest risk. Neither jobs with high demand and high control, such as teacher or engineer, nor those with low demand and low control, such as manual labor jobs, were associated with an increased risk of stroke compared with the low strain jobs.

Stress as a Risk Factor

The study, which appears in the journal *Neurology*, adds to the evidence that stress is harmful to your health and should be taken seriously, says stroke specialist Irene Katzan, MD. "This adds to the evidence that stress is a risk factor for stroke and, specifically in this study, stress related to your job," Dr. Katzan says.

Experts believe it's possible that stress may cause inflammation in the body. This then can lead to stroke or heart attack.

Simple Ways to De-Stress at Work

"For many of us, stress at work is inescapable. But there are strategies you can use to lessen the strain," Dr. Katzan says. The most important is to develop healthy eating habits and do some activity every day.

"Stress may lead to unhealthy behaviors," Dr. Katzan says.

"If your job is stressful, be mindful of your blood pressure, eat healthy foods and get exercise," Dr. Katzan says.

You also can take steps while on the job to take the tension down a notch. Here are some simple ways you can de-stress on the job:

- Breathe deeply to supply much-needed oxygen to the brain.

- Get up and move several times during the workday.

- Liven up your workspace with plants and soft colors.

- Focus on one thing at a time, and recognize it when you finish tasks.

Section 23.6

Alcohol and Stroke

This section includes text excerpted from "Beyond Hangovers:
Understanding Alcohol's Impact on Your Health," National Institute
on Alcohol Abuse and Alcoholism (NIAAA), October 2015.

Alcohol's Effects on the Heart

Americans know how prevalent heart disease is—about 1 in 12 of
us suffer from it. What we don't always recognize are the connections
heart disease shares with alcohol. On the one hand, researchers have
known for centuries that excessive alcohol consumption can damage
the heart. Drinking a lot over a long period of time or drinking too
much on a single occasion can put your heart—and your life—at risk.
On the other hand, researchers now understand that drinking moderate amounts of alcohol can protect the hearts of some people from
the risks of coronary artery disease.

Deciding how much, if any, alcohol is right for you can be compli-
cated. To make the best decision for yourself, you need to know the
facts and then consult your physician.

Know the Function of Heart

Your cardiovascular system consists of your heart, blood vessels,
and blood. This system works constantly—every second of your life—
delivering oxygen and nutrients to your cells, and carrying away carbon dioxide and other unnecessary material.

Your heart drives this process. It is a muscle that contracts and
relaxes over and over again, moving the blood along the necessary
path. Your heart beats about 100,000 times each day, pumping the
equivalent of 2,000 gallons of blood throughout your body.

The two sides, or chambers, of the heart receive blood and pump it
back into the body. The right ventricle of the heart pumps blood into
the lungs to exchange carbon dioxide from the cells for oxygen. The
heart relaxes to allow this blood back into its left chamber. It then
pumps the oxygen-rich blood to tissues and organs. Blood passing

through the kidneys allows the body to get rid of waste products. Electrical signals keep the heart pumping continuously and at the appropriate rate to propel this routine.

Know the Risks of Alcohol

Alcoholic Cardiomyopathy

Long-term heavy drinking weakens the heart muscle, causing a condition called *alcoholic cardiomyopathy*. A weakened heart droops and stretches and cannot contract effectively. As a result, it cannot pump enough blood to sufficiently nourish the organs. In some cases, this blood flow shortage causes severe damage to organs and tissues. Symptoms of cardiomyopathy include shortness of breath and other breathing difficulties, fatigue, swollen legs and feet, and irregular heartbeat. It can even lead to heart failure.

Arrhythmias

Both binge drinking and long-term drinking can affect how quickly a heart beats. The heart depends on an internal pacemaker system to keep it 10 pumping consistently and at the right speed. Alcohol disturbs this pacemaker system and causes the heart to beat too rapidly, or irregularly. These heart rate abnormalities are called *arrhythmias*. Two types of alcohol-induced arrhythmias are:

- Atrial Fibrillation—In this form of arrhythmia, the heart's upper, or atrial, chambers shudder weakly but do not contract. Blood can collect and even clot in these upper chambers. If a blood clot travels from the heart to the brain, a stroke can occur; if it travels to other organs such as the lungs, an embolism, or blood vessel blockage, occurs.

- Ventricular Tachycardia—This form of arrhythmia occurs in the heart's lower, or ventricular, chambers. Electrical signals travel throughout the heart's muscles, triggering contractions that keep blood flowing at the right pace. Alcohol-induced damage to heart muscle cells can cause these electrical impulses to circle through the ventricle too many times, causing too many contractions. The heart beats too quickly, and so does not fill up with enough blood between each beat. As a result, the rest of the body does not get enough blood. Ventricular tachycardia causes dizziness, lightheadedness, unconsciousness, cardiac arrest, and even sudden death.

Drinking to excess on a particular occasion, especially when you generally don't drink, can trigger either of these irregularities. In these cases, the problem is nicknamed "holiday heart syndrome," because people who don't usually drink may consume too much alcohol at parties during the holiday season.

Over the long-term, chronic drinking changes the course of electrical impulses that drive the heart's beating, which creates arrhythmia.

Strokes

A stroke occurs when blood cannot reach the brain. In about 80 percent of strokes, a blood clot prevents blood flow to the brain. These are called *ischemic strokes*. Sometimes, blood accumulates in the brain, or in the spaces surrounding it. This causes *hemorrhagic strokes.*

Both binge drinking and long-term heavy drinking can lead to strokes even in people without coronary heart disease. Studies show that people who binge drink are about 56 percent more likely than people who never binge drink to suffer an ischemic stroke over 10 years. Binge drinkers also are about 39 percent more likely to suffer any type of stroke than people who never binge drink.

In addition, alcohol exacerbates the problems that often lead to strokes, including hypertension, arrhythmias, and cardiomyopathy.

Hypertension

Chronic alcohol use, as well as binge drinking, can cause high blood pressure, or *hypertension*. Your blood pressure is a measurement of the pressure your heart creates as it beats, and the pressure inside your veins and arteries. Healthy blood vessels stretch like elastic as the heart pumps blood through them. Hypertension develops when the blood vessels stiffen, making them less flexible. Heavy alcohol consumption triggers the release of certain stress hormones that in turn constrict blood vessels. This elevates blood pressure. In addition, alcohol may affect the function of the muscles within the blood vessels, causing them to constrict and elevate blood pressure.

Know the Benefits of Alcohol

Research shows that healthy people who drink moderate amounts of alcohol may have a lower risk of developing coronary heart disease than nondrinkers. Moderate drinking is usually defined as no more than two drinks in a given day for men and one drink per day for women who are not pregnant or trying to conceive.

A variety of factors, including diet, genetics, high blood pressure, and age, can cause fat to build up in your arteries, resulting in coronary heart disease. An excess of fat narrows the coronary arteries, which are the blood vessels that supply blood directly to the heart. Clogged arteries reduce blood supply to the heart muscle, and make it easier for blood clots to form. Blood clots can lead to both strokes and heart attacks.

According to studies, drinking moderately can protect your heart from these conditions. Moderate drinking helps inhibit and reduce the buildup of fat in the arteries. It can raise the levels of HDL—or "good" cholesterol—in the blood, which wards off heart disease. It can help guard against heart attack and stroke by preventing blood clots from forming and by dissolving blood clots that do develop. Drinking moderately also may help keep blood pressure levels in check.

These benefits may not apply to people with existing medical conditions, or who regularly take certain medications. In addition, researchers discourage people from beginning to drink just for the health benefits. Rather, you can use this research to help you spark a conversation with your medical professional about the best path for you.

Section 23.7

Smoking and Stroke

This section includes text excerpted from "Smoking and Heart Disease and Stroke," Centers for Disease Control and Prevention (CDC), February 24, 2017.

Heart Disease and Stroke

Heart disease and stroke are cardiovascular (heart and blood vessel) diseases (CVDs).

Heart disease includes several types of heart conditions. The most common type in the United States is coronary heart disease (also known as coronary artery disease), which is narrowing of the blood vessels that carry blood to the heart. This can cause:

- Chest pain

- Heart attack (when blood flow to the heart becomes blocked and a section of the heart muscle is damaged or dies)

- Heart failure (when the heart cannot pump enough blood and oxygen to support other organs)

- Arrhythmia (when the heart beats too fast, too slow, or irregularly)

A stroke occurs when the blood supply to the brain is blocked or when a blood vessel in the brain bursts, causing brain tissue to die. Stroke can cause disability (such as paralysis, muscle weakness, trouble speaking, and memory loss) or death.

Smoking Is Related to Heart Disease and Stroke

Smoking is a major cause of cardiovascular disease (CVD) and causes one of every three deaths from CVD. Smoking can:

- Raise triglycerides (a type of fat in your blood)

- Lower "good" cholesterol/high-density lipoprotein (HDL)

- Make blood sticky and more likely to clot, which can block blood flow to the heart and brain

- Damage cells that line the blood vessels

- Increase the buildup of plaque (fat, cholesterol, calcium, and other substances) in blood vessels

- Cause thickening and narrowing of blood vessels

Breathing Secondhand Smoke and Heart Disease and Stroke

Breathing secondhand smoke also harms your health. Secondhand smoke is the smoke from burning tobacco products. Secondhand smoke also is smoke breathed out by a smoker.

Breathing secondhand smoke can cause coronary heart disease, including stroke and heart attack. Know the facts:

- Secondhand smoke causes nearly 34,000 early deaths from coronary heart disease each year in the United States among nonsmokers.

- Nonsmokers who breathe secondhand smoke at home or at work increase their risk of developing heart disease by 25–30 percent.

Secondhand smoke increases the risk for stroke by 20–30 percent.

- Each year, secondhand smoke exposure causes more than 8,000 deaths from stroke.

- Breathing secondhand smoke interferes with the normal functioning of the heart, blood, and vascular systems in ways that increase your risk of having a heart attack.

- Even briefly breathing secondhand smoke can damage the lining of blood vessels and cause your blood to become stickier. These changes can cause a deadly heart attack.

Preventing Heart Disease and Stroke

Stroke and heart disease are major causes of death and disability in the United States. Many people are at high risk for these diseases and don't know it. The good news is that many risk factors for heart disease and stroke can be prevented or controlled.

The federal government's Million Hearts® initiative aims to prevent 1 million heart attacks and strokes by 2017. It's important to know your risk for stroke and heart disease and to take action to reduce that risk. A good place to start is with the ABCS of heart health:

- **A**spirin: Aspirin may help reduce your risk for heart disease and stroke. But do not take aspirin if you think you are having a stroke. It can make some types of stroke worse. Before taking aspirin, talk to your doctor about whether aspirin is right for you.

- **B**lood pressure: Control your blood pressure.

- **C**holesterol: Manage your cholesterol.

- **S**moking: Quit smoking, or don't start.

In addition to your ABCS, several lifestyle choices can help protect your heart and brain health. These include the following:

- Avoid breathing secondhand smoke.

- Eat low-fat, low-salt foods most of the time and fresh fruits and vegetables.

- Maintain a healthy weight.

- Exercise regularly.

- Limit alcohol use.

- Get other health conditions (such as diabetes) under control.

Section 23.8

Illegal Substance Use and Stroke

This section contains text excerpted from the following
sources: Text in this section begins with excerpts from "Health
Consequences of Drug Misuse—Neurological Effects," National
Institute on Drug Abuse (NIDA), March 2017; Text beginning
with the heading "Bath Salts or Designer Cathinones (Synthetic
Stimulants)" is excerpted from "Drug Fact Sheet," Drug
Enforcement Administration (DEA), 2015.

All addictive drugs act in the brain to produce their euphoric effects.
However, some can also cause damage due to seizures, stroke, and
direct toxic effects on brain cells. Drug use can also lead to addiction,
a brain disorder that occurs when repeated drug use leads to changes
in the function of multiple brain circuits that control pleasures/reward,
stress, decision-making, impulse control, learning and memory, and
other functions. These changes make it harder for those with an addiction to experience pleasure in response to natural rewards—such as
food, sex, or positive social interactions—or to manage their stress,
control their impulses, and make the healthy choice to stop drug seeking and use.

Drugs that can cause neurological problems:

- ayahuasca

- cocaine

- DMT

- DXM

- GHB

- heroin

- inhalants

- ketamine

- khat

- kratom

- LSD

- marijuana

- MDMA

- mescaline (peyote)

- methamphetamine
- PCP
- prescription opioids
- prescription sedatives
- prescription stimulants
- psilocybin
- Rohypnol®

- salvia
- steroids (appearance- and performance-enhancing drugs)
- synthetic cannabinoids
- synthetic cathinones
- tobacco/nicotine

Bath Salts or Designer Cathinones (Synthetic Stimulants)

Synthetic stimulants that are marketed as "bath salts" are often found in a number of retail products. These synthetic stimulants are chemicals. The chemicals are synthetic derivatives of cathinone, a central nervous system stimulant, which is an active chemical found naturally in the khat plant. Mephedrone and MDPV (3-4 methylenedioxypyrovalerone) are two of the designer cathinones most commonly found in these "bath salt" products. Many of these products are sold over the Internet, in convenience stores, and in "head shops."

Effect on Body

Cathinone derivatives act as central nervous system stimulants causing rapid heart rate (which may lead to strokes and heart attacks), chest pains, nosebleeds, sweating, nausea, and vomiting.

Cocaine

Cocaine is an intense, euphoria-producing stimulant drug with strong addictive potential.

Effect on Body

Physiological effects of cocaine include increased blood pressure and heart rate, dilated pupils, insomnia, and loss of appetite. The widespread abuse of highly pure street cocaine has led to many severe adverse health consequences such as: strokes, ischemic heart conditions, cardiac arrhythmias, sudden cardiac arrest, convulsions, and death. In some users, the long-term use of inhaled cocaine has led to a unique respiratory syndrome, and chronic snorting of cocaine has led to the erosion of the upper nasal cavity.

Methamphetamine

Methamphetamine (meth) is a stimulant. The U.S. Food and Drug Administration (FDA)-approved brand-name medication is Desoxyn®.

Effect on Body

Taking even small amounts of meth can result in increased wakefulness, increased physical activity, decreased appetite, rapid breathing and heart rate, irregular heartbeat, increased blood pressure, and hyperthermia (overheating). High doses can elevate body temperature to dangerous, sometimes lethal, levels as well as cause convulsions and even cardiovascular collapse and death. Meth abuse may also cause extreme anorexia, memory loss, and severe dental problems.

Overdose Effects

High doses may result in death from stroke, heart attack, or multiple organ problems caused by overheating.

Steroids

Anabolic steroids are synthetically produced variants of the naturally occurring male hormone testosterone that are abused in an attempt to promote muscle growth, enhance athletic or other physical performance, and improve physical appearance. Testosterone, nandrolone, stanozolol, methandienone, and boldenone are some of the most frequently abused anabolic steroids.

Effect on Body

A wide range of adverse effects is associated with the use or abuse of anabolic steroids. These effects depend on several factors including: age, sex, the anabolic steroid used, amount used, and duration of use. In adolescents, anabolic steroid use can stunt the ultimate height that an individual achieves. In boys, steroid use can cause early sexual development, acne, and stunted growth. In adolescent girls and women, anabolic steroid use can induce permanent physical changes, such as deepening of the voice, increased facial and body hair growth, menstrual irregularities, male pattern baldness, and lengthening of the clitoris. In men, anabolic steroid use can cause shrinkage of the testicles, reduced sperm count, enlargement of the male breast tissue, sterility, and an increased risk of prostate cancer. In both men and women, anabolic steroid use can cause high cholesterol levels, which may increase the risk of coronary artery disease, strokes, and heart attacks. Anabolic steroid use can also cause acne and fluid retention. Oral preparations of anabolic steroids, in particular, can damage the liver. Abusers who inject steroids run the risk of contracting various infections due to non-sterile injection techniques, sharing of contaminated needles, and the use of steroid preparations manufactured in non-sterile environments. All these factors put users at risk for contracting viral infections such as human immunodeficiency virus infection and acquired immune deficiency syndrome (HIV/AIDS) or hepatitis B or C, and bacterial infections at the sight of injection. Abusers may also develop endocarditis, a bacterial infection that causes a potentially fatal inflammation of the heart lining.

Section 23.9

Traumatic Brain Injury (TBI) and Stroke

This section includes text excerpted from "Traumatic Brain Injury (TBI)," *Eunice Kennedy Shriver* National Institute of Child Health and Human Development (NICHD), December 1, 2012. Reviewed April 2017.

What Is Traumatic Brain Injury (TBI)?

Traumatic brain injury (TBI) is a sudden injury from an external force that affects the functioning of the brain. It can be caused by a bump or blow to the head (closed head injury) or by an object penetrating the skull (called a penetrating injury). Some TBIs result in mild, temporary problems, but a more severe TBI can lead to serious physical and psychological symptoms, coma, and even death.

TBI includes (but is not limited to) several types of injury to the brain:

- Skull fracture occurs when the skull cracks. Pieces of broken skull may cut into the brain and injure it, or an object such as a bullet may pierce the skull and enter the brain.

- Contusion is a bruise of the brain, in which swollen brain tissue mixes with blood released from broken blood vessels. A contusion can occur from the brain shaking back and forth against the skull, such as from a car collision or sports accident or in shaken baby syndrome.

- Intracranial hematoma occurs when damage to a major blood vessel in the brain or between the brain and the skull causes bleeding.

- Anoxia, absence of oxygen to the brain, causes damage to the brain tissue.

The most common form of TBI is concussion. A concussion can happen when the head or body is moved back and forth quickly, such as during a motor vehicle accident or sports injury. Concussions are often called "mild TBI" because they are usually not life-threatening. However, they still can cause serious problems, and research suggests that repeated concussions can be particularly dangerous.

A person who has a TBI may have some of the same symptoms as a person who has a non-traumatic brain injury. Unlike TBI, this type of injury is not caused by an external force, but is caused by an internal problem, such as a stroke or infection. Both types of injury can have serious, long-term effects on a person's cognition and functioning.

What Are Common Symptoms of TBI?

TBI symptoms vary depending on the extent of the injury and the area of the brain affected. Some symptoms appear immediately; others may appear several days or even weeks later. A person with TBI may or may not lose consciousness—loss of consciousness is not always a sign of severe TBI.

Symptoms of Mild TBI

A person with a mild TBI may experience:

- Headache

- Confusion
- Lightheadedness
- Dizziness
- Blurred vision
- Ringing in the ears
- Tiredness or sleepiness
- A bad taste in the mouth
- A change in sleep habits
- Behavior or mood changes
- Trouble with memory, concentration, attention, or thinking
- Loss of consciousness lasting a few seconds to minutes
- Sensitivity to light or sound
- Nausea or vomiting

Symptoms of Moderate or Severe TBI

A person with moderate or severe TBI may have some of the symptoms listed above. In addition, the person may experience any of the following:

- Headache that gets worse or won't go away
- Repeated vomiting or nausea
- Slurred speech
- Convulsions or seizures
- An inability to wake up from sleep
- Enlargement of the pupil (dark center) of one or both eyes
- Numbness or tingling of arms or legs
- Loss of coordination
- Increased confusion, restlessness, or agitation
- Loss of consciousness lasting a few minutes to hours

A person who suffers a blow to the head or another trauma that may have caused a TBI should seek medical attention.

How Many People Are Affected/at Risk for TBI?

According to the Centers for Disease Control and Prevention (CDC), approximately 1.7 million people experience a TBI in the United States each year. This number does not include injuries seen at military or Veterans Health Administration health facilities.

CDC data show that about 53,000 people in the United States die from TBI-related causes every year.

Anyone can experience TBI because it is caused by common events such as car crashes, sports injuries, and falls. However, certain groups of people are more likely to sustain a TBI. The age groups in which TBI is most common are:

• Children up to 4 years old

• Adolescents 15 to 19 years old

• Adults 65 and older

Within every age group, TBI rates are higher for males than for females.

In addition, active duty and reserve service members, who engage in dangerous training and operational activities in addition to combat, face a greater risk of TBI than their civilian peers.

What Causes a TBI?

A TBI is caused by an external force that injures the brain. It can occur when a person's head is hit, bumped, or jolted. It also can occur when an object, such as a bullet, pierces the skull, or when the body is shaken or hit hard enough to cause the brain to slam into the skull. The leading causes of TBI are falls, motor vehicle crashes and traffic-related incidents, collisions with an object, and assaults. Half of TBI incidents involve alcohol use.

Sports and recreational activities are also a significant cause of TBI, especially among young people. The activities associated with the greatest number of emergency department visits for TBI include bicycling, football, playground activities, basketball, and soccer.

In the military, the leading causes of TBI are bullets, fragments, blasts, falls, motor vehicle crashes, and assaults.

Preventing TBI

Some causes of TBI are avoidable. The list below offers some ways to help prevent TBI.

- Always wear a seatbelt when riding in a motor vehicle.

- Make sure a child in a car is protected with a child safety seat and/or seat belt.

- Never drive while under the influence of alcohol or drugs.

- Wear a helmet and make sure children wear the appropriate helmets for such activities as bike-riding, skateboarding, and playing certain sports.

- Make living areas safer for older people with measures such as removing rugs and other tripping hazards and improving lighting throughout the home.

- Install window guards to keep young children from falling out of windows, and use safety gates at the top and bottom of stairs when young children are around.

Another preventable cause of TBI is shaken baby syndrome (SBS). The syndrome can occur when an infant is shaken violently or hit. Nearly all victims of SBS suffer serious health consequences, and at least one of every four babies who are violently shaken dies. Preventing SBS involves helping people understand the dangers of shaking a baby, the risk factors and the triggers for SBS, and how to support overstressed parents and caregivers.

How Is a TBI Diagnosed?

To diagnose TBI, healthcare providers may use one or more tests that assess a person's physical injuries, brain and nerve functioning, and level of consciousness. Some of these tests are described below.

- **Glasgow Coma Scale (GCS):** The GCS measures a person's functioning in three areas: ability to speak, ability to open eyes, and ability to move. A healthcare provider rates a person's responses in these categories and calculates a total score. However, there may be no correlation between initial GCS score and the person's short- or long-term recovery or abilities.

- **Measurements for Level of TBI:** Healthcare providers sometimes rank the person's level of consciousness, memory loss, and GCS score.

  - A TBI is considered mild if:

  - The person was not unconscious or was unconscious for less than 30 minutes.

- Memory loss lasted less than 24 hours.
- The GCS was 13 to 15.
- A TBI is considered moderate if:
- The person was unconscious for more than 30 minutes and up to 24 hours.
- Memory loss lasted anywhere from 24 hours to 7 days.
- The GCS was 9 to 12.
- A TBI is considered severe if:
- The person was unconscious for more than 24 hours.
- Memory loss lasted more than 7 days.
- The GCS was 8 or lower.
- **Speech and language tests**
- **Imaging tests:** Healthcare providers may also use tests that take images of a person's brain. These include, but are not limited to:
  - Computerized tomography (CT)
  - Magnetic resonance imaging (MRI)
  - Intracranial pressure (ICP) monitoring

What Are the Treatments for TBI?

A variety of treatments can help promote recovery from the physical, emotional, and cognitive problems TBI may cause. The types and extent of treatments depend on the severity of the injury and its specific location in the brain.

Treatment for Mild TBI

Mild TBI, sometimes called concussion, may not require specific treatment other than rest. However, it is very important to follow a healthcare provider's instructions for complete rest and gradual return to normal activities after a mild TBI. In addition, alcohol and other drugs can slow recovery and increase the chances of re-injury.

Children and teens who may have sustained a concussion during sports should stop playing immediately. They should not return to play until a healthcare provider who is experienced in evaluating concussion confirms they are ready. Re-injury during recovery can slow healing and increase the chances of long-term problems. On rare occasions in which a person gets another concussion before healing from the first one, permanent brain damage and even death may result.

Emergency Treatment for TBI

In most cases, emergency care focuses on stabilizing the patient and promoting survival. This care may include ensuring adequate oxygen flow to the brain, controlling blood pressure, and preventing further injury to the head or neck. Once the patient is stable, other types of care for TBI and its effects can begin.

Surgery may be needed as part of emergency care to reduce additional damage to the brain tissues. Surgery may include:

- removing clotted blood

- repairing skull fractures

- relieving pressure in the skull

Medications

Medications may be used to treat symptoms of TBI and to lower some of the risks associated with it. These medications may include, but are not limited to:

- **Anti-anxiety medication** to lessen feelings of nervousness and fear

- **Anticoagulants** to prevent blood clots

- **Anticonvulsants** to prevent seizures

- **Antidepressants** to treat symptoms of depression and mood instability

- **Diuretics** to help remove fluid that can increase pressure inside the brain

- **Muscle relaxants** to reduce muscle spasms

- **Stimulants** to increase alertness and attention

Rehabilitation Therapies

Therapies can help someone with TBI relearn skills such as walking or cooking, or develop strategies for self-care, such as making lists of the steps involved in getting dressed. Rehabilitation can include several different kinds of therapy for physical, emotional, and cognitive difficulties. Depending on the injury, these treatments may be needed only briefly after the injury, occasionally throughout a person's life, or on an ongoing basis.

Types of rehabilitation therapy may include:

- **Physical therapy.** This treatment works to build physical strength, coordination, and flexibility.

- **Occupational therapy.** An occupational therapist helps a person learn or relearn how to perform daily tasks, such as getting dressed, cooking, and bathing.

- **Speech therapy.** This therapy works on the ability to form words and other communication skills as well as how to use special communication devices if necessary. Speech therapy can also include evaluation and treatment of swallowing disorders (dysphagia).

- **Psychological counseling.** A counselor can help a person learn coping skills, work on relationships, and improve general emotional well-being.

- **Vocational counseling.** This type of rehabilitation focuses on a person's ability to return to work, find appropriate opportunities, and deal with workplace challenges.

- **Cognitive therapy.** This includes activities designed to improve memory, attention, perception, learning, planning, and judgment. For many people with TBI, cognitive therapy is among the most common types of rehabilitation.

What Are the Possible Effects of a TBI?

The effects of TBI range in duration and seriousness, depending on the extent of the injury and its location. According to the CDC, nearly 45 percent of people who are hospitalized after a TBI have a related disability one year after the injury.

Immediate Problems

Sometimes, a person will have medical complications as a result of TBI, and the risk of these problems increases with the severity of the injury. Some complications of TBI include stroke, seizures, blood clots, contraction of a blood vessel, nerve damage, coma, and infections in the brain. The risks of many of these problems decrease as more time passes from the initial TBI and as the person's condition stabilizes.

Longer-Term Effects of TBI

TBI may cause problems with various brain functions. The types and extent of these problems depend on where the brain was injured. Possible problems from TBI include:

- **Cognition**, such as difficulty learning, remembering, making decisions, and reasoning

- **Senses**, such as double vision, a consistent bitter taste in the mouth or a loss of the sense of taste, ringing in the ears, and tingling or pain

- **Communication**, such as trouble talking, reading, writing, and explaining feelings or thoughts

- **Behavior**, including difficulty with social situations, relationships, and self-control, or aggression

- **Emotions**, including depression, anxiety, mood swings, and irritability

Degenerative Effects of TBI

Research suggests that having one or more TBIs may increase the risk of diseases that cause the degeneration, or breakdown, of brain cells. Some evidence indicates that TBI is associated with:

- Alzheimer disease, which impairs memory, emotions, and thinking skills

- Parkinson disease, which causes the loss of motor skills and control over motor skills

- Chronic traumatic encephalopathy, which often affects athletes involved in sports with head impacts, including boxing, football, and hockey, and causes problems with memory, thinking, and motor skills

Chapter 24

Stroke Prevention

Chapter Contents

Section 24.1—Preventing and Managing Diabetes.................... 268

Section 24.2—Preventing and Managing High
Blood Pressure.. 270

Section 24.3—Preventing and Managing High
Cholesterol.. 273

Section 24.4—Healthy Living Reduces Stroke Risk 276

Section 24.5—Quitting Smoking Reduces Stroke
Risk 277

Section 24.6—Even Modest Weight Loss Produces
Health Benefits... 281

Section 24.1

Preventing and Managing Diabetes

This section contains text excerpted from the following sources:
Text in this section begins with excerpts from "Diabetes, Heart
Disease, and Stroke," National Institute of Diabetes and Digestive
and Kidney Diseases (NIDDK), February 2017; Text under the
heading "Preventing Diabetes" is excerpted from "Preventing
Diabetes," Centers for Disease Control and Prevention (CDC),
November 9, 2016.

Having diabetes means that you are more likely to develop heart disease and have a greater chance of a stroke or a heart attack. People with diabetes are also more likely to have certain conditions, or risk factors, that increase the chances of having stroke or heart disease, such as high blood pressure or high cholesterol. If you have diabetes, you can protect your heart and health by managing your blood glucose, also called blood sugar, as well as your blood pressure and cholesterol. If you smoke, get help to stop.

Preventing Diabetes

Research studies have found that moderate weight loss and exercise can prevent or delay type 2 diabetes among adults at high-risk of diabetes. Find out more about the risk factors for type 2 diabetes, what it means to have prediabetes, and what you can do to prevent or delay diabetes.

What Are the Most Important Things to Do to Prevent Diabetes?

The Diabetes Prevention Program (DPP), a major federally funded study of 3,234 people at high risk for diabetes, showed that people can delay and possibly prevent the disease by losing a small amount of weight (5 to 7 percent of total body weight) through 30 minutes of physical activity 5 days a week and healthier eating.

When Should I Be Tested for Diabetes?

Anyone aged 45 years or older should consider getting tested for diabetes, especially if you are overweight. If you are younger than 45, but are overweight and have one or more additional risk factors, you should consider getting tested.

Additional risk factors include:

- Being overweight or obese.

- Having a parent, brother, or sister with diabetes.

- Being African American, American Indian, Asian American, Pacific Islander, or Hispanic American/Latino heritage.

- Having a prior history of gestational diabetes or birth of at least one baby weighing more than 9 pounds.

- Having high blood pressure measuring 140/90 or higher.

- Having abnormal cholesterol with high-density lipoprotein (HDL) ("good") cholesterol is 35 or lower, or triglyceride level is 250 or higher.

- Being physically inactive—exercising fewer than three times a week.

How Does Body Weight Affect the Likelihood of Developing Diabetes?

Being overweight or obese is a leading risk factor for type 2 diabetes. Being overweight can keep your body from making and using insulin properly, and can also cause high blood pressure. The Diabetes Prevention Program (DPP), a major federally funded study of 3,234 people at high risk for diabetes, showed that moderate diet and exercise of about 30 minutes or more, 5 or more days per week, or of 150 or more minutes per week, resulting in a 5 percent to 7 percent weight loss can delay and possibly prevent type 2 diabetes.

What Is Prediabetes?

People with blood glucose levels that are higher than normal but not yet in the diabetic range have "prediabetes." Doctors sometimes call this condition impaired fasting glucose (IFG) or impaired glucose tolerance (IGT), depending on the test used to diagnose it. Insulin resistance and prediabetes usually have no symptoms. You may have one or both conditions for several years without noticing anything.

If you have prediabetes, you have a higher risk of developing type 2 diabetes. In addition, people with prediabetes also have a higher risk of heart disease.

Progression to diabetes among those with prediabetes is not inevitable. Studies suggest that weight loss and increased physical activity among people with prediabetes prevent or delay diabetes and may return blood glucose levels to normal.

Section 24.2

Preventing and Managing High Blood Pressure

This section includes text excerpted from "Preventing Diseases—High Blood Pressure," National Center for Health Promotion and Disease Prevention (NCP), U.S. Department of Veterans Affairs (VA), February 22, 2016.

Why Is High Blood Pressure Dangerous?

Blood pressure is the force of blood pushing against your blood vessels. If blood pressure rises and stays high over time, it is called hypertension. If it is not controlled, high blood pressure can cause:

- Stroke
- Kidney problems
- Heart failure
- Heart attack
- Eye problems

Most people with high blood pressure feel healthy and don't have symptoms. The only way to know if you have high blood pressure is to have your blood pressure checked.

How Do You Get Checked for High Blood Pressure?

Checking your blood pressure is simple. Your provider places a fabric cuff around your upper arm and pumps it full of air. Your provider then listens to your heartbeat while the air is let out of the cuff.

Follow these steps to help your provider correctly measure your blood pressure:

- Wear a short-sleeved shirt or blouse.

- Empty your bladder.

- For at least 30 minutes before your appointment, don't:

  - smoke

  - do any vigorous activity

  - drink caffeine (in coffee, tea or cola)

- Sit down and relax with your feet on the floor and your back supported for at least 5 minutes before your blood pressure is checked.

- Don't talk while your blood pressure is being checked.

What Do Your Blood Pressure Numbers Mean?

Blood pressure is measured by two numbers.

The first (or top) number—"systolic"—is the pressure in your blood vessels when your heart beats. The second (or bottom) number—"diastolic"—is the pressure in your blood vessels between heartbeats.

If your blood pressure is normal, that's great! You should have it rechecked every year or so to be sure it stays within the normal range.

If your blood pressure is pre-high or high, it should be rechecked to determine whether you have hypertension. Ask your provider the following questions:

- When should I have my blood pressure checked again?

- Do I need treatment for high blood pressure?

What Can You Do to Prevent or Control High Blood Pressure?

- Quit smoking and/or chewing tobacco. Ask your provider for help with quitting.

- Achieve and maintain a healthy weight. If you are overweight, ask your provider for help with a plan to lose weight.
- Be physically active.
  - "Physical activity" includes any activity that raises your heart rate, such as brisk walking, working in the house or yard, or playing sports.
  - Do activity for 10 minutes or more at a time. Aim for at least 2 hours and 30 minutes of activity each week.
- Reduce salt (sodium) in your diet.
  - Read food labels. Choose and prepare foods that are low in sodium or are sodium-free.
  - Ask to see a registered dietitian if you need help with a plan.
- Limit alcohol.
  - Men should have no more than 2 drinks per day.
  - Women should have no more than 1 drink per day.

What Else Can You Do?

Always ask your provider what your blood pressure is and write it down. Keep track of your blood pressure numbers.

Your provider may prescribe medicine to help lower your blood pressure.

- Take your medicine every day, or as directed by your provider
- If your blood pressure numbers get lower, it's because your medicine is working. Don't stop it or take a lower dose unless your provider says you should.

Here are some questions to ask your provider:

- Is my blood pressure under good control?
- How often should I have my blood pressure checked?
- What is a healthy weight for me?
- Is it safe for me to start doing regular physical activity?

Section 24.3

Preventing and Managing High Cholesterol

This section includes text excerpted from "Preventing Diseases—High Cholesterol," National Center for Health Promotion and Disease Prevention (NCP), U.S. Department of Veterans Affairs (VA), February 22, 2016.

What Is High Cholesterol?

Cholesterol is a fat-like material that provides structure for your body's cells. Your liver makes most of the cholesterol your body needs, but you also get some from the foods you eat. Too much cholesterol can cause a sticky substance (plaque) to buildup in your blood vessels. This plaque can block blood vessels and cause strokes and heart attacks.

Most people with high cholesterol feel healthy and don't have symptoms. The only way to know if you have high cholesterol is to have your cholesterol checked.

You should have your cholesterol regularly checked if:

- You are a man 35 years or older; or

- You are a woman of any age or a younger man and have risk factors for stroke or heart disease such as:

  - Smoking

  - Diabetes

  - High blood pressure

  - Overweight

  - A family history of strokes or heart attacks before age 50 in male relatives or before age 60 in female relatives.

How Is Cholesterol Checked?

Cholesterol is checked with a blood test. The test works best if you don't eat or drink anything for at least 8 hours before the test.

What Do the Cholesterol Numbers Mean?

Your total cholesterol is made up of two types of cholesterol: LDL (low-density lipoproteins) and HDL (high-density lipoproteins).

- High levels of LDL increase your chances of heart disease. It is sometimes called the "bad cholesterol."

- High levels of HDL decrease your chances of heart disease. It is sometimes called the "good cholesterol."

Total Cholesterol Levels

Your provider will usually look at your total cholesterol first. Your total cholesterol should be under 200. If you already have heart disease or you have heart disease risk factors, such as smoking, diabetes, or high blood pressure, your provider will also look at your LDL and HDL results.

If your cholesterol is in the desirable range and you are healthy, have it checked again in 5 years.

If your cholesterol is borderline high or high, or you have heart disease, your next step depends on your LDL and HDL levels and your other conditions or risk factors. Ask your provider these questions:

- What should my cholesterol levels be?

- Do I need treatment for my cholesterol?

What Can You Do to Prevent or Control High Cholesterol?

Follow a Healthy Eating Plan

- Read food labels and limit foods high in saturated fat, *trans* fat, and cholesterol.

- Eat plenty of fruits, vegetables, low-fat dairy foods, and whole grains.

- Ask to see a registered dietitian if you need help with a plan.

Be Physically Active

- "Physical activity" includes any activity that raises your heart rate, such as brisk walking, working in the house or yard, or playing sports.

- Do activity for 10 minutes or more at a time. Aim for at least 2 hours and 30 minutes of activity each week.

Achieve and Maintain a Healthy Weight

If you are overweight, ask your provider for help with an eating and physical activity plan to lose weight

What Else Can You Do?

Always ask your provider what your cholesterol numbers are and write them down. Keep track with the log at the MyHealtheVet website: www.myhealth.va.gov.

Your provider may prescribe medicine to help lower your cholesterol.

- Take your medicine every day, or as directed by your provider.

- If your cholesterol numbers get lower, it's because your medicine is working. Don't stop it or take a lower dose unless your provider says you should.

Here are some questions to ask your provider:

- Is my cholesterol under good control?

- When should I have my cholesterol next checked?

- What is a healthy weight for me?

- Is it safe for me to start doing regular physical activity?

Section 24.4

Healthy Living Reduces Stroke Risk

This section includes text excerpted from "Preventing
Stroke: Healthy Living," Centers for Disease Control and
Prevention (CDC), January 17, 2017.

You can help prevent stroke by making healthy lifestyle choices.

No Smoking

Cigarette smoking greatly increases your chances of having a
stroke. If you don't smoke, don't start. If you do smoke, quitting will
lower your risk for stroke. Your doctor can suggest ways to help you
quit.

Limited Alcohol

Avoid drinking too much alcohol, which can raise your blood pressure. Men should have no more than two drinks per day, and women
only one.

Physical Activity

Physical activity can help you stay at a healthy weight and lower
your cholesterol and blood pressure levels. For adults, the Surgeon
General recommends 2 hours and 30 minutes of moderate-intensity
aerobic physical activity, such as a brisk walk, each week. Children
and teens should get 1 hour of physical activity every day.

Healthy Weight

Being overweight or obese increases your risk for stroke. To determine whether your weight is in a healthy range, doctors often calculate
your body mass index (BMI). If you know your weight and height, you
can calculate your BMI at CDC's Assessing Your Weight website (www.
cdc.gov/healthyweight/assessing/index.html). Doctors sometimes also
use waist and hip measurements to measure excess body fat.

Healthy Diet

Choosing healthy meal and snack options can help you prevent stroke. Be sure to eat plenty of fresh fruits and vegetables.

Eating foods low in saturated fats, trans fat, and cholesterol and high in fiber can help prevent high cholesterol. Limiting salt (sodium) in your diet can also lower your blood pressure. High cholesterol and high blood pressure increase your chances of having a stroke.

Section 24.5

Quitting Smoking Reduces Stroke Risk

This section contains text excerpted from the following sources: Text beginning with the heading "How Are Smoking Related to Heart Disease and Stroke?" is excerpted from "Smoking and Heart Disease and Stroke," Centers for Disease Control and Prevention (CDC), February 24, 2017; Text under the heading "Benefits of Quitting" is excerpted from "Benefits of Quitting," Centers for Disease Control and Prevention (CDC), March 17, 2016; Text under the heading "Strategies to Quit Smoking" is excerpted from "Strategies to Quit Smoking," National Heart, Lung, and Blood Institute (NHLBI), June 22, 2016.

How Are Smoking Related to Heart Disease and Stroke?

Smoking is a major cause of cardiovascular disease (CVD) and causes one of every three deaths from CVD. Smoking can:

- Make blood sticky and more likely to clot, which can block blood flow to the heart and brain

- Increase the buildup of plaque (fat, cholesterol, calcium, and other substances) in blood vessels

- Cause thickening and narrowing of blood vessels

- Raise triglycerides (a type of fat in your blood)

- Lower "good" cholesterol (HDL)

- Damage cells that line the blood vessels

Benefits of Quitting

- Quitting smoking at any age has benefits.

- The sooner you quit, the sooner your body can begin to heal.

- Tobacco smoke harms nonsmokers, too.

- Quitting smoking is the single best way to protect your family from secondhand smoke.

Reduced Risk for Various Health Issues

Some benefits of quitting smoking occur quickly; more occur over time. For example:

- Your risk for a heart attack drops sharply just 1 year after you quit smoking.

- After 2 to 5 years, your chance for stroke could fall to about the same as a nonsmoker's.

- Within 5 years of quitting, your chance of cancer of the mouth, throat, esophagus, and bladder is cut in half.

- Risks for other conditions—including ulcer, peripheral artery disease, and cancers of the larynx, lung, and cervix—are reduced after quitting.

- The risk of having a low birth weight baby drops to normal if you quit before pregnancy or during your first trimester.

Other Benefits of Quitting

- Health benefits for people with diabetes who quit smoking begin immediately and include having better control over blood sugar levels.

- If you quit smoking, you will breathe better and it will be easier to be active.

- By not smoking, you help protect family, friends, and coworkers from health risks associated with breathing secondhand smoke. These include an increased risk for heart disease and lung cancer among adults. For babies and children, risks include respiratory infections, ear infections, and sudden infant death syndrome (SIDS).

Strategies to Quit Smoking

Quitting smoking is possible, but it can be hard. Millions of people have successfully quit smoking and remain nonsmokers. Surveys of current adult smokers find that 70 percent say they want to quit.

There are a few ways to quit smoking, including quitting all at once (going "cold turkey") or slowly cutting back your number of cigarettes before quitting completely. Use the method that works best for you. Below are some strategies to help you quit.

Get Ready to Quit

If you want to quit smoking, try to get motivated. Make a list of your reasons for wanting to quit. Write a contract to yourself that outlines your plan for quitting.

If you've tried to quit smoking in the past, think about those attempts. What helped you during that time, and what made it harder?

Know what triggers you to smoke. For example, do you smoke after a meal, while driving, or when you're stressed? Develop a plan to handle each trigger.

Get Support

Set a quit date and let those close to you know about it. Ask your family and friends for support in your effort to quit smoking.

You also can get support from hotlines and websites.

Get Medicine and Use It Correctly

Talk with your doctor and pharmacist about medicines and over-the-counter products that can help you quit smoking. These medicines and products are helpful for many people.

You can buy nicotine gum, patches, and lozenges from a drug store. Other medicines that can help you quit smoking are available by prescription.

Learn New Skills and Behaviors

Try new activities to replace smoking. For example, instead of smoking after a meal, take a brisk walk in your neighborhood or around your office building. Try to be physically active regularly.

Take up knitting, carpentry, or other hobbies and activities that keep your hands busy. Try to avoid other people who smoke. Ask those you can't avoid to respect your efforts to stop smoking and not smoke around you.

279

Remove cigarettes, ashtrays, and lighters from your home, office, and car. Don't smoke at all—not even one puff. Also, try to avoid alcohol and caffeine. (People who drink alcohol are more likely to start smoking again after quitting.)

Be Prepared for Withdrawal and Relapse

Be prepared for the challenge of withdrawal. Withdrawal symptoms often lessen after only 1 or 2 weeks of not smoking, and each urge to smoke lasts only a few minutes.

You can take steps to cope with withdrawal symptoms. If you feel like smoking, wait a few minutes for the urge to pass. Remind yourself of the benefits of quitting. Don't get overwhelmed—take tasks one step at a time.

If you relapse (slip and smoke after you've quit), consider what caused the slip. Were you stressed out or unprepared for a situation that you associate with smoking? Make a plan to avoid or handle this situation in the future.

Getting frustrated with your slip will only make it harder to quit in the future. Accept that you slipped, learn from the slip, and recommit to quit smoking

If you start smoking regularly again, don't get discouraged. Instead, find out what you need to do to get back on track so you can meet your goals. Set a new quit date, and ask your family and friends to help you. Most people who smoke make repeated attempts to quit before doing so successfully.

Many smokers gain weight after they quit, but the average weight gain is 10 pounds or less. You can control weight gain by following a heart-healthy eating plan and being physically active. Remember the bright side—food smells and tastes better if you aren't smoking.

Section 24.6

Even Modest Weight Loss Produces Health Benefits

This section contains text excerpted from the following sources:
Text under the heading "Complications of Obesity" is excerpted
from "Overweight and Obesity—Signs, Symptoms, and
Complications," National Heart, Lung, and Blood Institute (NHLBI),
February 23, 2017; Text beginning with the heading "Losing
Weight" is excerpted from "Losing Weight," Centers for Disease
Control and Prevention (CDC), May 15, 2015.

Complications of Obesity

Obesity may cause the following complications:

- **Diseases of the heart and blood vessels** such as stroke, high blood pressure, atherosclerosis, and heart attacks

- **Metabolic Syndrome**

- **Type 2 diabetes**

- **High blood cholesterol** and high triglyceride levels in the blood

- **Respiratory problems** such as obstructive sleep apnea, asthma, and obesity hypoventilation syndrome

- **Back pain**

- **Non-alcoholic fatty liver disease (NAFLD)**

- **Osteoarthritis,** a chronic inflammation that damages the cartilage and bone in or around the affected joint. It can cause mild or severe pain and usually affects weight-bearing joints in people who are obese. It is a major cause of knee replacement surgery in patients who are obese for a long time.

- **Urinary incontinence,** the unintentional leakage of urine. Chronic obesity can weaken pelvic muscles, making it harder to maintain bladder control. While it can happen to both sexes, it usually affects women as they age.

- **Gallbladder disease**

- **Emotional health issues** such as low self-esteem or depression. This may commonly occur in children.

- **Cancers** of the esophagus, pancreas, colon, rectum, kidney, endometrium, ovaries, gallbladder, breast, or liver.

Losing Weight

What Is Healthy Weight Loss?

It's natural for anyone trying to lose weight to want to lose it very quickly. But evidence shows that people who lose weight gradually and steadily (about 1 to 2 pounds per week) are more successful at keeping weight off. Healthy weight loss isn't just about a "diet" or "program." It's about an ongoing lifestyle that includes long-term changes in daily eating and exercise habits.

To lose weight, you must use up more calories than you take in. Since one pound equals 3,500 calories, you need to reduce your caloric intake by 500–1000 calories per day to lose about 1 to 2 pounds per week.

Once you've achieved a healthy weight, by relying on healthful eating and physical activity most days of the week (about 60–90 minutes, moderate intensity), you are more likely to be successful at keeping the weight off over the long-term.

Losing weight is not easy, and it takes commitment. But if you're ready to get started, we've got a step-by-step guide to help get you on the road to weight loss and better health.

Even Modest Weight Loss Can Mean Big Benefits

The good news is that no matter what your weight loss goal is, even a modest weight loss, such as 5 to 10 percent of your total body weight, is likely to produce health benefits, such as improvements in blood pressure, blood cholesterol, and blood sugars.

For example, if you weigh 200 pounds, a 5 percent weight loss equals 10 pounds, bringing your weight down to 190 pounds. While this weight may still be in the "overweight" or "obese" range, this modest weight loss can decrease your risk factors for chronic diseases related to obesity.

So even if the overall goal seems large, see it as a journey rather than just a final destination. You'll learn new eating and physical activity habits that will help you live a healthier lifestyle. These habits may help you maintain your weight loss over time.

In addition to improving your health, maintaining a weight loss is likely to improve your life in other ways. For example, a study of participants in the National Weight Control Registry found that those who had maintained a significant weight loss reported improvements in not only their physical health, but also their energy levels, physical mobility, general mood, and self-confidence.

Keeping It Off

If you've recently lost excess weight, congratulations! It's an accomplishment that will likely benefit your health now and in the future. Now that you've lost weight, let's talk about some ways to maintain that success.

The following tips are some of the common characteristics among people who have successfully lost weight and maintained that loss over time.

Watch Your Diet

- **Follow a healthy and realistic eating pattern.** You have embarked on a healthier lifestyle, now the challenge is maintaining the positive eating habits you've developed along the way. In studies of people who have lost weight and kept it off for at least a year, most continued to eat a diet lower in calories as compared to their pre-weight loss diet.

- **Keep your eating patterns consistent.** Follow a healthy eating pattern regardless of changes in your routine. Plan ahead for weekends, vacations, and special occasions. By making a plan, it is more likely you'll have healthy foods on hand for when your routine changes.

- **Eat breakfast every day.** Eating breakfast is a common trait among people who have lost weight and kept it off. Eating a healthful breakfast may help you avoid getting "over-hungry" and then overeating later in the day.

Be Active

- **Get daily physical activity.** People who have lost weight and kept it off typically engage in 60–90 minutes of moderate intensity physical activity most days of the week while not exceeding calorie needs. This doesn't necessarily mean 60–90 minutes at one time. It might mean 20–30 minutes of physical activity three times a day. For example, a brisk walk in the morning, at lunch time, and in the evening. Some people may need to talk to their healthcare provider before participating in this level of physical activity.

Stay on Course

- **Monitor your diet and activity.** Keeping a food and physical activity journal can help you track your progress and spot trends. For example, you might notice that your weight creeps up during periods when you have a lot of business travel or when you have to work overtime. Recognizing this tendency can be a signal to try different behaviors, such as packing your own healthful food for the plane and making time to use your hotel's exercise facility when you are traveling. Or if working overtime, maybe you can use your breaks for quick walks around the building.

- **Monitor your weight.** Check your weight regularly. When managing your weight loss, it's a good idea to keep track of your weight so you can plan accordingly and adjust your diet and exercise plan as necessary. If you have gained a few pounds, get back on track quickly.

- **Get support from family, friends, and others.** People who have successfully lost weight and kept it off often rely on support from others to help them stay on course and get over any "bumps." Sometimes having a friend or partner who is also losing weight or maintaining a weight loss can help you stay motivated.

Part Four

Diagnosis and Treatment of Stroke

Chapter 25

After a Stroke: The First 24 Hours

Stroke is a medical emergency. Every minute counts when someone is having a stroke. The longer blood flow is cut off to the brain, the greater the damage. Immediate treatment can save people's lives and enhance their chances for successful recovery.

Ischemic strokes, the most common type of strokes, can be treated with a drug called tPA that dissolves blood clots obstructing blood flow to the brain. The window of opportunity to start treating stroke patients is three hours, but to be evaluated and receive treatment, patients need to get to the hospital within 60 minutes.

A five-year study by the National Institute of Neurological Disorders and Stroke (NINDS) found that some stroke patients who received tPA within three hours of the start of stroke symptoms were at least 30 percent more likely to recover with little or no disability after three months.

Don't wait for the symptoms of stroke to improve or worsen. If you believe you or someone else is having a stroke, call 911 immediately! Making the decision to call for medical help can make the difference

This chapter contains text excerpted from the following sources: Text in this chapter begins with excerpts from "Stroke—Frequently Asked Questions," NIHSeniorHealth, National Institute on Aging (NIA), February 2013. Reviewed April 2017; Text under the heading "Stroke Treatment" is excerpted from "Stroke— Stroke Treatment," Centers for Disease Control and Prevention (CDC), February 10, 2017.

in avoiding a lifelong disability and in greatly improving the chances for recovery.

Stroke Treatment

Your stroke treatment begins the moment emergency medical services (EMS) arrives to take you to the hospital. Once at the hospital, you may receive emergency care, treatment to prevent another stroke, rehabilitation to treat the side effects of stroke, or all three.

On the Way to the Hospital

If someone you know shows signs of stroke, call 9-1-1 right away.

Do not drive to the hospital or let someone else drive you. Call an ambulance so that medical personnel can begin life-saving treatment on the way to the emergency room. Stroke patients who are taken to the hospital in an ambulance may get diagnosed and treated more quickly than people who do not arrive in an ambulance.

The emergency workers may take you to a specialized stroke center to make sure you get the quickest possible diagnosis and treatment.

Your emergency treatment starts in the ambulance. The emergency workers may take you to a specialized stroke center to ensure that you receive the quickest possible diagnosis and treatment.

What Happens at the Hospital

At the hospital, health professionals will ask about your medical history and about the time your symptoms started. Brain scans will show what type of stroke you had. You may also work with a neurologist who treats brain disorders, a neurosurgeon that performs surgery on the brain, or a specialist in another area of medicine.

If you get to the hospital within 3 hours of the first symptoms of an ischemic stroke, you may get a type of medicine called a thrombolytic (a "clot-busting" drug) to break up blood clots. Tissue plasminogen activator (tPA) is a thrombolytic.

tPA improves the chances of recovering from a stroke. Studies show that patients with ischemic strokes who receive tPA are more likely to recover fully or have less disability than patients who do not receive the drug. Patients treated with tPA are also less likely to need long-term care in a nursing home. Unfortunately, many stroke victims don't get to the hospital in time for tPA treatment. This is why it's so important to recognize the signs and symptoms of stroke right away and call 9-1-1.

Medicine, surgery, or other procedures may be needed to stop the bleeding and save brain tissue. For example:

- Endovascular procedures. Endovascular procedures may be used to treat certain hemorrhagic strokes. The doctor inserts a long tube through a major artery in the leg or arm and then guides the tube to the site of the weak spot or break in a blood vessel. The tube is then used to install a device, such as a coil, to repair the damage or prevent bleeding.

- Surgical treatment. Hemorrhagic strokes may be treated with surgery. If the bleeding is caused by a ruptured aneurysm, a metal clip may be put in place to stop the blood loss.

What Happens Next

If you have had a stroke, you are at high risk for another stroke:

- 1 of 4 stroke survivors has another stroke within 5 years.
- The risk of stroke within 90 days of a Transient Ischemic Attack (TIA) may be as high as 17 percent, with the greatest risk during the first week.

That's why it's important to treat the underlying causes of stroke, including heart disease, high blood pressure, atrial fibrillation (fast, irregular heartbeat), high cholesterol, and diabetes. Your doctor may give you medications or tell you to change your diet, exercise, or adopt other healthy lifestyle habits. Surgery may also be helpful in some cases.

Chapter 26

Working with a Neurologist

Neurologists are medical doctors who specialize in diagnosing, treating, and managing disorders of the brain and nervous system, including the peripheral nerves that connect the brain to organs and muscles throughout the body. Their extensive training includes an undergraduate degree, four years of medical school, a one-year internship, and a minimum of three years of specialty training. In addition, many neurologists train in subspecialties, such as specific diseases or disorders that affect particular body systems. Because of the complexity of the brain and nervous system, which influence and control so many bodily functions, neurologists must be extremely detail-oriented and attuned to even the smallest signs of neurological problems.

What Do Neurologists Do?

Neurologists do not perform surgery but rather treat disorders through the use of medication, physical therapy, and rehabilitation. However, the neurosurgeons who do perform surgeries always work with neurologists to ensure the best possible outcome for the patient, so consulting is another important role for a neurologist. And when patients require ongoing treatment, the neurologist is often the principal care provider. Some of the disorders treated by neurologists include:

- headaches
- pain

- stroke

- brain tumors

- sleep disorders

- epilepsy

- brain and spinal cord injuries

- Parkinson disease

- seizure disorders

- Alzheimer disease

- multiple sclerosis

- amyotrophic lateral sclerosis (ALS, or Lou Gehrig disease)

How Do Neurologists Diagnose Disorders?

As is the case with most doctors, the first thing a neurologist will do is perform an examination of the patient. This includes a review of the person's medical history and a discussion of the current condition, followed by a neurological exam. This will generally include an assessment of the patient's vision, hearing, reflexes, strength, and coordination. Often, additional tests will be required, such as:

- **Magnetic resonance imaging (MRI).** This test uses a magnetic field and radio waves to get an accurate picture of the brain.

- **Computer-assisted tomography (CAT scan).** Here X-rays and a computer are used to create 3-D images of various body parts.

- **Electroencephalogram (EEG).** This records electrical activity in the brain and is used to diagnose physical brain disorders.

- **Electromyogram (EMG).** An EMG records electrical activity in muscles and nerves to help determine the cause of pain, numbness, or weakness.

- **Transcranial Doppler (TCD).** This test measures blood flow in the vessels in the brain using sound waves. It can detect blockages or constrictions that may be causing symptoms.

- **Neurosonography.** Here ultra-high-frequency sounds waves analyze the flow of blood in the vessels in or leading to the brain.

- **Cerebrospinal fluid analysis.** Also called a lumbar puncture or spinal tap, this procedure tests for blood, infection, or other abnormalities in the brain, spinal cord, and nerves.

- **Evoked potentials.** These tests record the brain's response to various types of stimulation in order to diagnose problems with eyesight, hearing, dizziness, or numbness.

- **Sleep studies.** Here the patient usually spends the night in a sleep lab with sensors placed on the scalp. These record brain waves and electrical activity, as well as such functions as heart rate, blood oxygen levels, and breathing, to help determine the cause of sleep disorders.

How Do Neurologists Treat Disorders?

Because of the wide range of neurological disorders, treatments can vary considerably depending on the nature of the disease and the parts of the body that are affected. In the case of stroke, treatment options depend on whether the diagnosis is ischemic stroke or hemorrhagic stroke.

Ischemic strokes result from an obstruction (clot) in a vessel supplying blood to the brain. Treatment options for ischemic stroke generally include:

- **Medication.** A drug called a tissue plasminogen activator (tPA) is injected into a vein in the arm to dissolve the clot that is restricting blood flow to the brain. For this treatment to be most effective, it's important for the medication to be given as soon as possible after the stroke occurs. In addition, an anticoagulant, such as heparin, may be administered to help prevent more blood clots from forming.

- **Mechanical thrombectomy.** Here a catheter is inserted into an artery leading to the brain and a wire-cage device called a stent retriever is used to capture and remove the clot and restore blood flow to the brain. The procedure is most beneficial if it is performed within six hours of the onset of stroke symptoms, and it can only be used on patients who have a clot in one of the large arteries in the brain.

Hemorrhagic strokes occur when a vessel ruptures and allows blood to flow into the brain where it compresses the brain tissue. Treatment options for hemorrhagic stroke usually include:

- **Emergency treatment.** Emergency care is vital for a patient with hemorrhagic stroke in order to control bleeding and reduce pressure in the brain. Medication can be used to reduce blood pressure or slow the bleeding. Patients who are taking blood thinners will likely be given drugs to counteract their effects.

- **Mechanical repair.** A catheter may be inserted through an artery in the arm or leg and guided to the site of the rupture in the brain. Then the doctor places a coil or other device through the catheter to help repair the problem. In some cases, though, surgery may be required to repair the problem.

How to Choose a Neurologist

Obviously, in an emergency situation patients don't get to choose their doctors, but often there's time to consider which neurologist might be the best physician to work with. Here are some tips:

- **Referrals.** Your primary care doctor will likely recommend a neurologist that he or she works with and knows to be good. Family and friends might also have recommendations.

- **Research.** Make the effort to research the neurologist's credentials, experience, and patient satisfaction surveys and ratings. This information is generally available online, as are records of malpractice claims and disciplinary actions.

- **Meet.** Request an introductory visit with the neurologist. Discuss your case and ask about his or her experience treating your condition, as well as possible treatment plans.

- **Consider.** Think about what you've learned, and take into account your impressions of the neurologist at your meeting. It's important not only that the doctor be qualified but also that you feel comfortable with him or her.

- **Don't forget the hospital.** In addition to researching the neurologist, be sure to do your homework about the hospital or treatment facility. Again, get recommendations when possible and research the facility online, paying special attention to its neurology unit.

- **Insurance.** It's also important to be sure the neurologist, facility, and expected treatment are compatible with your insurance plan in order to incur the least out-of-pocket expense.

Rehabilitation

Whatever treatment is required, stroke patients generally need rehabilitation care to facilitate their recovery and help prevent future strokes. This could include follow-up visits with a neurologist or other doctor, medication, and physical or occupational therapy, as well as lifestyle counseling and modification.

When to See a Neurologist

You might need to see a neurologist if you have:

- severe or recurring headaches
- seizures
- dizziness
- numbness
- chronic pain
- weakness
- difficulty moving
- vision problems
- difficulty with memory
- sleep problems

Questions to Ask Your Neurologist after a Stroke

- What kind of stroke did I have?
- What are my treatment options?
- What medication will I need to take?
- What are the medication's side effects?
- What rehabilitation services will I need?
- What healthcare providers will be on the team?
- What lifestyle changes will I need to make?
- What can I do to help prevent a recurrence?
- Should I plan for follow-up visits?

References

1. Caplan, Louis. "Stroke Is Best Managed by Neurologists," *Stroke*, November 6, 2003.

2. "How Is Stroke Treated?" National Institutes of Health, January 27, 2017.

3. "Neurologists and Neurosurgeons Explained," Lifenph.com, n.d.

4. "Quick Stroke Treatment for Saving the Brain," American Stroke Association, n.d.

5. "What does a Neurologist do?" Sokanu.com, n.d.

6. "Working with Your Doctor," American Academy of Neurology, n.d.

Chapter 27

Diagnosing Stroke

Chapter Contents

Section 27.1—How a Stroke Is Diagnosed.................................. 298

Section 27.2—Blood Tests for Stroke... 301

Section 27.3—Cerebral Angiography.. 305

Section 27.4—Echocardiogram.. 308

Section 27.5—Electrocardiogram (EKG) 312

Section 27.6—Computerized Tomography (CT) Scan.............. 313

Section 27.7—Magnetic Resonance Imaging (MRI)................. 316

Section 27.8—Ultrasound.. 319

Section 27.1

How a Stroke Is Diagnosed

This section includes text excerpted from "Stroke—How
Is a Stroke Diagnosed?" National Heart, Lung, and Blood
Institute (NHLBI), January 27, 2017.

Your doctor will diagnose a stroke based on your signs and symptoms, your medical history, a physical exam, and test results.

Your doctor will want to find out the type of stroke you've had, its cause, the part of the brain that's affected, and whether you have bleeding in the brain.

If your doctor thinks you've had a transient ischemic attack (TIA), he or she will look for its cause to help prevent a future stroke.

Medical History and Physical Exam

Your doctor will ask you or a family member about your risk factors for stroke. Examples of risk factors include high blood pressure, smoking, heart disease, and a personal or family history of stroke. Your doctor also will ask about your signs and symptoms and when they began.

During the physical exam, your doctor will check your mental alertness and your coordination and balance. He or she will check for numbness or weakness in your face, arms, and legs; confusion; and trouble speaking and seeing clearly.

Your doctor will look for signs of carotid artery disease, a common cause of ischemic stroke. He or she will listen to your carotid arteries with a stethoscope. A whooshing sound called a bruit may suggest changed or reduced blood flow due to plaque buildup in the carotid arteries.

Diagnostic Tests and Procedures

Your doctor may recommend one or more of the following tests to diagnose a stroke or TIA.

Brain Computed Tomography

A brain computed tomography scan, or brain CT scan, is a painless test that uses X-rays to take clear, detailed pictures of your brain. This test often is done right after a stroke is suspected.

A brain CT scan can show bleeding in the brain or damage to the brain cells from a stroke. The test also can show other brain conditions that may be causing your symptoms.

Magnetic Resonance Imaging

Magnetic resonance imaging (MRI) uses magnets and radio waves to create pictures of the organs and structures in your body. This test can detect changes in brain tissue and damage to brain cells from a stroke.

An MRI may be used instead of, or in addition to, a CT scan to diagnose a stroke.

Computed Tomography Arteriogram and Magnetic Resonance Arteriogram

A CT arteriogram (CTA) and magnetic resonance arteriogram (MRA) can show the large blood vessels in the brain. These tests may give your doctor more information about the site of a blood clot and the flow of blood through your brain.

Carotid Ultrasound

Carotid ultrasound is a painless and harmless test that uses sound waves to create pictures of the insides of your carotid arteries. These arteries supply oxygen-rich blood to your brain.

Carotid ultrasound shows whether plaque has narrowed or blocked your carotid arteries.

Your carotid ultrasound test may include a Doppler ultrasound. Doppler ultrasound is a special test that shows the speed and direction of blood moving through your blood vessels.

Carotid Angiography

Carotid angiography is a test that uses dye and special X-rays to show the insides of your carotid arteries.

For this test, a small tube called a catheter is put into an artery, usually in the groin (upper thigh). The tube is then moved up into one of your carotid arteries.

Your doctor will inject a substance (called contrast dye) into the carotid artery. The dye helps make the artery visible on X-ray pictures.

Heart Tests

Echocardiography

Echocardiography, or echo, is a painless test that uses sound waves to create pictures of your heart.

The test gives information about the size and shape of your heart and how well your heart's chambers and valves are working.

Echo can detect possible blood clots inside the heart and problems with the aorta. The aorta is the main artery that carries oxygen-rich blood from your heart to all parts of your body.

EKG (Electrocardiogram)

An EKG is a simple, painless test that records the heart's electrical activity. The test shows how fast the heart is beating and its rhythm (steady or irregular). An EKG also records the strength and timing of electrical signals as they pass through each part of the heart.

An EKG can help detect heart problems that may have led to a stroke. For example, the test can help diagnose atrial fibrillation or a previous heart attack.

Section 27.2

Blood Tests for Stroke

This section contains text excerpted from the following
sources: Text in this section begins with excerpts from
"Stroke—How Is a Stroke Diagnosed?" National Heart, Lung,
and Blood Institute (NHLBI), January 27, 2017; Text under
the heading "Types of Blood Tests" is excerpted from "Blood
Tests—Types of Blood Tests," National Heart, Lung, and Blood
Institute (NHLBI), January 6, 2012. Reviewed April 2017.

Your doctor may use blood tests to help diagnose a stroke.

A blood glucose test measures the amount of glucose (sugar) in
your blood. Low blood glucose levels may cause symptoms similar to
those of a stroke.

A platelet count measures the number of platelets in your blood.
Blood platelets are cell fragments that help your blood clot. Abnormal
platelet levels may be a sign of a bleeding disorder (not enough clotting)
or a thrombotic disorder (too much clotting).

Your doctor also may recommend blood tests to measure how long
it takes for your blood to clot. Two tests that may be used are called
prothrombin time (PT) and partial thromboplastin time (PTT) tests.
These tests show whether your blood is clotting normally.

Types of Blood Tests

Some of the most common blood tests are:

- A complete blood count (CBC)

- Blood chemistry tests

- Blood enzyme tests

- Blood tests to assess heart disease risk

Complete Blood Count

The CBC is one of the most common blood tests. It's often done as
part of a routine checkup.

The CBC can help detect blood diseases and disorders, such as anemia, infections, clotting problems, blood cancers, and immune system disorders. This test measures many different parts of your blood, as discussed in the following paragraphs.

Red Blood Cells

Red blood cells carry oxygen from your lungs to the rest of your body. Abnormal red blood cell levels may be a sign of anemia, dehydration (too little fluid in the body), bleeding, or another disorder.

White Blood Cells

White blood cells are part of your immune system, which fights infections and diseases. Abnormal white blood cell levels may be a sign of infection, blood cancer, or an immune system disorder.

A CBC measures the overall number of white blood cells in your blood. A CBC with differential looks at the amounts of different types of white blood cells in your blood.

Platelets

Platelets are blood cell fragments that help your blood clot. They stick together to seal cuts or breaks on blood vessel walls and stop bleeding.

Abnormal platelet levels may be a sign of a bleeding disorder (not enough clotting) or a thrombotic disorder (too much clotting).

Hemoglobin

Hemoglobin is an iron-rich protein in red blood cells that carries oxygen. Abnormal hemoglobin levels may be a sign of anemia, sickle cell anemia, thalassemia, or other blood disorders.

If you have diabetes, excess glucose in your blood can attach to hemoglobin and raise the level of hemoglobin A1c.

Hematocrit

Hematocrit is a measure of how much space red blood cells take up in your blood. A high hematocrit level might mean you're dehydrated. A low hematocrit level might mean you have anemia. Abnormal hematocrit levels also may be a sign of a blood or bone marrow disorder.

Mean Corpuscular Volume

Mean corpuscular volume (MCV) is a measure of the average size of your red blood cells. Abnormal MCV levels may be a sign of anemia or thalassemia.

Blood Chemistry Tests / Basic Metabolic Panel

The basic metabolic panel (BMP) is a group of tests that measures different chemicals in the blood. These tests usually are done on the fluid (plasma) part of blood. The tests can give doctors information about your muscles (including the heart), bones, and organs, such as the kidneys and liver.

The BMP includes blood glucose, calcium, and electrolyte tests, as well as blood tests that measure kidney function. Some of these tests require you to fast (not eat any food) before the test, and others don't. Your doctor will tell you how to prepare for the test(s) you're having.

Blood Glucose

Glucose is a type of sugar that the body uses for energy. Abnormal glucose levels in your blood may be a sign of diabetes.

For some blood glucose tests, you have to fast before your blood is drawn. Other blood glucose tests are done after a meal or at any time with no preparation.

Calcium

Calcium is an important mineral in the body. Abnormal calcium levels in the blood may be a sign of kidney problems, bone disease, thyroid disease, cancer, malnutrition, or another disorder.

Electrolytes

Electrolytes are minerals that help maintain fluid levels and acid-base balance in the body. They include sodium, potassium, bicarbonate, and chloride.

Abnormal electrolyte levels may be a sign of dehydration, kidney disease, liver disease, heart failure, high blood pressure, or other disorders.

Kidneys

Blood tests for kidney function measure levels of blood urea nitrogen (BUN) and creatinine. Both of these are waste products that the kidneys filter out of the body. Abnormal BUN and creatinine levels may be signs of a kidney disease or disorder.

Blood Enzyme Tests

Enzymes are chemicals that help control chemical reactions in your body. There are many blood enzyme tests. This section focuses on blood enzyme tests used to check for heart attack. These include troponin and creatine kinase (CK) tests.

Troponin

Troponin is a muscle protein that helps your muscles contract. When muscle or heart cells are injured, troponin leaks out, and its levels in your blood rise.

For example, blood levels of troponin rise when you have a heart attack. For this reason, doctors often order troponin tests when patients have chest pain or other heart attack signs and symptoms.

Creatine Kinase

A blood product called CK-MB is released when the heart muscle is damaged. High levels of CK-MB in the blood can mean that you've had a heart attack.

Blood Tests to Assess Heart Disease Risk

A lipoprotein panel is a blood test that can help show whether you're at risk for coronary heart disease (CHD). This test looks at substances in your blood that carry cholesterol.

A lipoprotein panel gives information about your:

- Total cholesterol.

- Low-density lipoprotein, or LDL ("bad") cholesterol. This is the main source of cholesterol buildup and blockages in the arteries.

- High-density lipoprotein, or HDL ("good") cholesterol. This type of cholesterol helps decrease blockages in the arteries.

- Triglycerides. Triglycerides are a type of fat in your blood.

A lipoprotein panel measures the levels of LDL and HDL cholesterol and triglycerides in your blood. Abnormal cholesterol and triglyceride levels may be signs of increased risk for CHD.

Most people will need to fast for 9 to 12 hours before a lipoprotein panel.

Blood Clotting Tests

Blood clotting tests sometimes are called a coagulation panel. These tests check proteins in your blood that affect the blood clotting process. Abnormal test results might suggest that you're at risk of bleeding or developing clots in your blood vessels.

Your doctor may recommend these tests if he or she thinks you have a disorder or disease related to blood clotting.

Blood clotting tests also are used to monitor people who are taking medicines to lower the risk of blood clots. Warfarin and heparin are two examples of such medicines.

Section 27.3

Cerebral Angiography

"Cerebral Angiography," © 2017 Omnigraphics.
Reviewed April 2017.

What Is Cerebral Angiography?

Cerebral angiography is a minimally invasive medical diagnostic test that is performed using X-rays and a contrast dye to create images of blood vessels in the brain. During this test, a catheter is inserted in the body to carry the contrast dye to the brain. The catheter makes it possible to perform diagnosis and any necessary treatment during the same procedure. Therefore, use of cerebral angiography may eliminate the need for surgery.

Uses of Cerebral Angiography

Cerebral angiography is used to identify or diagnose certain abnormalities in the brain, such as:

- Blood clot

- Brain tumor
- Inflammation or narrowing of blood vessels
- Aneurysm or stroke
- Tears in artery walls

The test is also used to help identify the cause of physical symptoms such as:

- Severe or frequent headaches
- Slurred speech
- Frequent or persistent dizziness
- Blurred or double vision
- Weakness or numbness in the body
- Loss of coordination or balance

How Cerebral Angiography Works

To conduct cerebral angiography, a doctor or other healthcare provider inserts a thin, hollow tube called a catheter into an artery in the arm or leg. This is done through a small incision in the skin. The catheter is guided through the artery using X-ray imaging. When the catheter reaches the area of the body that is to be examined, a contrast dye is injected through the catheter. This dye enables the creation of X-ray images of the area.

Preparing for Cerebral Angiography

Your doctor or healthcare provider will provide instructions on how to prepare for the test. Generally, preparation includes not eating or drinking anything after midnight on the day of the procedure. You may be instructed to withhold any medications you normally take. Cerebral angiography is usually an outpatient procedure, meaning that you will not have to stay overnight in a hospital. Recovery after cerebral angiography can last several hours. You may be required to have a friend accompany you to the procedure in order to ensure your safe travel back home afterwards.

Risks

Any medical procedure that uses a catheter in the body includes certain risks, such as:

- Damage to blood vessels
- Bruising or bleeding at the catheter introduction site
- Infection
- Blood clot formation
- Plaque dislodging from blood vessel walls and disrupting normal blood flow
- Internal bleeding, although this is a very rare occurrence

It is important to notify your doctor immediately if you experience any of these symptoms after receiving a cerebral angiograph:

- Weakness or numbness in the muscles of your face, arms or legs
- Slurred speech
- Changes in vision
- Chest pain
- Dizziness
- Difficulty breathing
- Rash or sign of infection
- Loss of normal use of the arm or leg where the catheter was inserted

References

1. "Cerebral Angiography," Cleveland Clinic, January 25, 2016.
2. "Cerebral Angiography," HealthLine, n.d.
3. "Cerebral Angiography," RadiologyInfo.org, July 13, 2016.
4. Levy, Jason. "Cerebral Angiography," MedLinePlus, July 3, 2016.

Section 27.4

Echocardiogram

This section includes text excerpted from "Echocardiography,"
National Heart, Lung, and Blood Institute (NHLBI),
October 31, 2011. Reviewed April 2017.

What Is Echocardiography?

Echocardiography, or echo, is a painless test that uses sound waves to create moving pictures of your heart. The pictures show the size and shape of your heart. They also show how well your heart's chambers and valves are working.

Echo also can pinpoint areas of heart muscle that aren't contracting well because of poor blood flow or injury from a previous heart attack. A type of echo called Doppler ultrasound shows how well blood flows through your heart's chambers and valves.

Echo can detect possible blood clots inside the heart, fluid buildup in the pericardium (the sac around the heart), and problems with the aorta. The aorta is the main artery that carries oxygen-rich blood from your heart to your body.

Doctors also use echo to detect heart problems in infants and children.

Who Needs Echocardiography?

Your doctor may recommend echo if you have signs or symptoms of heart problems.

For example, shortness of breath and swelling in the legs are possible signs of heart failure. Heart failure is a condition in which your heart can't pump enough oxygen-rich blood to meet your body's needs. Echo can show how well your heart is pumping blood.

Echo also can help your doctor find the cause of abnormal heart sounds, such as heart murmurs. Heart murmurs are extra or unusual sounds heard during the heartbeat. Some heart murmurs are harmless, while others are signs of heart problems.

Your doctor also may use echo to learn about:

- The size of your heart. An enlarged heart might be the result of high blood pressure, leaky heart valves, or heart failure. Echo also can detect increased thickness of the ventricles (the heart's lower chambers). Increased thickness may be due to high blood pressure, heart valve disease, or congenital heart defects.

- Heart muscles that are weak and aren't pumping well. Damage from a heart attack may cause weak areas of heart muscle. Weakening also might mean that the area isn't getting enough blood supply, a sign of coronary heart disease.

- Heart valve problems. Echo can show whether any of your heart valves don't open normally or close tightly.

- Problems with your heart's structure. Echo can detect congenital heart defects, such as holes in the heart. Congenital heart defects are structural problems present at birth. Infants and children may have echo to detect these heart defects.

- Blood clots or tumors. If you've had a stroke, you may have echo to check for blood clots or tumors that could have caused the stroke.

Your doctor also might recommend echo to see how well your heart responds to certain heart treatments, such as those used for heart failure.

Types of Echocardiography

There are several types of echo—all use sound waves to create moving pictures of your heart. This is the same technology that allows doctors to see an unborn baby inside a pregnant woman.

Unlike X-rays and some other tests, echo doesn't involve radiation.

Transthoracic Echocardiography

Transthoracic echo is the most common type of echocardiogram test. It's painless and noninvasive. "Noninvasive" means that no surgery is done and no instruments are inserted into your body.

This type of echo involves placing a device called a transducer on your chest. The device sends special sound waves, called ultrasound, through your chest wall to your heart. The human ear can't hear ultrasound waves.

309

As the ultrasound waves bounce off the structures of your heart, a computer in the echo machine converts them into pictures on a screen.

Stress Echocardiography

Stress echo is done as part of a stress test. During a stress test, you exercise or take medicine (given by your doctor) to make your heart work hard and beat fast. A technician will use echo to create pictures of your heart before you exercise and as soon as you finish.

Some heart problems, such as coronary heart disease, are easier to diagnose when the heart is working hard and beating fast.

Transesophageal Echocardiography

Your doctor may have a hard time seeing the aorta and other parts of your heart using a standard transthoracic echo. Thus, he or she may recommend transesophageal echo, or TEE.

During this test, the transducer is attached to the end of a flexible tube. The tube is guided down your throat and into your esophagus (the passage leading from your mouth to your stomach). This allows your doctor to get more detailed pictures of your heart.

Fetal Echocardiography

Fetal echo is used to look at an unborn baby's heart. A doctor may recommend this test to check a baby for heart problems. When recommended, the test is commonly done at about 18 to 22 weeks of pregnancy. For this test, the transducer is moved over the pregnant woman's belly.

Three-Dimensional Echocardiography

A three-dimensional (3D) echo creates 3D images of your heart. These detailed images show how your heart looks and works.

During transthoracic echo or TTE, 3D images can be taken as part of the process used to do these types of echo.

Doctors may use 3D echo to diagnose heart problems in children. They also may use 3D echo for planning and overseeing heart valve surgery.

Researchers continue to study new ways to use 3D echo.

What Does Echocardiography Show?

Echo shows the size, structure, and movement of various parts of your heart. These parts include the heart valves, the septum (the wall separating the right and left heart chambers), and the walls of the heart chambers. Doppler ultrasound shows the movement of blood through your heart.

Your doctor may use echo to:

- Diagnose heart problems

- Guide or determine next steps for treatment

- Monitor changes and improvement

- Determine the need for more tests

Echo can detect many heart problems. Some might be minor and pose no risk to you. Others can be signs of serious heart disease or other heart conditions. Your doctor may use echo to learn about:

- The size of your heart. An enlarged heart might be the result of high blood pressure, leaky heart valves, or heart failure. Echo also can detect increased thickness of the ventricles (the heart's lower chambers). Increased thickness may be due to high blood pressure, heart valve disease, or congenital heart defects.

- Heart muscles that are weak and aren't pumping well. Damage from a heart attack may cause weak areas of heart muscle. Weakening also might mean that the area isn't getting enough blood supply, a sign of coronary heart disease.

- Heart valve problems. Echo can show whether any of your heart valves don't open normally or close tightly.

- Problems with your heart's structure. Echo can detect congenital heart defects, such as holes in the heart. Congenital heart defects are structural problems present at birth. Infants and children may have echo to detect these heart defects.

- Blood clots or tumors. If you've had a stroke, you may have echo to check for blood clots or tumors that could have caused the stroke.

What Are the Risks of Echocardiography?

Transthoracic and fetal echo have no risks. These tests are safe for adults, children, and infants.

If you have a TEE, some risks are associated with the medicine given to help you relax. For example, you may have a bad reaction to the medicine, problems breathing, and nausea (feeling sick to your stomach).

Your throat also might be sore for a few hours after the test. Rarely, the tube used during TEE causes minor throat injuries.

Stress echo has some risks, but they're related to the exercise or medicine used to raise your heart rate, not the echo. Serious complications from stress tests are very uncommon.

Section 27.5

Electrocardiogram (EKG)

This section contains text excerpted from the following sources: Text in this section begins with excerpts from "Electrocardiogram," National Heart, Lung, and Blood Institute (NHLBI), December 9, 2016; Text under the heading "How EKG Is Used" is excerpted from "VA Electrocardiogram (EKG) Learn More," U.S. Department of Veterans Affairs (VA), February 2, 2013. Reviewed April 2017.

An electrocardiogram, also called an ECG or EKG, is a simple, painless test that detects and records your heart's electrical activity. An EKG can show how fast your heart is beating, whether the rhythm of your heartbeats is steady or irregular, and the strength and timing of the electrical impulses passing through each part of your heart. You may have an EKG as part of a routine exam to screen for heart disease. This test also is used to detect and study heart problems such as heart attacks, arrhythmia or irregular heartbeat, and heart failure. Results from this test also may suggest other heart disorders.

An EKG may be recorded in a doctor's office, an outpatient facility, in a hospital before major surgery, or as part of stress testing. For the test, you will lie still on a table. A nurse or technician will attach up to 12 electrodes to the skin on your chest, arms, and legs. Your skin may need to be shaved to help the electrodes stick. The electrodes are connected by wires to a machine that records your heart's electrical activity on graph paper or on a computer. After the test, the electrodes will be removed.

An EKG has no serious risks. EKGs don't give off electrical charges such as shocks. You may develop a slight rash where the electrodes were attached to your skin. This rash usually goes away on its own without treatment.

How EKG Is Used

EKGs are used in one of two ways:

1. **Screening**—to determine if you have a certain condition even before you have symptoms

2. **Diagnosing**—used if you have signs, symptoms, or some other reason to think heart problems may be present

Your healthcare provider may recommend additional tests based on the results of your EKG.

Section 27.6

Computerized Tomography (CT) Scan

This section includes text excerpted from "Computed Tomography (CT)," National Institute of Biomedical Imaging and Bioengineering (NIBIB), December 9, 2016.

What Is a Computed Tomography (CT) Scan?

The term "computed tomography," or CT, refers to a computerized X-ray imaging procedure in which a narrow beam of X-rays is aimed at a patient and quickly rotated around the body, producing signals that are processed by the machine's computer to generate cross-sectional images—or "slices"—of the body. These slices are called tomographic images and contain more detailed information than conventional X-rays. Once a number of successive slices are collected by the machine's computer, they can be digitally "stacked" together to form a three-dimensional image of the patient that allows for easier identification and location of basic structures as well as possible tumors or abnormalities.

How Does CT Work?

Unlike a conventional X-ray—which uses a fixed X-ray tube—a CT scanner uses a motorized X-ray source that rotates around the circular opening of a donut-shaped structure called a gantry. During a CT scan, the patient lies on a bed that slowly moves through the gantry while the X-ray tube rotates around the patient, shooting narrow beams of X-rays through the body. Instead of film, CT scanners use special digital X-ray detectors, which are located directly opposite the X-ray source. As the X-rays leave the patient, they are picked up by the detectors and transmitted to a computer.

Each time the X-ray source completes one full rotation, the CT computer uses sophisticated mathematical techniques to construct a 2D image slice of the patient. The thickness of the tissue represented in each image slice can vary depending on the CT machine used, but usually ranges from 1–10 millimeters. When a full slice is completed, the image is stored and the motorized bed is moved forward incrementally into the gantry. The X-ray scanning process is then repeated to produce another image slice. This process continues until the desired number of slices is collected.

Image slices can either be displayed individually or stacked together by the computer to generate a 3D image of the patient that shows the skeleton, organs, and tissues as well as any abnormalities the physician is trying to identify. This method has many advantages including the ability to rotate the 3D image in space or to view slices in succession, making it easier to find the exact place where a problem may be located.

When Would I Get a CT Scan?

CT scans can be used to identify disease or injury within various regions of the body. For example, CT has become a useful screening tool for detecting possible tumors or lesions within the abdomen. A CT scan of the heart may be ordered when various types of heart disease or abnormalities are suspected. CT can also be used to image the head in order to locate injuries, tumors, clots leading to stroke, hemorrhage, and other conditions. It can image the lungs in order to reveal the presence of tumors, pulmonary embolisms (blood clots), excess fluid, and other conditions such as emphysema or pneumonia. A CT scan is particularly useful when imaging complex bone fractures, severely eroded joints, or bone tumors since it usually produces more detail than would be possible with a conventional X-ray.

What Is a CT Contrast Agent?

As with all X-rays, dense structures within the body—such as bone—are easily imaged, whereas soft tissues vary in their ability to stop X-rays and, thus, may be faint or difficult to see. For this reason, intravenous (IV) contrast agents have been developed that are highly visible in an X-ray or CT scan and are safe to use in patients. Contrast agents contain substances that are better at stopping X-rays and, thus, are more visible on an X-ray image. For example, to examine the circulatory system, a contrast agent based on iodine is injected into the bloodstream to help illuminate blood vessels. This type of test is used to look for possible obstructions in blood vessels, including those in the heart. Oral contrast agents, such as barium-based compounds, are used for imaging the digestive system, including the esophagus, stomach, and GI tract.

Are There Risks?

CT scans can diagnose possibly life-threatening conditions such as hemorrhage, blood clots, or cancer. An early diagnosis of these conditions could potentially be life-saving. However, CT scans use X-rays, and all X-rays produce ionizing radiation. Ionizing radiation has the potential to cause biological effects in living tissue. This is a risk that increases with the number of exposures added up over the life of an individual. However, the risk of developing cancer from radiation exposure is generally small.

A CT scan in a pregnant woman poses no known risks to the baby if the area of the body being imaged isn't the abdomen or pelvis. In general, if imaging of the abdomen and pelvis is needed, doctors prefer to use exams that do not use radiation, such as MRI or ultrasound. However, if neither of those can provide the answers needed, or there is an emergency or other time constraint, CT may be an acceptable alternative imaging option.

In some patients, contrast agents may cause allergic reactions, or in rare cases, temporary kidney failure. IV contrast agents should not be administered to patients with abnormal kidney function since they may induce a further reduction of kidney function, which may sometimes become permanent.

Children are more sensitive to ionizing radiation and have a longer life expectancy and, thus, a higher relative risk for developing cancer than adults. Parents may want to ask the technologist or doctor if their machine settings have been adjusted for children.

Section 27.7

Magnetic Resonance Imaging (MRI)

This section contains text excerpted from the following sources:
Text beginning with the heading "What Is Magnetic Resonance
Imaging (MRI)?" is excerpted from "Magnetic Resonance
Imaging (MRI)," National Institute of Biomedical Imaging and
Bioengineering (NIBIB), May 4, 2013. Reviewed April 2017; Text
under the heading "More Sensitive Stroke Detection" is excerpted
from "More Sensitive Stroke Detection," National Institutes
of Health (NIH), August 20, 2015.

What Is Magnetic Resonance Imaging (MRI)?

MRI is a noninvasive imaging technology that produces three dimensional detailed anatomical images without the use of damaging radiation. It is often used for disease detection, diagnosis, and treatment monitoring. It is based on sophisticated technology that excites and detects the change in the direction of the rotational axis of protons found in the water that makes up living tissues.

How Does MRI Work?

MRIs employ powerful magnets which produce a strong magnetic field that forces protons in the body to align with that field. When a radiofrequency current is then pulsed through the patient, the protons are stimulated, and spin out of equilibrium, straining against the pull of the magnetic field. When the radiofrequency field is turned off, the MRI sensors are able to detect the energy released as the protons realign with the magnetic field. The time it takes for the protons to realign with the magnetic field, as well as the amount of energy released, changes depending on the environment and the chemical nature of the molecules. Physicians are able to tell the difference between various types of tissues based on these magnetic properties.

To obtain an MRI image, a patient is placed inside a large magnet and must remain very still during the imaging process in order not to blur the image. Contrast agents (often containing the element Gadolinium) may be given to a patient intravenously before or during the

MRI to increase the speed at which protons realign with the magnetic field. The faster the protons realign, the brighter the image.

What Is MRI Used For?

MRI scanners are particularly well suited to image the non-bony parts or soft tissues of the body. They differ from computed tomography (CT), in that they do not use the damaging ionizing radiation of X-rays. The brain, spinal cord and nerves, as well as muscles, ligaments, and tendons are seen much more clearly with MRI than with regular X-rays and CT; for this reason MRI is often used to image knee and shoulder injuries.

In the brain, MRI can differentiate between white matter and grey matter and can also be used to diagnose aneurysms and tumors. Because MRI does not use X-rays or other radiation, it is the imaging modality of choice when frequent imaging is required for diagnosis or therapy, especially in the brain. However, MRI is more expensive than X-ray imaging or CT scanning.

One kind of specialized MRI is functional Magnetic Resonance Imaging (fMRI). This is used to observe brain structures and determine which areas of the brain "activate" (consume more oxygen) during various cognitive tasks. It is used to advance the understanding of brain organization and offers a potential new standard for assessing neurological status and neurosurgical risk.

Are There Risks?

Although MRI does not emit the damaging ionizing radiation that is found in X-ray and CT imaging, it does employ a strong magnetic field. The magnetic field extends beyond the machine and exerts very powerful forces on objects of iron, some steels, and other magnetizable objects; it is strong enough to fling a wheelchair across the room. Patients should notify their physicians of any form of medical or implant prior to an MR scan.

When having an MRI scan, the following should be taken into consideration:

- People with implants, particularly those containing iron—pacemakers, vagus nerve stimulators, implantable cardioverter-defibrillators, loop recorders, insulin pumps, cochlear implants, deep brain stimulators, and capsules from capsule endoscopy should not enter an MRI machine.

- Noise—loud noise commonly referred to as clicking and beeping, as well as sound intensity up to 120 decibels in certain MR scanners, may require special ear protection.

- Nerve stimulation—a twitching sensation sometimes results from the rapidly switched fields in the MRI.

- Contrast agents—patients with severe renal failure who require dialysis may risk a rare but serious illness called nephrogenic systemic fibrosis that may be linked to the use of certain gadolinium-containing agents, such as gadodiamide and others. Although a causal link has not been established, current guidelines in the United States recommend that dialysis patients should only receive gadolinium agents when essential, and that dialysis should be performed as soon as possible after the scan to remove the agent from the body promptly.

- Pregnancy—while no effects have been demonstrated on the fetus, it is recommended that MRI scans be avoided as a precaution especially in the first trimester of pregnancy when the fetus' organs are being formed and contrast agents, if used, could enter the fetal bloodstream.

- Claustrophobia—people with even mild claustrophobia may find it difficult to tolerate long scan times inside the machine. Familiarization with the machine and process, as well as visualization techniques, sedation, and anesthesia provide patients with mechanisms to overcome their discomfort. Additional coping mechanisms include listening to music or watching a video or movie, closing or covering the eyes, and holding a panic button. The open MRI is a machine that is open on the sides rather than a tube closed at one end, so it does not fully surround the patient. It was developed to accommodate the needs of patients who are uncomfortable with the narrow tunnel and noises of the traditional MRI and for patients whose size or weight make the traditional MRI impractical. Newer open MRI technology provides high quality images for many but not all types of examinations.

More Sensitive Stroke Detection

Researchers at the National Institute of Neurological Disorders and Stroke (NINDS) have found that magnetic resonance imaging (MRI) can provide a more sensitive diagnosis than computed tomography (CT) for the most common type of stroke, called ischemic stroke.

The researchers studied more than 350 patients who arrived in the emergency room with suspected strokes to determine whether MRI or CT was better for rapid diagnosis. Doctors face an urgent need to swiftly distinguish between acute ischemic stroke, which is caused by clots in blood vessels, and hemorrhagic stroke, which is caused by bleeding into the brain, because the two types of stroke are treated in very different ways.

Standard CT uses X-rays which are passed through the body at different angles and processed by a computer as cross-sectional images, or slices of the internal structure of the body or organ. Standard MRI uses computer-generated radio waves and a powerful magnet to produce detailed slices or three-dimensional images of body structures and nerves. A contrast dye may be used in both imaging techniques to enhance visibility of certain areas or tissues.

Results of the NINDS study showed that standard MRI is superior to standard CT in diagnosing acute stroke, particularly acute ischemic stroke. That is very good news for patients, says NINDS Deputy Director Walter J. Koroshetz, M.D., noting that brain injury from ischemic stroke often can be avoided if clot-busting therapy is administered within three hours of stroke onset.

Section 27.8

Ultrasound

This section includes text excerpted from "Ultrasound,"
National Institute of Biomedical Imaging and
Bioengineering (NIBIB), July 2016.

What Is Medical Ultrasound?

Medical ultrasound falls into two distinct categories: diagnostic and therapeutic.

Diagnostic ultrasound is a noninvasive diagnostic technique used to image inside the body. Ultrasound probes, called transducers, produce sound waves that have frequencies above the threshold of human hearing (above 20KHz), but most transducers in current use operate at much higher frequencies (in the megahertz (MHz) range). Most diagnostic ultrasound probes are placed on the skin. However, to optimize image quality, probes may be placed inside the body via the gastrointestinal tract, vagina, or blood vessels. In addition, ultrasound is sometimes used during surgery by placing a sterile probe into the area being operated on.

Diagnostic ultrasound can be further sub-divided into anatomical and functional ultrasound. Anatomical ultrasound produces images of internal organs or other structures. Functional ultrasound combines information such as the movement and velocity of tissue or blood, softness or hardness of tissue, and other physical characteristics, with anatomical images to create "information maps." These maps help doctors visualize changes/differences in function within a structure or organ.

Therapeutic ultrasound also uses sound waves above the range of human hearing but does not produce images. Its purpose is to interact with tissues in the body such that they are either modified or destroyed. Among the modifications possible are: moving or pushing tissue, heating tissue, dissolving blood clots, or delivering drugs to specific locations in the body. These destructive, or ablative, functions are made possible by use of very high-intensity beams that can destroy diseased or abnormal tissues such as tumors. The advantage of using ultrasound therapies is that, in most cases, they are noninvasive. No incisions or cuts need to be made to the skin, leaving no wounds or scars.

How Does It Work?

Ultrasound waves are produced by a transducer, which can both emit ultrasound waves, as well as detect the ultrasound echoes reflected back. In most cases, the active elements in ultrasound transducers are made of special ceramic crystal materials called piezoelectrics. These materials are able to produce sound waves when an electric field is applied to them, but can also work in reverse, producing an electric field when a sound wave hits them. When used in an ultrasound scanner, the transducer sends out a beam of sound waves into the body. The sound waves are reflected back to the transducer by boundaries between tissues in the path of the beam (e.g., the boundary between fluid and soft tissue or tissue and bone). When these echoes hit the transducer, they generate electrical signals that are sent to the ultrasound scanner. Using the speed of sound and the time of each echo's return, the scanner calculates the distance from the transducer to the tissue boundary. These distances are then used to generate two-dimensional images of tissues and organs.

During an ultrasound exam, the technician will apply a gel to the skin. This keeps air pockets from forming between the transducer and the skin, which can block ultrasound waves from passing into the body.

What Is Ultrasound Used For?

Diagnostic ultrasound. Diagnostic ultrasound is able to noninvasively image internal organs within the body. However, it is not good for imaging bones or any tissues that contain air, like the lungs. Under some conditions, ultrasound can image bones (such as in a fetus or in small babies) or the lungs and lining around the lungs, when they are filled or partially filled with fluid. One of the most common uses of ultrasound is during pregnancy, to monitor the growth and development of the fetus, but there are many other uses, including imaging the heart, blood vessels, eyes, thyroid, brain, breast, abdominal organs, skin, and muscles. Ultrasound images are displayed in either 2D, 3D, or 4D (which is 3D in motion).

Functional ultrasound. Functional ultrasound applications include Doppler and color Doppler ultrasound for measuring and visualizing blood flow in vessels within the body or in the heart. It can also measure the speed of the blood flow and direction of movement. This is done using color-coded maps called color Doppler imaging. Doppler ultrasound is commonly used to determine whether plaque buildup inside the carotid arteries is blocking blood flow to the brain.

Another functional form of ultrasound is elastography, a method for measuring and displaying the relative stiffness of tissues, which can be used to differentiate tumors from healthy tissue. This information can be displayed as either color-coded maps of the relative stiffness; black-and-white maps that display high-contrast images of tumors compared with anatomical images; or color-coded maps that are overlayed on the anatomical image. Elastography can be used to test for liver fibrosis, a condition in which excessive scar tissue builds up in the liver due to inflammation.

Ultrasound is also an important method for imaging interventions in the body. For example, ultrasound-guided needle biopsy helps physicians see the position of a needle while it is being guided to a selected target, such as a mass or a tumor in the breast. Also, ultrasound is used for real-time imaging of the location of the tip of a catheter as it is inserted in a blood vessel and guided along the length of the vessel. It can also be used for minimally invasive surgery to guide the surgeon with real-time images of the inside of the body.

Therapeutic or interventional ultrasound. Therapeutic ultrasound produces high levels of acoustic output that can be focused on specific targets for the purpose of heating, ablating, or breaking up tissue. One type of therapeutic ultrasound uses high-intensity beams of sound that are highly targeted, and is called High Intensity Focused Ultrasound (HIFU). HIFU is being investigated as a method for modifying or destroying diseased or abnormal tissues inside the body (e.g., tumors) without having to open or tear the skin or cause damage to the surrounding tissue. Either ultrasound or MRI is used to identify and target the tissue to be treated, guide and control the treatment in real time, and confirm the effectiveness of the treatment. HIFU is currently U.S. Food and Drug Administration (FDA) approved for the treatment of uterine fibroids, to alleviate pain from bone metastases, and most recently for the ablation of prostate tissue. HIFU is also being investigated as a way to close wounds and stop bleeding, to break up clots in blood vessels, and to temporarily open the blood brain barrier so that medications can pass through.

Are There Risks?

Diagnostic ultrasound is generally regarded as safe and does not produce ionizing radiation like that produced by X-rays. Still, ultrasound is capable of producing some biological effects in the body under specific settings and conditions. For this reason, the FDA requires that diagnostic ultrasound devices operate within acceptable limits. The FDA, as well as many professional societies, discourage the casual use of ultrasound and recommend that it be used only when there is a true medical need.

Chapter 28

Stroke Treatment

Treatment for a stroke depends on whether it is ischemic or hemorrhagic. Treatment for a transient ischemic attack (TIA) depends on its cause, how much time has passed since symptoms began, and whether you have other medical conditions.

Strokes and TIAs are medical emergencies. If you have stroke symptoms, call 9-1-1 right away. Do not drive to the hospital or let someone else drive you. Call an ambulance so that medical personnel can begin life-saving treatment on the way to the emergency room. During a stroke, every minute counts.

Once you receive immediate treatment, your doctor will try to treat your stroke risk factors and prevent complications by recommending heart-healthy lifestyle changes.

Treating an Ischemic Stroke or Transient Ischemic Attack

An ischemic stroke or TIA occurs if an artery that supplies oxygen-rich blood to the brain becomes blocked. Often, blood clots cause the blockages that lead to ischemic strokes and TIAs. Treatment for an ischemic stroke or TIA may include medicines and medical procedures.

This chapter includes text excerpted from "Stroke—How Is a Stroke Treated?" National Heart, Lung, and Blood Institute (NHLBI), January 27, 2017.

Medicines

If you have a stroke caused by a blood clot, you may be given a clot-dissolving, or clot-busting, medication called tissue plasminogen activator (tPA). A doctor will inject tPA into a vein in your arm. This type of medication must be given within 4 hours of symptom onset. Ideally, it should be given as soon as possible. The sooner treatment begins, the better your chances of recovery. Thus, it's important to know the signs and symptoms of a stroke and to call 9-1-1 right away for emergency care.

If you can't have tPA for medical reasons, your doctor may give you antiplatelet medicine that helps stop platelets from clumping together to form blood clots or anticoagulant medicine (blood thinner) that keeps existing blood clots from getting larger. Two common medicines are aspirin and clopidogrel.

Medical Procedures

If you have carotid artery disease, your doctor may recommend a carotid endarterectomy or carotid artery angioplasty. Both procedures open blocked carotid arteries.

Researchers are testing other treatments for ischemic stroke, such as intra-arterial thrombolysis and mechanical clot removal in cerebral ischemia (MERCI).

In intra-arterial thrombolysis, a long flexible tube called a catheter is put into your groin (upper thigh) and threaded to the tiny arteries of the brain. Your doctor can deliver medicine through this catheter to break up a blood clot in the brain.

MERCI is a device that can remove blood clots from an artery. During the procedure, a catheter is threaded through a carotid artery to the affected artery in the brain. The device is then used to pull the blood clot out through the catheter.

Treating a Hemorrhagic Stroke

A hemorrhagic stroke occurs if an artery in the brain leaks blood or ruptures. The first steps in treating a hemorrhagic stroke are to find the cause of bleeding in the brain and then control it. Unlike ischemic strokes, hemorrhagic strokes aren't treated with antiplatelet medicines and blood thinners because these medicines can make bleeding worse.

If you're taking antiplatelet medicines or blood thinners and have a hemorrhagic stroke, you'll be taken off the medicine. If high blood pressure is the cause of bleeding in the brain, your doctor may prescribe medicines to lower your blood pressure. This can help prevent further bleeding.

Surgery also may be needed to treat a hemorrhagic stroke. The types of surgery used include aneurysm clipping, coil embolization, and arteriovenous malformation (AVM) repair.

Aneurysm Clipping and Coil Embolization

If an aneurysm (a balloon-like bulge in an artery) is the cause of a stroke, your doctor may recommend aneurysm clipping or coil embolization.

Aneurysm clipping is done to block off the aneurysm from the blood vessels in the brain. This surgery helps prevent further leaking of blood from the aneurysm. It also can help prevent the aneurysm from bursting again. During the procedure, a surgeon will make an incision (cut) in the brain and place a tiny clamp at the base of the aneurysm. You'll be given medicine to make you sleep during the surgery. After the surgery, you'll need to stay in the hospital's intensive care unit for a few days.

Coil embolization is a less complex procedure for treating an aneurysm. The surgeon will insert a tube called a catheter into an artery in the groin. He or she will thread the tube to the site of the aneurysm. Then, a tiny coil will be pushed through the tube and into the aneurysm. The coil will cause a blood clot to form, which will block blood flow through the aneurysm and prevent it from bursting again. Coil embolization is done in a hospital. You'll be given medicine to make you sleep during the surgery.

Arteriovenous Malformation (AVM) Repair

If an AVM is the cause of a stroke, your doctor may recommend an AVM repair. (An AVM is a tangle of faulty arteries and veins that can rupture within the brain.) AVM repair helps prevent further bleeding in the brain.

Doctors use several methods to repair AVMs. These methods include:

- Injecting a substance into the blood vessels of the AVM to block blood flow

- Surgery to remove the AVM

- Using radiation to shrink the blood vessels of the AVM

Treating Stroke Risk Factors

After initial treatment for a stroke or TIA, your doctor will treat your risk factors. He or she may recommend heart-healthy lifestyle changes to help control your risk factors.

Heart-healthy lifestyle changes may include:

- Heart-healthy eating
- Aiming for a healthy weight
- Managing stress
- Physical activity
- Quitting smoking

If heart-healthy lifestyle changes aren't enough, you may need medicine to control your risk factors.

Chapter 29

Surgical Procedures Used in the Treatment of Stroke

Chapter Contents

Section 29.1—Brain Aneurysm Repair 328

Section 29.2—Carotid Artery Angioplasty and
Stent Placement 337

Section 29.3—Carotid Endarterectomy 346

Section 29.1

Brain Aneurysm Repair

This section includes text excerpted from "FDA
Executive Summary," U.S. Food and Drug
Administration (FDA), April 17, 2015.

Aneurysm Treatment Methods

While aneurysm occurrence can be relatively common, the treatment methods prescribed have been the subject of controversy for a number of years. With the advent of the less invasive endovascular treatments there has been an increase in the number of unruptured aneurysms that are being treated rather than followed, but a consensus has yet to be reached as to which aneurysms are best treated with which method.

Surgical Clipping

Aneurysms, both ruptured and unruptured, may be treated via craniotomy (brain surgery) by surgical clip ligation and microsurgical clips placed on the aneurysm neck in order to remove the aneurysm from the circulation and prevent possible rupture (or if the aneurysm had already ruptured, to prevent re-rupture). Some feel that surgical clipping is still the best option for particular aneurysms types. The advantage with this technique is that it can provide immediate aneurysm occlusion and has been shown to provide positive results for patients with large and giant aneurysms and the immediate occlusion reduces the risk of subarachnoid hemorrhage (SAH). As part of the International Subarachnoid Aneurysm Trial (ISAT) that compared open surgery to endovascular coiling, clipping was shown to have a lower annual risk of rebleeding in previously ruptured aneurysms, 3.6 percent and 4.2 percent for clipping and coiling respectively at 7 year follow up. It has also been shown that clipped aneurysms are 4 times less likely to be retreated than with endovascular treatment. It is important to note however, that clipped aneurysms are much less likely to have follow-up imaging.

While there are some clear benefits to surgical clipping there are also some concerns. There was a higher mortality rate associated with open surgery, 10.7 percent and 13.8 percent for traditional coiling and surgical clipping respectively. Patient age has been shown to be a strong indicator of poor surgical outcome. This phenomenon is most easily attributed to the inherent trauma that any open surgical procedure carries. It has also been shown that surgical clipping carries an increased risk of seizures both in the short- and long-term follow up. It was showed that 4.1 percent of surgical patients (compared to 2.5 percent of the interventional patients) had seizures associated with rebleed after receiving treatment for their aneurysm. Surgical clipping is also not immune to interaction with perforators. While open surgery allows for visualization of perforators that may not be visible on angiography, there still is a risk of unintentionally clipping a perforator which will cause immediate occlusion and could significantly affect a patient's outcome.

Coiling

Endovascular treatment methods offer a less invasive method to treat intracranial aneurysms. For traditional coiling a catheter, typically inserted in the femoral artery, is tracked through the vasculature to the aneurysm where coils are placed inside the body of the aneurysm to promote occlusion. The first endovascular method was performed using detachable embolic coils which were placed through a guide catheter into the aneurysm to promote occlusion. The number of coils used varied depending on the size of the aneurysm. An early trial included 15 patients all of which showed significant benefit from the procedure. Subsequent to this first trial, several larger studies have investigated the benefit of coiling for aneurysm repair. The largest of these investigations was the ISAT which studied 2143 patients treated with either surgical clipping or coiling. This study found that while there was a small increased risk of recurrent bleeding from coiling, 1.0 percent and 0.3 percent for coiling and clipping respectively, a decreased risk of death was observed at 5 years for patients treated endovascularly, 10.7 percent and 13.8 percent for coiling and clipping.

A study retrospectively investigated the treatment of 173 patients with unruptured aneurysms (202 total aneurysms) over a 12 year period, all treated with traditional coiling. Aneurysms in this study were primarily small (<7 mm) and medium (7–12 mm) in size, 43.5 percent and 37.1 percent respectively, and were most frequently found in the in the internal carotid artery (ICA), 43.1 percent. Of the 202 aneurysms, 57.5 percent demonstrated complete occlusion following the procedure. This outcome was significantly higher for small sized aneurysms (71.6%). Giant aneurysms (>25 mm) resulted in the poorest initial occlusion rate at 10.5 percent rising only slightly to 11.8 percent at follow up. Morbidity and mortality rates for the 173 patients were relatively low, 3.5 percent and 0.5 percent, respectively. The most common complication found in this study was thromboembolic events with 3 percent of these patients suffering a stroke. This study also noted a strong dependence on neck size and occlusion rate. Aneurysms with narrow necks had an occlusion rate of 77.1 percent while the rate for wide-neck aneurysms was 35.8 percent. These results suggest that not all aneurysms types may be best suited for treatment with traditional coiling.

A prospective study was performed to investigate the use of detachable coils in 169 aneurysms. This study focused almost exclusively on smaller aneurysms (<8 mm) with aneurysms most frequently occurring in the ICA (35%). Immediate occlusion was seen in 56 percent of the aneurysms with that number rising to 79 percent at follow up. Of the 148 aneurysms that reached complete occlusion, 20 (14%) required retreatment within the first 3–40 months after treatment. This study showed almost no connection between retreatment rate and anatomical location but did show a slight dependence on neck size, with wide-neck (defined the by dome to neck ratio < 2) having a higher probability of requiring retreatment. Although traditional coiling is less invasive than surgical clipping, the possible need for retreatment is another important factor when deciding on a treatment method.

Balloon-Assisted Coiling

One of the concerns associated with coiling is the possibility of coils protruding into the arterial lumen and occluding flow in the parent artery. To help mitigate this risk, a procedure referred to as Balloon-Assisted Coiling (BAC), also known as the Remodeling Technique (RT), was developed. During this technique, a balloon is inflated inside the parent artery after a microcatheter used to deliver the coils is placed inside the neck of the aneurysms. The coils are then detached with the balloon inflated to allow the clinician to more tightly pack the aneurysm without the risk of coils protruding into the lumen.

A study investigated BAC as part of the Analysis of Treatment by Endovascular approach of Nonruptured Aneurysms (ATENA Trial). This was a prospective trial that included 649 patients harboring

739 unruptured aneurysms. The majority of these aneurysms (54.5%) were treated with traditional coiling, while (37.3%) were treated using BAC. Of 739 unruptured aneurysms, 91.9 percent were located in the anterior circulation with only 60 (8.1%) aneurysms in the posterior circulation. Aneurysm size was classified using the following groupings: 1 to 3 mm (17.7%), 4 to 6 mm (41.1%), 7 to 10 mm (29.1%), and 11 to 15 mm (12%). Aneurysms greater than 15 mm were listed as part of the exclusion criteria. Postoperative evaluation of aneurysm occlusion (evaluated by a core laboratory) showed that 59.0 percent had complete occlusion, 21.7 percent had some neck remnant (i.e., flow still present in a portion of the aneurysm neck) and 19.3 percent had aneurysm remnant (i.e., flow still present in the dome of the aneurysm). When comparing the number of complications between traditional coiling and BAC, this study showed an increased percentage of patients had thromboembolic complications with coiling as compared to BAC (7.3 percent compared to 5.5 percent respectively). While this information helps to support use of the BAC technique for anterior aneurysm, little is known about the efficacy in the posterior portion of the neurovasculature because of the small number of subjects with aneurysms in the posterior neurovasculature.

A review article discussed some of the differing opinions on the safety and effectiveness of BAC, such as complication rates and thrombus events as well as the treatment of wide-neck aneurysms (neck > 4 mm). One of the studies included in this review indicated there was increased risk of procedure related complications with BAC, 14.1 percent as opposed to 3.0 percent seen with traditional coiling. A study had shown that complication rates are similar, 10.8 percent and 11.7 percent for BAC and traditional coiling respectively. Another study showed that the rate of thrombus events is also comparable between these two techniques (14 percent and 9 percent for BAC and traditional coiling respectively). For treating wide-neck (> 4 mm) aneurysms a retrospective study by Chalouhi et al. found that SAC had higher occlusion rate then BAC, 75.4 percent versus 50 percent respectively, as well as a lower retreatment rate, 4.3 percent and 15.6 percent.

The apparent disagreement between studies using BAC suggests that additional studies are required to fully understand the complete benefit/risk profile associated with BAC.

Stent-Assisted Coiling (SAC)

In conjunction with detachable coil technology, SAC utilizes a stent placed across the opening of the aneurysms to aid in coil packing which in turn promotes occlusion. Similar to BAC, these stents act as a rigid structure that helps prevent protrusion of the coils into the parent vessel. The only SAC systems approved by the U.S. Food and Drug Administration (FDA) are through the humanitarian device exemption (HDE) process where the regulatory determination for approval is an assessment of the risks and probable benefits of the device which is different than the evidence required to provide a reasonable assurance that the device is safe and effective for its intended use under the PMA regulatory path.

One development in SAC came with the introduction of self-expandable stents. Previous stent iterations required the use of a balloon for placement of the stent (similar to the original cardiac stents) which limited use to regions of the neurovasculature that could be accessed using balloon catheters, and the devices had reduced stent flexibility. Self-expanding stents are constructed from nitinol, a shape memory alloy that eliminates the requirement for a balloon, thus improving tractability and removing the risk of rupturing the parent vessel through balloon overexpansion. These stents were also relatively large in diameter which made delivery into some of the smaller vessel in the neurovasculature more difficult. Subsequent device iterations allowed for greater access to new portions of the neurovasculature. Nonetheless, long-term follow-up for devices used in these regions remains unavailable and therefore, effectiveness of this technique has not been established.

One of the first studies to investigate the use of SAC for the treatment of intracranial aneurysms utilized coronary balloon expandable stents in sections of the internal carotid, vertebral, and basilar arteries. Of the 10 patients treated in this study there were no permanent periprocedural complications. Greater than 90 percent occlusion was seen in all 8 of the patients treated with both a stent and detachable coils (2 patients were treated with stenting alone). In-stent stenosis was noted on follow up angiography for at least one of the patients. This study demonstrated the technical feasibility of using stents to aid in the coiling of intracranial aneurysms but the authors at the time noted that while immediate results were positive, long-term effects were still unknown.

A study demonstrated the use of a specifically designed intracranial microstents (Neurofrom) for use with both ruptured and unruptured wide-necked intracranial aneurysms. This study included 48 patients with 49 aneurysms (32 of which were unruptured). Eight of the stent deployments failed. Forty-one aneurysms were stented then coiled, six were treated with stent only, and one aneurysm was coiled and then stented. The mortality rate for this trial was 8.9 percent with four patients (7%) experiencing a thromboembolic event with an overall complication rate of 10.7 percent. Complete occlusion was reported in 35 (66%) of the patients treated. These early findings suggested that a device could provide possible benefit to a previously under-severed patient population could be achieved. This device was approved by the FDA under HDE.

In one of the first studies that investigated the use of SAC specifically for wide-neck intracranial aneurysms, twenty-two patients harboring 23 aneurysms (16 unruptured) were treated with SAC. These aneurysms were primarily located in the ICA (60%). Immediate occlusion was reported in 43 percent of the aneurysms studied in this trial. Interestingly, this study reported infrequent in-stent thrombosis even when patients were not given antithrombolytics due to the presence of SAH. The authors also reported no evidence of stent-related thromboembolic complications during the follow up period. While this study again highlights the utilization of SAC for the treatment of wide-neck aneurysms, the authors assert that longer periods of follow-up are required before a better understanding of the safety and efficacy can be reached. As this technology has been further developed, SAC has been shown to have a lower recurrence rate (i.e., flow returning to the aneurysm dome) compared to coiling alone. Clinical outcomes of 1137 patients with 1325 aneurysms were retrospectively analyzed. Of these aneurysms 206 (16.5%) were treated with stents while the remaining aneurysms (1109) were treated with coiling alone. A significantly higher recurrence rate was seen in the patients treated with coiling alone versus those treated with stents. A study suggested that one factor reducing recurrence rates in SAC is improvements to arterial wall reconstruction at the aneurysm neck. This study is affected by the technological development in stent design that occurred over the course of enrollment, which caused variation in the results. Although tighter packing of coils is more difficult with SAC than coiling alone, follow-up results show SAC to have a better long-term occlusion rate.

Flow Diverters

One of the developments in the treatment of aneurysms has been flow diversion technology. One flow diverter is approved by FDA. Flow diverters function by reducing the blood flow from the parent artery into the aneurysm. While similar in concept to a stent used for SAC, flow diverters have a significantly higher mesh density preventing flow in the parent artery from entering the aneurysm thus eliminating the need for a coil. This reduction in flow is designed to promote blood stasis, endothelial growth across the neck, and occlusion of the aneurysm. Typically when an aneurysm is treated with either coils, stent-assisted coils, or surgical clipping, aneurysm occlusion occurs very rapidly which will protect against bleeding or rebleeding. Alternatively, a complete occlusion was observed in only 49 percent of patients at 3 months and 95 percent of patients at 6 months post procedure. Although a portion of the slower occlusion progression may be attributed to the antiplatelet regimen prescribed to patients, this progression is slower in flow diverters where the aneurysm is left empty. This latent occlusion has been cited as a potential major safety risk because of the possibility for aneurysm rupture during this time.

One common flow diverter described in the literature is the Pipeline Embolization Device (PED, ev3). One study conducted on PED included 53 patients harboring 63 aneurysms who were enrolled in this multicenter trial. All of the aneurysms treated were wide-neck which was defined as a dome-to-neck ratio of <2 or a neck size > 4 mm. The majority of the aneurysms included in this study were located along the anterior circulation (87%). Due to the inherent nature of flow diversion which works endoluminally, immediate occlusion was only seen in 5 aneurysms (8%) all of which were < 10 mm in their maximum dimension. At 6-month of follow-up 93 percent (26 of the 28 available aneurysms, not all patients were available at follow up) had complete occlusion with this percentage rising slightly at 12 months to 94.4 percent (17 of the 18 available aneurysms).

A second study called the Pipeline Embolization Device for the Intracranial Treatment of Aneurysm Trial (PITA) investigated 31 patients harboring 31 aneurysms with all but two located in the anterior circulation. These aneurysms were primarily small, <10 mm (64.5%) and only 2 cases (6.5%) > 25 mm. While PED is intended to be used without adjunctive coiling, 16 of 31 aneurysms included in this trial used coils in addition to the PED. At follow-up (180 days) 93.3 percent of the aneurysms had been fully occluded with no reported device migrations. Mild in-stent stenosis (25%–50%) was reported in one case. This trial demonstrates the technical feasibility of flow diverters. It should also be noted that this study involved adjunctive coiling, an off-label use in the United States; additional testing will be important to demonstrate a reasonable assurance of safety and effectiveness.

A study reported on early experiences with another flow diverter technology called SILK flow diverter in 70 patients as part of a prospective multicenter study outside the United States (OUS). Primarily the patients in this study presented with either wide-neck or fusiform aneurysms (91%). Immediately after treatment only 7 (10%) had complete occlusion of their aneurysm with occlusion rates rising to 49 percent at follow-up. Follow-up angiography was specified at one month after stoppage of antiplatelet therapy (median of 119 days of follow-up). Similar to early experience with SAC systems, there were 15 reports (21%) of deployment related complications. The morbidity and mortality rates for this trial were 4 percent and 8 percent respectively (4 deaths and 2 cases of permanent neurological deficit).

As discussed above, these improving angiographic outcomes using flow diverter technology are in contrast to what is typically seen with coiling procedures. As reported earlier, coiling procedures have demonstrated favorable immediate occlusion results but reports also note high recurrence rates especially for large (>10 mm) and wide-neck aneurysms. The ability of flow diverters to produce endothelial growth across the aneurysm neck is an important factor in providing long-term aneurysm occlusion. Flow diverters also by design do not typically require manipulation of the aneurysm sack which reduces the risk of rupture.

A meta-analysis of the literature was performed that included 29 studies with a total of 1654 aneurysms treated with flow diverters. This analysis showed that 76 percent of these aneurysms achieved complete occlusion at 6 months with procedure related morbidity and mortality as low as 5 percent and 4 percent respectively. One of the major concerns with flow diverters is the risk of rupture due to the latency of occlusion. It has been estimated that the risk for SAH after treatment with a flow diverter could be between 2 and 4 percent and the rate of SAH and intraparenchymal hemorrhage decreases after the first 30 days post treatment.

Although flow diverters are becoming more prevalent, safety and effectiveness data is limited for use in both the anterior circulation and posterior circulation, regions of the brain that are outside the approved labeling of approved devices. The PED device is only indicated for use in ICA from the petrous to the superior hypophyseal segment while the SAC systems (all with HDE approval) are approved for all locations in the neurovasculature. The use of the PED in other regions of the neurovasculature has not been shown to demonstrate a reasonable assurance of safety and effectiveness. In addition, the risk of occluding perforator arteries exists. Specifically, occlusion of perforating vessels can lead to infarcts which can significantly impact patient function. A study investigated 32 posterior aneurysms to evaluate the safety associated with the use of these types of devices. This study showed complete occlusion of the target aneurysm in 86 percent of the patients at 6 months with 100 percent occlusion seen in those patients followed > 2 years. The authors note that higher clinical perforator infarction in basilar artery compared to the carotid may be seen with the PED. In this study perforator occlusion was seen in 3 patients (14%). While no deaths or poor neurological outcomes were reported, this investigation highlights the fact that flow diverters can produce varying results based on the target aneurysm location and aneurysm location may be a factor in deciding the best course of treatment.

Other Treatment Approaches

Pharmacotherapy may include prescribed drugs that lower your blood pressure or reduce the impact of the heart's contraction and minimizing the risk of a rupture. Another approach may be drug therapies with ongoing observations, and periodic assessment to track the aneurysm status. Additional approaches reported in the literature include the development and use of precipitates, second generation stents of various designs, aneurysm liners, liquid polymers, hydrogels, aneurysm neck protection, and microanastomoses, bioactive manipulations to endovascular devices.

Section Review

When deciding on a treatment method for aneurysms, there are a number of factors that can be considered such as size, morphology, anatomical location, rupture rate as well as patient age. A number of treatment strategies exist, each involving specific benefit/risk considerations.

Coiling is a less invasive approach than open surgery for treating aneurysms. There is a risk of increased bleeding with coiling versus clipping but the long-term mortality rate has been shown to be lower. Not all aneurysms types may be appropriate for coiling as wide-neck aneurysm (> 4 mm) have been shown to have a lower occlusion rate.

Balloon-assisted coiling is a method to increase the coil packing density without leaving a permanent implant in the parent vessel. Studies suggest that complications rates for BAC and traditional coiling are similar. However the disagreement for thrombus events, complication rates, and occlusion rates suggests that this method still requires further evaluation before the associated benefits and risks are better understood.

Stent-assisted coiling provides another approach to treat wide-neck aneurysms but the impact of stents placed in the neurovasculature is still unknown. Published literature has also stated that longer term follow-up is still required to better understand all of the benefits and risks associated with this device type.

Similar to SAC, the effect of flow diverters on the surrounding vasculature (e.g., perforators) is still not completely understood. Understanding the impact of flow diverter technologies in specific sections of the neurovasculature will help to further examine the benefit risk ratio in other areas of the neurovasculature.

Section 29.2

Carotid Artery Angioplasty and Stent Placement

This section includes text excerpted from "Stents," National Heart, Lung, and Blood Institute (NHLBI), December 17, 2013. Reviewed April 2017.

What Is a Stent?

A stent is a small mesh tube that's used to treat narrow or weak arteries. Arteries are blood vessels that carry blood away from your heart to other parts of your body.

A stent is placed in an artery as part of a procedure called percutaneous coronary intervention (PCI), also known as coronary angioplasty. PCI restores blood flow through narrow or blocked arteries. A stent helps support the inner wall of the artery in the months or years after PCI.

Doctors also may place stents in weak arteries to improve blood flow and help prevent the arteries from bursting.

Stents usually are made of metal mesh, but sometimes they're made of fabric. Fabric stents, also called stent grafts, are used in larger arteries.

Some stents are coated with medicine that is slowly and continuously released into the artery. These stents are called drug-eluting stents. The medicine helps prevent the artery from becoming blocked again.

How Are Stents Used?

For the Coronary Arteries

Doctors may use stents to treat coronary heart disease (CHD). CHD is a disease in which a waxy substance called plaque builds up inside the coronary arteries. These arteries supply your heart muscle with oxygen-rich blood.

When plaque builds up in the arteries, the condition is called atherosclerosis.

Plaque narrows the coronary arteries, reducing the flow of oxygen-rich blood to your heart. This can lead to chest pain or discomfort called angina.

The buildup of plaque also makes it more likely that blood clots will form in your coronary arteries. If blood clots block a coronary artery, a heart attack will occur.

Doctors may use percutaneous coronary intervention (PCI), and stents to treat CHD. During PCI, a thin, flexible tube with a balloon or other device on the end is threaded through a blood vessel to the narrow or blocked coronary artery.

Once in place, the balloon is inflated to compress the plaque against the wall of the artery. This restores blood flow through the artery, which reduces angina and other CHD symptoms.

Unless an artery is too small, a stent usually is placed in the treated portion of the artery during PCI. The stent supports the artery's inner wall. It also reduces the chance that the artery will become narrow or blocked again. A stent also can support an artery that was torn or injured during PCI.

Even with a stent, there's about a 10–20 percent chance that an artery will become narrow or blocked again in the first year after PCI. When a stent isn't used, the risk can be as much as 10 times as high. Research has shown that as time goes by, people who have coronary artery stents are in less danger of risks from the surgery but more prone to the risks of chronic diseases, such as type 2 diabetes and renal failure.

For the Carotid Arteries

Doctors also may use stents to treat carotid artery disease. This is a disease in which plaque builds up in the arteries that run along each side of your neck. These arteries, called carotid arteries, supply oxygen-rich blood to your brain.

The buildup of plaque in the carotid arteries limits blood flow to your brain and puts you at risk for a stroke.

Doctors use stents to help support the carotid arteries after they're widened with PCI. Researchers continue to explore the risks and benefits of carotid artery stenting.

For Other Arteries

Plaque also can narrow other arteries, such as those in the kidneys and limbs. Narrow kidney arteries can affect kidney function and lead to severe high blood pressure.

Narrow arteries in the limbs, a condition called peripheral artery disease (P.A.D.), can cause pain and cramping in the affected arm or leg. Severe narrowing can completely cut off blood flow to a limb, which could require surgery.

To relieve these problems, doctors may do PCI on a narrow kidney, arm, or leg artery. They often will place a stent in the affected artery during the procedure. The stent helps support the artery and keep it open.

For the Aorta in the Abdomen or Chest

The aorta is a major artery that carries oxygen-rich blood from the left side of the heart to the body. This artery runs through the chest and down into the abdomen.

Over time, some areas of the aorta's walls can weaken. These weak areas can cause a bulge in the artery called an aneurysm. An aneurysm in the aorta can burst, leading to serious internal bleeding. When aneurysms occur, they're usually in the abdominal aorta.

To help avoid a burst, doctors may place a fabric stent in the weak area of the abdominal aorta. The stent creates a stronger inner lining for the artery.

Aneurysms also can develop in the part of the aorta that runs through the chest. Doctors also use stents to treat these aneurysms. How well the stents work over the long-term still isn't known.

To Close Off Aortic Tears

Another problem that can occur in the aorta is a tear in its inner wall. If blood is forced into the tear, it will widen.

The tear can reduce blood flow to the tissues that the aorta serves. Over time, the tear can block blood flow through the artery or burst. If this happens, it usually occurs in the chest portion of the aorta.

Researchers are developing and testing new kinds of stents that will prevent blood from flowing into aortic tears. A stent placed within the torn area of the aorta might help restore normal blood flow and reduce the risk of a burst aorta.

How Are Stents Placed?

Doctors place stents in arteries as part of a procedure called PCI. To place a stent, your doctor will make a small opening in a blood vessel in your groin (upper thigh), arm, or neck.

Through this opening, your doctor will thread a thin, flexible tube called a catheter. The catheter will have a deflated balloon at its tip.

A stent is placed around the deflated balloon. Your doctor will move the tip of the catheter to the narrow section of the artery or to the aneurysm or aortic tear site.

Special X-ray movies will be taken of the tube as it's threaded through your blood vessel. These movies will help your doctor position the catheter.

For Arteries Narrowed by Plaque

Your doctor will use special dye to help show narrow or blocked areas in the artery. He or she will then move the catheter to the area and inflate the balloon.

As the balloon inflates, it pushes the plaque against the artery wall. This widens the artery and helps restore blood flow. The fully extended balloon also expands the stent, pushing it into place in the artery.

The balloon is deflated and pulled out along with the catheter. The stent remains in your artery. Over time, cells in your artery grow to cover the mesh of the stent. They create an inner layer that looks like the inside of a normal blood vessel.

Coronary Artery Stent Placement

A very narrow artery, or one that's hard to reach with a catheter, may require more steps to place a stent. At first, your doctor may use a small balloon to expand the artery. He or she then removes the balloon.

The small balloon is replaced with a larger balloon that has a collapsed stent around it. At this point, your doctor can follow the standard process of compressing the plaque and placing the stent.

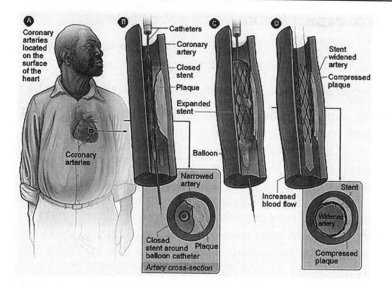

Figure 29.1. *Coronary Artery Stent Placement*

Figure A shows the location of the heart and coronary arteries. Figure B shows the deflated balloon catheter and closed stent inserted into the narrow coronary artery. The inset image shows a cross-section of the artery with the inserted balloon catheter and closed stent. In figure C, the balloon is inflated, expanding the stent and compressing the plaque against the artery wall. Figure D shows the stent-widened artery. The inset image shows a cross-section of the compressed plaque and stent-widened artery.

Doctors use a special filter device when doing PCI and stent placement on the carotid arteries. The filter helps keep blood clots and loose pieces of plaque from traveling to the brain during the procedure.

For Aortic Aneurysms

The procedure to place a stent in an artery with an aneurysm is very similar to the one described above. However, the stent used to treat an aneurysm is different. It's made out of pleated fabric instead of metal mesh, and it often has one or more tiny hooks.

The stent is expanded to fit tight against the artery wall. The hooks latch on to the wall of the artery, holding the stent in place.

The stent creates a new inner lining for that portion of the artery. Over time, cells in the artery grow to cover the fabric. They create an inner layer that looks like the inside of a normal blood vessel.

341

What to Expect before a Stent Procedure

Most stent procedures require an overnight stay in a hospital and someone to take you home. Talk with your doctor about:

- when to stop eating and drinking before coming to the hospital
- what medicines you should or shouldn't take on the day of the procedure
- when to come to the hospital and where to go

If you have diabetes, kidney disease, or other conditions, ask your doctor whether you need to take any extra steps during or after the procedure to avoid complications.

Before the procedure, your doctor may talk to you about medicines you'll likely need to take after the stent is placed. These medicines help prevent blood clots from forming in the stent.

You'll need to know how long you should take these medicines and why they're important.

What to Expect during a Stent Procedure

For Arteries Narrowed by Plaque

This procedure usually takes about an hour. It might take longer if stents are inserted into more than one artery during the procedure.

Before the procedure starts, you'll get medicine to help you relax. You'll be on your back and awake during the procedure. This allows you to follow your doctor's instructions.

Your doctor will numb the area where the catheter will be inserted. You won't feel the doctor threading the catheter, balloon, or stent inside the artery. You may feel some pain when the balloon is expanded to push the stent into place.

For Aortic Aneurysms

Although this procedure takes only a few hours, it often requires a 2- to 3-day hospital stay.

Before the procedure, you'll be given medicine to help you relax. If your doctor is placing the stent in your abdominal aorta, you may receive medicine to numb your stomach area. However, you'll be awake during the procedure.

If your doctor is placing the stent in the chest portion of your aorta, you'll likely receive medicine to make you sleep during the procedure.

Once you're numb or asleep, your doctor will make a small cut in your groin (upper thigh). He or she will insert a catheter into the blood vessel through this cut.

Sometimes two cuts (one in the groin area of each leg) are needed to place fabric stents that come in two parts. You will not feel the doctor threading the catheter, balloon, or stent into the artery.

What to Expect after a Stent Procedure

Recovery

After either type of stent procedure (for arteries narrowed by plaque or aortic aneurysms), your doctor will remove the catheter from your artery. The site where the catheter was inserted will be bandaged.

A small sandbag or other type of weight may be put on top of the bandage to apply pressure and help prevent bleeding. You'll recover in a special care area, where your movement will be limited.

While you're in recovery, a nurse will check your heart rate and blood pressure regularly. The nurse also will look to see whether you're bleeding from the insertion site.

Eventually, a small bruise and sometimes a small, hard "knot" will appear at the insertion site. This area may feel sore or tender for about a week.

You should let your doctor know if:

- You have a constant or large amount of bleeding at the insertion site that can't be stopped with a small bandage.

- You have any unusual pain, swelling, redness, or other signs of infection at or near the insertion site.

Common Precautions after a Stent Procedure

Blood Clotting Precautions

After a stent procedure, your doctor will likely recommend that you take aspirin and another anticlotting medicine. These medicines help prevent blood clots from forming in the stent. A blood clot can lead to a heart attack, stroke, or other serious problems.

If you have a metal stent, your doctor may recommend aspirin and another anticlotting medicine for at least 1 month. If your stent is coated with medicine, your doctor may recommend aspirin and another anticlotting medicine for 12 months or more. Your doctor will work with you to decide the best course of treatment.

Your risk of blood clots significantly increases if you stop taking the anticlotting medicine too early. Taking these medicines for as long as your doctor recommends is important. He or she may recommend lifelong treatment with aspirin.

If you're considering surgery for some other reason while you're on these medicines, talk to your doctor about whether it can wait until after you've stopped the medicine. Anticlotting medicines may increase the risk of bleeding.

Also, anticlotting medicines can cause side effects, such as an allergic rash. Talk to your doctor about how to reduce the risk of these side effects.

Other Precautions

You should avoid vigorous exercise and heavy lifting for a short time after the stent procedure. Your doctor will let you know when you can go back to your normal activities.

Metal detectors used in airports and other screening areas don't affect stents. Your stent shouldn't cause metal detectors to go off.

If you have an aortic fabric stent, your doctor will likely recommend follow up imaging tests (for example, chest X-ray) within the first year of having the procedure. After the first year, he or she may recommend yearly imaging tests.

Lifestyle Changes

Stents help prevent arteries from becoming narrow or blocked again in the months or years after PCI. However, stents aren't a cure for atherosclerosis or its risk factors.

Making lifestyle changes can help prevent plaque from building up in your arteries again. Talk with your doctor about your risk factors for atherosclerosis and the lifestyle changes you'll need to make.

Lifestyle changes may include changing your diet, quitting smoking, being physically active, losing weight, and reducing stress. You also should take all medicines as your doctor prescribes. Your doctor may suggest taking statins, which are medicines that lower blood cholesterol levels.

What Are the Risks of Having a Stent?

Risks Related to Percutaneous Coronary Intervention

Percutaneous coronary intervention (PCI), the procedure used to place stents, is a medical procedure that is commonly known as coronary angioplasty. PCI carries a small risk of serious complications, such as:

- Bleeding from the site where the catheter was inserted into the skin

- Damage to the blood vessel from the catheter

- Arrhythmias (irregular heartbeats)

- Damage to the kidneys caused by the dye used during the procedure

- An allergic reaction to the dye used during the procedure

- Infection

Another problem that can occur after PCI is too much tissue growth within the treated portion of the artery. This can cause the artery to become narrow or blocked again. When this happens, it's called restenosis.

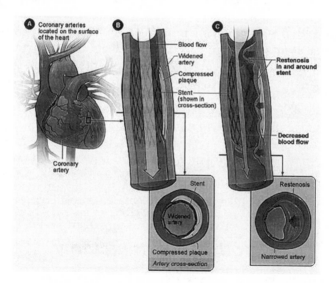

Figure 29.2. *Restenosis of a Stent-Widened Coronary Artery*

Figure A shows the coronary arteries located on the surface of the heart. Figure B shows a stent-widened artery with normal blood flow. The inset image shows a cross-section of the stent-widened artery. In figure C, tissue grows through and around the stent over time. This causes a partial blockage of the artery and abnormal blood flow. The inset image shows a cross-section of the tissue growth around the stent.

Using drug-eluting stents can help prevent this problem. These stents are coated with medicine to stop excess tissue growth.

Treating the tissue around the stent with radiation also can delay tissue growth. For this procedure, the doctor threads a wire through a catheter to the stent. The wire releases radiation and stops cells around the stent from growing and blocking the artery.

Risks Related to Stents

About 1–2 percent of people who have stented arteries develop a blood clot at the stent site. Blood clots can cause a heart attack, stroke, or other serious problems. The risk of blood clots is greatest during the first few months after the stent is placed in the artery.

Your doctor will likely recommend that you take aspirin and another anticlotting medicine, such as clopidogrel, for at least 1 month or up to a year or more after having a stent procedure. These medicines help prevent blood clots.

The length of time you need to take anticlotting medicines depends on the type of stent you have. Your doctor may recommend lifelong treatment with aspirin.

Stents coated with medicine may raise your risk of dangerous blood clots. (These stents often are used to keep clogged heart arteries open.) However, research hasn't proven that these stents increase the chances of having a heart attack or dying, if used as recommended.

Section 29.3

Carotid Endarterectomy

This section includes text excerpted from "Questions and Answers about Carotid Endarterectomy," National Institute of Neurological Disorders and Stroke (NINDS), March 21, 2016.

What Is a Carotid Endarterectomy?

A carotid endarterectomy is a surgical procedure in which a doctor removes fatty deposits blocking one of the two carotid arteries, the main supply of blood for the brain. Carotid artery problems become more common as people age. The disease process that causes the buildup of fat and other material inside the artery walls is called atherosclerosis, popularly known as "hardening of the arteries." The fatty deposit is called plaque; the narrowing of the artery is called stenosis. The degree of stenosis is usually expressed as a percentage of the normal diameter of the opening.

Why Is Surgery Performed?

Carotid endarterectomy is performed to prevent stroke. Two large clinical trials supported by the National Institute of Neurological Disorders and Stroke (NINDS) have identified specific individuals for whom the surgery is beneficial when performed by surgeons and in institutions that can match the standards set in those studies. The surgery has been found highly beneficial for persons who have already had a stroke or experienced the symptoms of a stroke and have a severe stenosis of 70 to 99 percent. In this group, surgery reduces the estimated 2-year risk of stroke or death by more than 80 percent, from greater than 1 in 4 to less than 1 in 10.

For patients who have already had transient or mild stroke symptoms due to moderate carotid stenosis (50 to 69 percent), surgery reduces the 5-year risk of stroke or death by 6.5 percent. The failure rate for ipsilateral stroke or death for the medical group is 22.2 percent, and for the surgery group is 15.7 percent from greater than 1 in 4 to less than 1 in 7. Individuals who have already had stroke symptoms, and who have carotid stenosis greater than 50 percent, may wish to consider surgery to prevent future stroke. Based on findings of the North American Symptomatic Carotid Endarterectomy Trial (NASCET) trial, patients with moderate (50 to 69 percent) stenosis are now better able to make more informed decisions.

In another trial (Asymptomatic Carotid Atherosclerosis Study, or ACAS), the procedure has also been found highly beneficial for persons who are symptom-free but have a carotid stenosis of 60 to 99 percent. In this group, the surgery reduces the estimated 5-year risk of stroke by more than one-half, from about 1 in 10 to less than 1 in 20.

The Carotid Revascularization Endarterectomy vs. Stenting Trial (CREST) compared carotid endarterectomy surgery to carotid artery stenting and found no significance between the procedures regarding the 4-year rate of stroke or death in patients with or without a previous stroke. The pivotal differences were the lower rate of stroke following surgery and the lower rate of heart attack following stenting.

The study also found that the age of the patient made a difference with a larger benefit for stenting, the younger the age of the patient. At age 69 and younger, stenting results were slightly better. Conversely, for patients older than 70, surgical benefits were slightly superior to stenting, with larger benefit for surgery, the older the patient.

What Is a Stroke?

A stroke occurs when blood flow is cut off from part of the brain. In the same way that a person suffering a loss of blood to the heart can be said to be having a "heart attack," a person with a loss of blood to the brain can be said to be having a *"brain attack."* There are two kinds of stroke, hemorrhagic and ischemic. Hemorrhagic strokes are caused by bleeding within the brain. Ischemic strokes, which are far more common, are caused by a blockage of blood flow in an artery in the head or neck leading to the brain. Some ischemic strokes are due to stenosis, or narrowing of arteries due to the buildup of plaque, fatty deposits and blood clots along the artery wall. A vascular disease that can cause stenosis is atherosclerosis, in which deposits of plaque build up along the inner wall of large and medium-sized arteries, decreasing blood flow. Atherosclerosis in the carotid arteries, two large arteries in the neck that carry blood to the brain, is a major risk factor for ischemic stroke.

What Are the Symptoms of a Stroke?

Symptoms of stroke include:

- Sudden numbness, weakness, or paralysis of face, arm or leg, especially on one side of the body.

- Sudden confusion, trouble talking or understanding speech.

- Sudden trouble seeing in one or both eyes.

- Sudden trouble walking, loss of balance, or coordination.

- Sudden severe headache with no known cause (often described as the worst headache in a person's life).

Symptoms may last a few moments and then disappear. When they disappear within 24 hours or less, they are called a transient ischemic attacks (TIA).

How Important Is a Blockage as a Cause of Stroke?

A blockage of a blood vessel is the most frequent cause of stroke and is responsible for about 80 percent of the approximately 700,000 strokes in the United States each year. Stroke is the leading cause of adult disability in the United States with 2 million of the 3 million Americans who have survived a stroke sustaining some permanent disability. The overall cost of stroke to the nation is $40 billion a year.

How Many Carotid Endarterectomies Are Performed Each Year?

An estimated 140,000 carotid endarterectomies were performed in the United States in 2009, according to the National Hospital Discharge Survey (NHDS). The procedure was first described in the mid-1950s. It began to be used increasingly as a stroke prevention measure in the 1960s and 1970s. Its use peaked in the mid-1980s when more than 100,000 operations were performed each year. At that time, several authorities began to question the trend and the risk-benefit ratio for some groups, and the use of the procedure dropped precipitously. The NINDS-supported NASCET and ACAS trials were launched in the mid-1980s to identify the specific groups of people with carotid artery disease who would clearly benefit from the procedure.

What Are the Risk Factors and How Risky Is the Surgery?

Important risk factors in addition to the degree of stenosis include, gender, diabetes, the type of stroke symptoms, and blockage of the carotid artery on the opposite side. Without other complicating illnesses, age alone is not a worrisome risk factor. Risk factors can affect patients in two ways. They can, particularly in combination, greatly increase a person's risk of having a stroke. In addition, these risk factors can increase the likelihood of surgical complications.

How Is Carotid Artery Disease Diagnosed?

In some cases, the disease can be detected during a normal checkup by a physician. In other cases further testing is needed. Some of the tests a physician can use or order include ultrasound imaging, arteriography, and magnetic resonance angiography (MRA). Frequently these procedures are carried out in a stepwise fashion: from a doctor's evaluation of signs and symptoms to ultrasound, MRA, and arteriography for increasingly difficult cases.

- **History and physical exam.** A doctor will ask about symptoms of a stroke such as numbness or muscle weakness, speech or vision difficulties, or lightheadedness. Using a stethoscope, a doctor may hear a rushing sound, called a bruit in the carotid artery. Unfortunately, dangerous levels of disease sometimes fail to make a sound, and some blockages with a low risk can make the same sound.

- **Ultrasound imaging.** This is a painless, noninvasive test in which sound waves above the range of human hearing are sent into the neck. Echoes bounce off the moving blood and the tissue in the artery and can be formed into an image. Ultrasound is fast, risk-free, relatively inexpensive, and painless compared to MRA and arteriography.

- **Arteriography.** This can be used to confirm the findings of ultrasound imaging which can be uncertain in some cases. Arteriography is an X-ray of the carotid artery taken when a special dye is injected into the artery. A burning sensation may be felt when the dye is injected. An arteriogram is more expensive and carries its own small risk of causing a stroke.

  - **Magnetic Resonance Angiography (MRA).** This is an imaging technique that avoids most of the risks associated with arteriography. An MRA is a type of image that uses magnetism instead of X-rays to create an image of the carotid arteries.

What Is "Best Medical Therapy" for Stroke Prevention?

The mainstay of stroke prevention is risk factor management: smoking cessation, treatment of high blood pressure, and control of blood sugar levels among persons with diabetes. Additionally, physicians may prescribe aspirin, warfarin, or ticlopidine for some individuals.

Chapter 30

Medications Used to Treat Stroke

Chapter Contents

Section 30.1—Tissue Plasminogen Activator (tPA)
and Thrombolytic Therapy 352

Section 30.2—Antiplatelets and Anticoagulants 355

Section 30.3—Blood Pressure-Lowering Drugs......................... 357

Section 30.4—Taking Statins after Stroke Reduces
Risk of Death 369

Section 30.1

Tissue Plasminogen Activator (tPA) and Thrombolytic Therapy

This section contains text excerpted from the following sources:
Text under the heading "Tissue Plasminogen Activator (tPA)" is
excerpted from "Stroke—Stroke Treatment," Center for Disease
Control and Prevention (CDC), March 27, 2017; Text beginning
with the heading "Use of tPA" is excerpted from "Stroke: Percent of
Acute Ischemic Stroke Patients for Whom IV T-PA Was Initiated
at the Hospital within 3 Hours (Less than or Equal to 180 Minutes)
of Time Last Known Well," Agency for Healthcare Research
and Quality (AHRQ), U.S. Department of Health and Human
Services (HHS), October 2015.

Tissue Plasminogen Activator (tPA)

Tissue plasminogen activator (tPA) is a thrombolytic. tPA improves
the chances of recovering from a stroke. Studies show that patients
with ischemic strokes who receive tPA are more likely to recover fully
or have less disability than patients who do not receive the drug.
Patients treated with tPA are also less likely to need long-term care
in a nursing home. Unfortunately, many stroke victims don't get to
the hospital in time for tPA treatment.

Use of tPA

The administration of thrombolytic agents to carefully screened,
eligible patients with acute ischemic stroke has been shown to be
beneficial in several clinical trials. These included two positive randomized controlled trials in the United States: the National Institute
of Neurological Disorders and Stroke (NINDS) Studies, Part I and
Part II. Based on the results of these studies, the U.S. Food and Drug
Administration (FDA) approved the use of intravenous recombinant
tissue plasminogen activator (IV r-TPA or tPA) for the treatment of
acute ischemic stroke when given within 3 hours of stroke symptom
onset. A large meta-analysis controlling for factors associated with
stroke outcome confirmed the benefit of IV tPA in patients treated

within 3 hours of symptom onset. While controversy still exists among some specialists, the major society practice guidelines developed in the United States all recommend the use of IV tPA for eligible patients. Physicians with experience and skill in stroke management and the interpretation of computed tomography (CT) scans should supervise treatment.

The European Cooperative Acute Stroke Study (ECASS) III trial indicated that intravenous r-TPA can be given safely to, and can improve outcomes for, carefully selected patients treated 3 to 4.5 hours after stroke; however, as the NINDS investigators concluded, the earlier that IV thrombolytic therapy is initiated, the better the patient outcome. Therefore, the target for IV tPA initiation remains within 3 hours of time last known well. The administration of IV thrombolytic therapy beyond 3 hours of stroke symptom onset has not been FDA approved.

Additional Information Supporting Need for the Measure

- Thrombolytic therapy is one of the most promising treatments for acute ischemic stroke. The majority of strokes are due to blockage of an artery in the brain by a blood clot. Prompt treatment with clot dissolving (thrombolytic) drugs can restore blood flow before major brain damage has occurred. In the United States, Canada, and most European countries, alteplase/recombinant tissue plasminogen activator (r-tPA) has been approved for use within three hours of stroke symptom onset. Successful treatment is likely to improve neurological outcomes for ischemic stroke patients at three months and later; however, intracranial hemorrhage is a serious complication of therapy and may be fatal.

- Clinical practice guidelines for intravenous thrombolysis with r-tPA cite the NINDS r-tPA Stroke Study (1995), which partially supported the approval of r-tPA by the FDA. The NINDS trial was conducted in two consecutive parts. Part A trials in the 1980s studied very low doses of thrombolytic therapy, given daily by intravenous route for several days. The onset of treatment occurred anytime from 5 to 14 days post symptom onset. Part A trials did not collect data on functional outcome. Part B trials from the 1990s and later used a single large dose of thrombolytic drug (80 to 100 mg r-tPA), given intravenously

353

(IV) or intra-arterially (IA) within three, six, nine, or 24 hours of stroke. The primary end point in Part B of the study was a favorable outcome, defined as complete or nearly complete neurological recovery 3 months after stroke. Favorable outcomes were achieved in 31 percent to 50 percent of patients treated with r-tPA, as compared to 20 percent to 38 percent of patients given placebo. The benefit was similar one year after stroke. The major risk of treatment was symptomatic intracranial hemorrhage which occurred in 6.4 percent of patients treated with r-tPA and 0.6 percent of patients given placebo.

- In 2008, European Cooperative Acute Stroke Study (ECASS)-3, a multi-center, prospective, randomized, placebo-controlled trial, studied the administration of r-tPA between three and 4.5 hours of stroke symptom onset. The trial enrolled 418 patients treated with r-tPA per the current dosing guidelines (i.e., 0.9 mg/kg [maximum of 90 mg] with 10 percent given as an initial IV bolus and the remainder infused over one hour) and compared them with 403 who were given placebo. The frequency of the primary efficacy outcome (i.e., modified Rankin Scale score of 0 to 1 at 90 days after treatment) was significantly greater with r-tPA (52.4%) than with placebo (45.2 percent; odds ratio [OR] 1.34, 95 percent confidence interval [CI] 1.02 to 1.76; risk ratio 1.16, 95 percent CI 1.01 to 1.34; P=0.04). The point estimate for the degree of benefit seen in ECASS-3 (OR for global favorable outcome, 1.28, 95 percent CI 1.00 to 1.65) was less than the point estimate of benefit found in the pool of patients enrolled for 0 to 3 hours after stroke symptom onset in the NINDS study (OR 1.9, 95% CI 1.2 to 2.9).

Section 30.2

Antiplatelets and Anticoagulants

This section includes text excerpted from "Anticoagulants,"
LiverTox®, National Institutes of Health (NIH), March 9, 2017.

Antithrombotic agents are separated into those drugs that decrease the synthesis of coagulation factors or interrupt the coagulation cascade (anticoagulants) and those that inhibit platelet function (antiplatelet agents). A third class of agents are the thrombolytic drugs, which act to promote dissolution of thromboses after they have formed. The antithrombotic agents are rare causes of clinically apparent acute liver injury.

Anticoagulants are used largely for the prevention and treatment of venous thromboses, although they have some activity against arterial thromboses. Their major clinical use is prevention and treatment of deep vein thrombosis in high risk persons (such as after hip or knee replacement surgery or with prolonged immobilization), prevention and treatment of pulmonary embolism, and prevention of arterial embolism in patients with atrial fibrillation.

The anticoagulant agents in clinical use and their year of approval include heparin and its low molecular weight derivatives (dalteparin: 1994, enoxaparin: 1993, and tinzaparin: 2000), direct thrombin inhibitors such as dabigatran (2010) and desirudin (2003), factor Xa inhibitors such as fondaparinux (2001), rivaroxaban (2011) apixaban (2012) and edoxaban (2015), and warfarin (1967), a vitamin K antagonist.

Antiplatelet agents are effective for the prevention and treatment of arterial thromboses (which are platelet rich). Aspirin is an irreversible inhibitor of cyclooxygenase 1, which blocks platelet activation and aggregation for the life of the platelet. Aspirin is an irreversible inhibitor of cyclooxygenase 1, which blocks platelet activation and aggregation for the life of the platelet. Aspirin is commonly used for treatment and prevention of coronary, cerebrovascular and other arterial thromboses (myocardial infarction, stroke, peripheral vascular disease). Dipyridamole blocks adenosine uptake which results in inhibition of platelet aggregation; it is used with or without aspirin for secondary prevention of myocardial infarction or stroke. The thienopyridines inhibit the major adenosine diphosphate receptor on platelets which blocks their activation and aggregation; these agents are also used for secondary prevention of coronary and cerebrovascular thrombosis. Ticagrelor is a platelet aggregation inhibitor with activity similar to the thienopyridines that is used with aspirin (<100 mg daily) as secondary prevention of arterial thrombosis with acute coronary syndrome. Finally, the glycoprotein IIb/IIIa receptor blockers have an immediate effect in preventing platelet aggregation blocking the action of fibrinogen and von Willebrand factor on these platelet receptors; these agents are administered intravenously and are used to attain immediate platelet inhibition in acute coronary syndrome or percutaneous coronary artery intervention. They have not been convincingly linked to instances of clinically apparent acute liver injury.

The antiplatelet drugs in current use and their year of approval include aspirin, dipyridamole (a pyrimidopyrimidine derivative: 1961), the thienopyridines including ticlopidine (1991), clopidogrel (1997), and prasugrel (2009), ticagrelor (an agent with activity similar to the thienopyridines: 2011), and the intravenously administered glycoprotein IIb/IIIa receptor blockers including abciximab and eptifibatide.

Thrombolytic drugs include tissue plasminogen activators (tPA: alteplase, reteplase and tenecteplase), anistreplase, streptokinase and urokinase. These agents are administered intravenously immediately or soon after arterial or venous thromboses or emboli. These agents have not been definitely linked to instances of acute liver injury. Because of their highly restricted use, they are not discussed in LiverTox.

Other antithrombotic agents include defibrotide, which is a complex mixture of single stranded polydeoxyribonucleotides derived from porcine intestinal mucosa that has antithrombotic and profibrinolytic activity and is used in the treatment of severe sinusoidal obstruction syndrome after hematopoietic cell transplantation. Finally, anagrelide is an antithrombotic agent that inhibits the production of platelets, thereby reducing platelet counts, which is used to treat essential thrombocytosis and other causes of thombocythemia associated with an increased rate of arterial or venous thromboses.

Section 30.3

Blood Pressure-Lowering Drugs

This section includes text excerpted from "High Blood Pressure—Medicines to Help You," U.S. Food and Drug Administration (FDA), December 18, 2014.

High Blood Pressure Is a Serious Illness

High blood pressure is often called a "silent killer" because many people have it but do not know it. Some people do not feel sick at first. Over time, people who do not get treated for high blood pressure can get very sick or even die.

High blood pressure can cause:

- stroke

- kidney failure

- blindness and

- heart attacks.

There are life-saving medicines people can take every day to help control their high blood pressure. People who eat healthy foods, exercise, and take their medicines every day can control their blood pressure.

Take Your Blood Pressure Medicines

It is important to take your blood pressure medicines every day. Take your medicines even when your blood pressure comes down— even when you do not feel bad. Do not stop taking your medicine until your doctor says that it is OK.

Most people who take high blood pressure medicines do not get any side effects. Like all medicines, high blood pressure medicines can sometimes cause side effects. Some people have common problems like headaches, dizziness or an upset stomach. These problems are small compared to what could happen if you do not take your medicine.

Understanding Your Blood Pressure—What Do the Numbers Mean?

When you have your blood pressure taken, you are told 2 numbers, like 120/80. Both numbers are important.

The first number is your pressure when your heart beats (**systolic pressure**).

The second number is your pressure when your heart relaxes (**diastolic pressure**).

High Blood Pressure Medicines

Use this section to help you talk to your doctor about your blood pressure medicines. Ask your doctor about the risks of taking your medicine. This section only talks about some of the risks. Tell your doctor about any problems you are having. Also, tell your doctor if you are pregnant, nursing or planning to get pregnant. Your doctor will help you find the medicine that is best for you.

The different kinds of blood pressure medicines are listed below. The drugs are listed in groups. The brand names and generic names are given for the drugs in each group. Find your drug. Then read some basic information about your kind of drug.

Types of High Blood Pressure Medicines

Angiotension-Converting Enzyme (ACE) Inhibitors

Table 30.1. Angiotension-Converting Enzyme (ACE) Inhibitors

Brand Name	Generic Name
Aceon	Perindopril
Accupril	Quinapril
Altace	Ramipril
Capoten	Captopril
Lotensin	Benazepril
Mavik	Trandolapril
Monopril	Fosinopril
Prinivil	Lisinopril
Univasc	Moexipril
Vasotec	Enalapril
	Enalaprilat
Zestril	Lisinopril

Warnings

- Women who are pregnant should talk to their doctor about the risks of using these drugs late in pregnancy.
- People who have kidney or liver problems, diabetes, or heart problems should talk to their doctor about the risks of using ACE drugs.
- People taking diuretics (water pills) should talk to their doctor about the risks of using ACE drugs.

Common Side Effects

- Cough
- Dizziness
- Feeling tired
- Headache
- Problems sleeping
- Fast heart beat

Warning Signs

Call your doctor if you have any of these signs:

- Chest pain
- Problems breathing or swallowing
- Swelling in the face, eyes, lips, tongue, or legs

Beta Blockers

Table 30.2. Beta Blockers

Brand Name	Generic Name
Bystolic	Nebivolol
	Timolol
Coreg	Carvedilol
Corgard	Nadolol
Inderal	Propranolol
Inderal LA	Propranolol
	Betaxolol

Table 30.2. Continued

Brand Name	Generic Name
Levatol	Penbutolol
Lopressor	Metoprolol
Sectral	Acebutolol
Tenormin	Atenolol
Toprol XL	Metoprolol
Trandate	Labetalol
	Pindolol
Zebeta	Bisoprolol

Warnings

- Do not use these drugs if you have slow heart rate, heart block or shock.

- Women who are pregnant or nursing should talk to their doctor before they start using beta blockers.

- The elderly and people who have kidney or liver problems, asthma, diabetes or overactive thyroid should talk to their doctor about the specific risks of using any of these beta blockers.

Common Side Effects

- Feeling tired

- Upset stomach

- Headache

- Dizziness

- Constipation/diarrhea

- Feeling lightheaded

Warning Signs

Call your doctor if you have any of these signs:

- Chest pain

- Problems breathing

- Slow or irregular heartbeat

- Swelling in the hands, feet, or legs

Calcium Channel Blockers (CCBs)

Table 30.3. Calcium Channel Blockers

Brand Name	Generic Name
Norvasc	Amlodipine
Cleviprex	Clevidipine
Cardizem	Diltiazem
Dilacor XR	Diltiazem
Tiazac	Diltiazem
Plendil	Felodipine
DynaCirc CR	Isradipine
Cardene	Nicardipine
Adalat CC	Nifedipine
Procardia	Nifedipine
	Nimodipine
Sular	Nisoldipine
Calan	Verapamil
Covera HS	Verapamil
Isoptin	Verapamil
Verelan	Verapamil

Warnings

- Do not use calcium channel blockers if you have a heart condition or if you are taking nitrates, quinidine, or fentanyl.

- People who have liver or kidney problems should talk to their doctor about the specific risks of using any calcium channel blocker.

- Women who are pregnant or nursing should talk to their doctor before they start using these drugs.

Common Side Effects

- Feeling drowsy
- Headache
- Upset stomach
- Ankle swelling
- Feeling flushed (warm)

Warning Signs

Call your doctor if you have any of these signs:

- Chest pain
- Serious rashes
- Swelling of the face, eyes, lips, tongue, arms, or legs
- Fainting
- Irregular heartbeat

Peripherally Acting Alpha-Adrenergic Blockers

Table 30.4. Peripherally Acting Alpha-Adrenergic Blockers

Brand Name	Generic Name
Cardura	Doxazosin
Dibenzyline	Phenoxybenzamine
Minipress	Prazosin
Hytrin	Terazosin

Warnings

- The elderly and people who have liver problems should talk to their doctor about the risks of using these drugs.

Common Side Effects

- Dizziness
- Feeling tired
- Feeling lightheaded
- Vision problems
- Swelling of the hands, feet, ankles, or legs
- Decreased sexual ability

Warning Signs

Call your doctor if you have any of these signs:

- Chest pain
- Irregular heartbeat
- Painful erection in men

Vasodilators

Table 30.5. Vasodilators

Brand Name	Generic Name
	Hydralazine
	Minoxidil

Warnings

- Do not use these drugs if you are also taking bisulfates.

- Women who are pregnant or nursing should talk to their doctor before they start using these drugs.

- People who have diabetes, heart disease, or uremia (buildup of waste in your blood) should talk to their doctor about the risks of using any of these drugs.

- People taking diuretics (water pills), insulin, phenytoin, cortico-steroids, estrogen, warfarin, or progesterone should talk to their doctor about the risks of using any of these drugs.

Common Side Effects

- Headache

- Upset stomach

- Dizziness

- Growth in body hair

Warning Signs

Call your doctor if you have any of these signs:

- Fever

- Fast heartbeat

- Fainting

- Chest pain

- Problems breathing

- Sudden weight gain

Angiotension II Antagonists

Table 30.6. Angiotension II Antagonists

Brand Name	Generic Name
Atacand	Candesartan
Avapro	Irbesartan
Benicar	Olmesartan
Cozaar	Losartan
Diovan	Valsartan
Edarbi	Azilsartan
Micardis	Telmisartan
Teveten	Eprosartan

Warnings

- Do not use these drugs if you are pregnant or nursing

- People who have kidney disease, liver disease, low blood volume, or low salt in their blood should talk to their doctor about the risks of taking these drugs.

- People taking diuretics (water pills) should talk to their doctor about the risks of taking these drugs.

Common Side Effects

- Sore throat

- Sinus problems

- Heartburn

- Dizziness

- Diarrhea

- Back pain

Warning Signs

Call your doctor if you have any of these signs:

- Problems breathing

- Fainting

- Swelling of the face, throat, lips, eyes, hands, feet, ankles, or legs

Centrally-Acting Alpha Adrenergics

Table 30.7. Centrally-Acting Alpha Adrenergics

Brand Name	Generic Name
Catapres	Clonidine
Tenex	Guanfacine

Warnings

- Women who are pregnant or nursing should talk to their doctor before using these drugs.

- People with heart disease, recent heart attack, or kidney disease should talk to their doctor before using these drugs.

- Drinking alcohol may make side effects worse.

Common Side Effects

- Dizziness

- Dry mouth

- Upset stomach

- Feeling drowsy or tired

Warning Signs

Call your doctor if you have any of these signs:

- Fainting

- Slow or irregular heartbeat

- Fever

- Swollen ankles or feet

Renin Inhibitors

Table 30.8. Renin Inhibitors

Brand Name	Generic Name
Tekturna	Aliskiren

Warnings

- Women who are pregnant or planning to become pregnant should talk to their doctor before using this drug.

- People with kidney problems should talk to their doctor before using this drug.
- Tell your doctor if you are taking water pills (diuretics), high blood pressure medicines, heart medicines, or medicines to treat a fungus.

Common Side Effects

- Diarrhea

Warning Signs

Call your doctor if you have any of these signs:

- Low blood pressure
- Swelling of the face, throat, lips, eyes or tongue

Combination Medicines

Table 30.9. Combination Medicines

Brand Name	Generic Name
Diovan HCT	hydrochlorothiazide and valsartan
Exforge	amlodipine and valsartan
Exforge HCT	amlodipine, valsartan, and hydrochlorothiazide
Hyzaar	hydrochlorothiazide and losartan
Lotrel	benazepril and amlodipine
Tarka	verapamil and trandolapril
Tribenzor	olmesartan, amlodipine and hydrochlorothiazide
Vaseretic	enalapril and hydrochlorothiazide

- These medicines are made up of 2 different kinds of blood pressure medicines.
- Look for the generic names of these drugs

Warnings and Side Effects

The warnings and side effects for these drugs will be the same as those listed earlier for both generic drugs.

Other Combination Medicines

Table 30.10. Other Combination Medicines

Brand Name	Generic Name
Caduet	Amlodipine and Atorvastatin

Caduet is used to treat people who have both high blood pressure and high cholesterol.

Warnings

- Do not take Caduet if you are pregnant or planning to become pregnant.
- Do not take Caduet if you are breastfeeding.
- Do not take Caduet if you have liver problems.

Common Side Effects

- Swelling of the legs or ankles (edema)
- Muscle or joint pain
- Headache
- Diarrhea or constipation
- Feeling dizzy
- Feeling tired or sleepy
- Gas
- Rash
- Nausea
- Stomach pain
- Fast or irregular heartbeat
- Face feels hot or warm (flushing)

Warning Signs

Call your doctor if you have any of these signs:

- Muscle problems like weakness, tenderness, or pain that happens without a good reason (like exercise or injury)

- Brown or dark-colored urine
- Skin or eyes look yellow (jaundice)
- Feel more tired than usual

Diuretics (Sometimes Called "Water Pills")

Table 30.11. Diuretics

Brand Name	Generic Name
Aldactazide Aldactone	Spironolactone
Demadex	Torsemide
Diuril	Chlorothiazide
Enduron	Methyclothiazide
Microzide Oretic	Hydrochlorothiazide
Lasix	Furosemide
	Indapamide
Saluron	Hydroflumethiazide
Thalitone	Chlorthalidone
Zaroxolyn	Metolazone

Warnings

- Tell your doctor if you are breastfeeding. These medicines may pass into your breast milk.
- Do not use these medicines if you have problems making urine.
- People with kidney or liver problems, pregnant women, and the elderly should talk to their doctor about the risks of using diuretics.

Common Side Effects

- Dizziness
- Frequent urination
- Headache
- Feeling thirsty
- Muscle cramps
- Upset stomach

Warning Signs

Call your doctor if you have any of these signs:

- Severe rash

- Problems breathing or swallowing

- Hyperuricemia (Gout)

Section 30.4

Taking Statins after Stroke Reduces Risk of Death

This section includes text excerpted from "Controlling Cholesterol with Statins," U.S. Food and Drug Administration (FDA), February 16, 2017.

You go to the gym faithfully, and try to watch your diet. But after your annual physical, you find out that your blood cholesterol is surprisingly high. Your doctor calls you back to discuss taking a medication known as a statin.

What Are Statins? How Do They Work?

Statins are a class of medicines used to lower cholesterol in the blood. Most of the cholesterol in your blood is made by the liver. Statins work by reducing the amount of cholesterol made by the liver and by helping the liver remove cholesterol that is already in the blood.

According to James P. Smith, M.D., M.S., deputy director of the Division of Metabolism and Endocrinology at the U.S. Food and Drug Administration (FDA), "An important first step is to have a discussion with your healthcare provider about your risk of having a stroke or heart disease, how a statin would reduce that risk, and any side effects that you should consider."

Why Is It Important to Keep Cholesterol Levels in the Blood Low?

Your body needs cholesterol, but too much of it in your blood can lead to buildup on the walls of your arteries (this buildup is called "plaque"), putting you at higher risk for stroke or heart disease. According to the Centers for Disease Control and Prevention (CDC), heart disease is the leading cause of death for both men and women in the United States.

Frequently Asked Questions

I've Heard about "Good" and "Bad" Cholesterol. What's the Difference?

Cholesterol is carried in the bloodstream on different types of particles, called lipoproteins. The majority is carried on low-density lipoprotein (LDL) particles and is sometimes referred to as "bad" cholesterol, because high levels of LDL particles can lead to stroke and heart disease. High-density lipoprotein (HDL) particles, on the other hand, carry cholesterol back to the liver for removal from the body. Since people with higher levels of HDL-cholesterol tend to have a lower risk of heart disease, this is sometimes referred to as "good" cholesterol. Your healthcare provider should help you interpret what your numbers mean for your cardiovascular health.

I Thought a Healthy Diet and Regular Exercise Would Keep My Cholesterol in Check. Not So?

"A heart-healthy diet, regular physical activity, and maintaining a healthy weight are all very important components of a lifestyle that can help lower cholesterol and reduce the risk of stroke and heart disease" says Smith. "But other factors that are out of our control, such as genetics, also play a role. For many people, cholesterol simply cannot be lowered enough by lifestyle changes alone."

For people who are at increased risk of having a stroke or heart attack, statins may be recommended even when cholesterol levels might not seem too high. "Statins have a well-established track record for reducing the risk for strokes and heart attacks," Smith says. "Whether or not a statin is appropriate for a specific patient should involve a conversation between the patient and his or her healthcare provider."

I've Heard That There Are Some Risks to Taking Statins. Should I Be Worried?

Statins are typically very well tolerated. Two risks that patients may be aware of are muscle-related complaints and an increased risk of developing type 2 diabetes. "Muscle complaints are quite common even among people not taking statins, so it is important to have your healthcare provider evaluate any symptoms before stopping your medication," Smith explains. "It is rare for statins to cause serious muscle problems."

Similarly, the risk of developing diabetes as a result of a statin is small. "The benefits of statins in reducing strokes and heart attacks should generally outweigh this small increased risk," Smith says.

I've Heard You Shouldn't Drink Grapefruit Juice If You're Taking a Statin. Is That True?

Grapefruit juice and fresh grapefruit can affect the way some medicines work. That's true with certain statins, too—but only some of them. In addition, other medications can also interact with statins. Smith advises patients ensure that their healthcare provider and pharmacist know about all the prescription and non-prescription medications they take.

Chapter 31

Stroke Recovery

Stroke Recovery Steps

Stroke is a life-changing event. How long it takes you to recover depends on many factors, including the type of stroke you had, the area of your brain affected, and the amount of brain injury. The recovery process begins at the hospital as soon as you are medically stable. Often, this is within a day of having the stroke. Your doctor will talk to you about next steps. This will involve changes in your everyday habits, medicines, rehabilitation, or surgeries to lower the risk of another stroke.

Step One: Educate Yourself about Stroke Recovery

The first step is to learn all you can about your condition and what to expect during recovery.

Ask your doctor, nurses, or physical or occupational therapist questions about your treatment and rehabilitation. Other stroke survivors can also help with practical tips.

This chapter includes text excerpted from "Heart Disease and Stroke—Stroke Recovery Steps," Office on Women's Health (OWH), U.S. Department of Health and Human Services (HHS), January 24, 2017.

Step Two: Take Steps to Prevent Another Stroke

If you've had a stroke, you're at high risk of having another. As you recover from your stroke, take steps to prevent a second one:

- Identify and control your stroke risk factors

- Continue with your treatment plan. After a stroke, your doctor will work with you on a treatment plan. Your plan is designed to help you recover from your stroke and prevent another stroke. Even if you feel better, do not stop taking a medicine without talking to your doctor first.

Step Three: Figure out What Rehabilitation Services You Will Need

Stroke rehabilitation is a program to help you recover from stroke. Almost all stroke survivors benefit from rehabilitation. However, many women do not join a rehabilitation program for reasons that are not clear. Many women are older at the time of their stroke and often go to assisted-living facilities or hospice after a stroke rather than to a rehabilitation program.

Under the Affordable Care Act (ACA), most insurance plans must cover stroke rehabilitation, although you may need to pay a copayment, coinsurance, and meet your deductible first. Find out what your insurance will cover, and what benefits you can receive from government programs or from your employer.

After a stroke, you will often recover some function in the first few months. This is part of the body's natural healing process. Women who get stroke rehabilitation:

- Relearn skills and abilities that were damaged or lost

- Regain as much independence as possible

- Learn to cope with any remaining limitations

Also, think about what, if anything, you will need from caregivers at home and what they are able to provide. Who is available to help with your care? How much time can they spend taking care of you? Can they provide financial support?

Step Four: Set Goals for Your Recovery

Set realistic, measurable goals for recovery in each area of your life your stroke affected. Keep in mind that stroke recovery is usually fast in the first few months. Then it may slow down. Having goals will help to motivate you to keep making progress.

Write down your long-term goals and create a timeline for achieving them. Break each one down into steps to make short-term goals.

Step Five: Follow through on Your Plan

A stroke can often make you feel powerless. Part of recovery is figuring out how to live as independently as possible. Know that you are likely to face challenges as you adjust to the differences in how your body works.

The road to stroke recovery is often a long one, but focusing on your progress can help you reach your goals.

Part Five

Poststroke Complications and Rehabilitation

Chapter 32

Cognitive Problems Caused by Stroke

Chapter Contents

Section 32.1—Agnosia 380

Section 32.2—Right Hemisphere Brain Damage...................... 382

Section 32.3—Vascular Dementia... 385

Section 32.4—Multi-Infarct Dementia (MID) 391

Section 32.1

Agnosia

This section includes text excerpted from "Agnosia," Genetic and
Rare Diseases Information Center (GARD), National Center
for Advancing Translational Sciences (NCATS), April 22, 2011.
Reviewed April 2017.

Agnosia is characterized by an inability to recognize and identify
objects and/or persons. Symptoms may vary, according to the area of
the brain that is affected. It can be limited to one sensory modality
such as vision or hearing; for example, a person may have difficulty in
recognizing an object as a cup or identifying a sound as a cough. Agnosia can result from strokes, traumatic brain injury, dementia, a tumor,
developmental disorders, overexposure to environmental toxins (e.g.,
carbon monoxide poisoning), or other neurological conditions. Visual
agnosia may also occur in association with other underlying disorders.
People with agnosia may retain their cognitive abilities in other areas.
Treatment of primary agnosia is symptomatic and supportive; when
it is caused by an underlying disorder, treatment of the disorder may
reduce symptoms and help prevent further brain damage.

Symptoms of Agnosia

People with primary visual agnosia may have one or several impairments in visual recognition without impairment of intelligence, motivation, and/or attention. Vision is almost always intact and the mind
is clear. Some affected individuals do not have the ability to recognize
familiar objects. They can see objects, but are unable to identify them
by sight. However, objects may be identified by touch, sound, and/or
smell. For example, affected individuals may not be able to identify a
set of keys by sight, but can identify them upon holding them in their
hands.

Some researchers separate visual agnosia into two broad categories: apperceptive agnosia and associative agnosia. *Apperceptive
agnosia* refers to individuals who cannot properly process what they
see, meaning they have difficulty identifying shapes or differentiating

between different objects (visual stimuli). Affected individuals may not be able to recognize that pictures of the same object from different angles are of the same object. Affected individuals may be unable to copy (e.g., draw a picture) of an object. *Associative agnosia* refers to people who cannot match an object with their memory. They can accurately describe an object and even draw a picture of the object, but are unable to state what the object is or is used for. However, if told verbally what the object is, an affected individual will be able to describe what it is used for.

In some cases, individuals with primary visual agnosia cannot identify familiar people (prosopagnosia). They can see the person clearly and can describe the person (e.g., hair and eye color), but cannot identify the person by name. People with prosopagnosia may identify people by touch, smell, speech, or the way that they walk (gait). In some rare cases, affected individuals cannot recognize their own face.

Some people have a form of primary visual agnosia associated with the loss of the ability to identify their surroundings (loss of environmental familiarity agnosia). Symptoms include the inability to recognize familiar places or buildings. Affected individuals may be able to describe a familiar environment from memory and point to it on a map.

Simultanagnosia is a characterized by the inability to read and the inability to view one's surroundings as a whole. The affected individual can see parts of the surrounding scene, but not the whole. There is an inability to comprehend more than one part of a visual scene at a time or to coordinate the parts.

In rare cases, people with primary visual agnosia may not be able to recognize or point to various parts of the body (autotopagnosia). Symptoms may also include loss of the ability to distinguish left from right.

Causes of Agnosia

Primary visual agnosia occurs as a result of damage to the brain. Symptoms develop due to the inability to retrieve information from those damaged areas that are associated with visual memory. Lesions may occur as a result of stroke, traumatic brain injury, tumor, or overexposure to dangerous environmental toxins (e.g., carbon monoxide poisoning). In some cases, the cause of the brain damage may not be known. Symptoms may vary, according to the area of the brain that is affected.

Visual agnosia may also occur in association with other underlying disorders (secondary visual agnosia) such as Alzheimer disease, agenesis of the corpus callosum, Mitochondrial Encephalomyopathy,

Lactic Acidosis, and Stroke-Like Episodes (MELAS), and other diseases that result in progressive dementia. Disorders that may precede the development of primary visual agnosia (and may be useful in identifying an underlying cause of some forms of this disorder) include Alzheimer disease, Pick disease, and a rare disorder called Balint syndrome.

Diagnosis of Agnosia

A variety of psychophysical tests can be conducted to pinpoint the nature of the visual process that is disrupted in an individual. Brain damage that causes visual agnosia may be identified through imaging techniques, including computed tomography (CT scan) and magnetic resonance imaging (MRI).

Section 32.2

Right Hemisphere Brain Damage

What Is Right Hemisphere Brain Damage?

Right hemisphere brain damage (RHD) is damage to the right side of the brain. The brain is made up of two sides or hemispheres. Each hemisphere is responsible for different body functions and skills. In most people, the left side of the brain contains the person's language functions. The right side contributes to a number of functions, such as attention, memory, reasoning, and problem solving (all of which contribute to effective communication). Damage to the right hemisphere of the brain may lead to disruption of these cognitive processes, resulting in unique cognitive and communication problems. In many cases, the person with right brain damage is not aware of the problems that he or she is experiencing (anosognosia).

What Are Some Signs or Symptoms of Right Hemisphere Brain Damage?

Cognitive-communication problems that can occur from RHD include difficulty with the following:

- **Attention:** Difficulty concentrating on a task or focusing on what is said or seen.

- **Perception:** Visual perception deficits causing a person to have difficulty perceiving and processing any information on the left visual field (left-sided neglect). For example, individuals with RHD may have difficulty with reading words on the left side of a page, eating food on the left side of their plate, or acknowledging the left side of their body.

- **Reasoning and problem solving:** Difficulty identifying that there is a problem (e.g., ran out of medication) and generating solutions (e.g., call the pharmacy).

- **Memory:** Difficulty recalling previously learned information and learning new information.

- **Social communication (pragmatics):** Difficulty interpreting abstract language such as metaphors, making inferences, and understanding jokes; and problems understanding nonverbal cues and following the rules of communication (e.g., saying inappropriate things, not using facial expressions, talking at the wrong time).

- **Organization:** Difficulty with systematically arranging information and planning, which is often reflected in communication difficulties, such as trouble telling a story with events in the right order, giving directions, or maintaining a topic during conversation.

- **Insight:** Difficulty recognizing problems and their impact on daily functioning.

- **Orientation:** Difficulty recalling the date, time, or place. The individual may also be disoriented to self, meaning that he/she cannot correctly recall personal information, such as birth date, age, or family names.

What Causes Right Hemisphere Brain Damage?

The causes of right hemisphere brain damage include stroke, tumors, infection, and traumatic brain injury (TBI).

How Are Cognitive-Communication Problems Following Right Hemisphere Brain Damage Diagnosed?

A speech-language pathologist (SLP) will complete a variety of formal and informal evaluation procedures. Specifically, the person's language (comprehension and expression) and cognitive processes (attention, memory, reasoning, problem solving) will be examined. The nature and severity of the cognitive-communication problem will depend on the extent of damage to the brain.

What Treatment Is Available for Individuals with Right Hemisphere Brain Damage?

A person with right hemisphere brain damage should see an SLP, a professional trained to work with people with communication disorders, in addition to his or her doctor. The SLP will work with the person and develop a treatment plan designed to improve his or her cognitive-communication abilities.

How Can I Communicate More Effectively with a Person with Right Hemisphere Brain Damage?

- Ask questions and use reminders to keep the individual on topic.
- Avoid sarcasm, metaphors, etc., when speaking to the individual.
- Provide a consistent routine every day.
- Break down instructions into small steps and repeat directions as needed.
- Decrease distractions when communicating.
- Provide appropriate supervision to ensure the person's safety.
- Stand to the person's right side and place objects to the person's right if he or she is experiencing left-side neglect.
- Use calendars, clocks, and notepads to remind the person of important information.

Section 32.3

Vascular Dementia

This section includes text excerpted from "Dementia: Hope through Research," National Institute of Neurological Disorders and Stroke (NINDS), September 2013. Reviewed April 2017.

The Basics of Dementia

Dementia is the loss of cognitive functioning, which means the loss of the ability to think, remember, or reason, as well as behavioral abilities, to such an extent that it interferes with a person's daily life and activities. Signs and symptoms of dementia result when once-healthy neurons (nerve cells) in the brain stop working, lose connections with other brain cells, and die. While everyone loses some neurons as they age, people with dementia experience far greater loss.

Researchers are still trying to understand the underlying disease processes involved in the disorders. Scientists have some theories about mechanisms that may lead to different forms of dementias, but more research is needed to better understand if and how these mechanisms contribute to the development of dementia.

While dementia is more common with advanced age (as many as half of all people age 85 or older may have some form of dementia), it is not a normal part of aging. Many people live into their 90s and beyond without any signs of dementia.

Memory loss, though common, is not the only sign of dementia. For a person to be considered to have dementia, he or she must meet the following criteria:

- Two or more core mental functions must be impaired. These functions include memory, language skills, visual perception, and the ability to focus and pay attention. These also include cognitive skills such as the ability to reason and solve problems.

- The loss of brain function is severe enough that a person cannot do normal, everyday tasks.

In addition, some people with dementia cannot control their emotions. Their personalities may change. They can have delusions, which

385

are strong beliefs without proof, such as the idea that someone is stealing from them. They also may hallucinate, seeing or otherwise experiencing things that are not real.

Types of Dementia

Various disorders and factors contribute to the development of dementia. Neurodegenerative disorders such as Alzheimer disease (AD), frontotemporal disorders, and Lewy body dementia result in a progressive and irreversible loss of neurons and brain functions. Currently, there are no cures for these progressive neurodegenerative disorders.

However, other types of dementia can be halted or even reversed with treatment. Normal pressure hydrocephalus, for example, often resolves when excess cerebrospinal fluid in the brain is drained via a shunt and rerouted elsewhere in the body. Cerebral vasculitis responds to aggressive treatment with immunosuppressive drugs. In rare cases, treatable infectious disorders can cause dementia. Some drugs, vitamin deficiencies, alcohol abuse, depression, and brain tumors can cause neurological deficits that resemble dementia. Most of these causes respond to treatment.

Some types of dementia disorders are mentioned below.

- Tauopathies

- Corticobasal degeneration (CBD)

- Frontotemporal disorders (FTD)

- Behavioral variant frontotemporal dementia

- Primary progressive aphasia (PPA)

- Frontotemporal dementia with parkinsonism linked to chromosome 17 (FTDP-17)

- Pick disease

- Progressive supranuclear palsy (PSP)

- Argyrophilic grain disease

Vascular Dementia and Vascular Cognitive Impairment

Vascular dementia and vascular cognitive impairment (VCI) are caused by injuries to the vessels supplying blood to the brain. These disorders can be caused by brain damage from multiple strokes or any injury to the small vessels carrying blood to the brain. Dementia risk can be significant even when individuals have suffered only small strokes. Vascular dementia and VCI arise as a result of risk factors that similarly increase the risk for cerebrovascular disease (stroke), including atrial fibrillation, hypertension, diabetes, and high cholesterol. Vascular dementia also has been associated with a condition called amyloid angiopathy, in which amyloid plaques accumulate in the blood-vessel walls, causing them to break down and rupture. Symptoms of vascular dementia and VCI can begin suddenly and progress or subside during one's lifetime.

Some types of vascular dementia include:

Cerebral autosomal dominant arteriopathy with subcortical infarcts and leukoencephalopathy (CADASIL). This inherited form of cardiovascular disease results in a thickening of the walls of small- and medium-sized blood vessels, eventually stemming the flow of blood to the brain. It is associated with mutations of a specific gene called *Notch3*, which gives instructions to a protein on the surface of the smooth muscle cells that surround blood vessels. CADASIL is associated with multi-infarct dementia, stroke, migraine with aura (migraine preceded by visual symptoms), and mood disorders. The first symptoms can appear in people between ages 20 and 40. Many people with CADASIL are undiagnosed. People with first-degree relatives who have CADASIL can be tested for genetic mutations to the *Notch3* gene to determine their own risk of developing CADASIL.

Multi-infarct dementia. This type of dementia occurs when a person has had many small strokes that damage brain cells. One side of the body may be disproportionally affected, and multi-infarct dementia may impair language or other functions, depending on the region of the brain that is affected. Doctors call these "local" or "focal" symptoms, as opposed to the "global" symptoms seen in AD that tend to affect several functions and both sides of the body. When the strokes occur on both sides of the brain, however, dementia is more likely than when stroke occurs on one side of the brain. In some cases, a single stroke can damage the brain enough to cause dementia. This so-called single-infarct dementia is more common when stroke affects the left side of the brain—where speech centers are located—and/or when it involves the hippocampus, the part of the brain that is vital for memory.

Subcortical vascular dementia, also called Binswanger disease. This is a rare form of dementia that involves extensive microscopic damage to the small blood vessels and nerve fibers that make up white matter, the "network" part of the brain believed to be critical for relaying messages between regions. The symptoms of Binswanger are related to the disruption of subcortical neural circuits involving short-term memory, organization, mood, attention, decision making, and appropriate behavior. A characteristic feature of this disease is psychomotor slowness, such as an increase in the time it takes for a person to think of a letter and then write it on a piece of paper.

Other symptoms include urinary incontinence that is unrelated to a urinary tract condition, trouble walking, clumsiness, slowness, lack of facial expression, and speech difficulties. Symptoms tend to begin after age 60, and they progress in a stepwise manner. People with subcortical vascular disease often have high blood pressure, a history of stroke, or evidence of disease of the large blood vessels in the neck or heart valves. Treatment is aimed at preventing additional strokes and may include drugs to control blood pressure.

Risk Factors for Dementia

The following risk factors can increase a person's chance of developing one or more kinds of dementia. Some of these factors can be modified, while others cannot.

- **Age.** The risk goes up with advanced age.

- **Alcohol use.** Most studies suggest that drinking large amounts of alcohol increases the risk of dementia, while drinking a moderate amount may be protective.

- **Atherosclerosis.** The accumulation of fats and cholesterol in the lining of arteries, coupled with an inflammatory process that leads to a thickening of the vessel walls (known as atherosclerosis), can hinder blood from getting to the brain, which can lead to stroke or another brain injury. For example, high levels of low-density lipoprotein (LDL, or "bad" cholesterol) can raise the risk for vascular dementia. High LDL levels also have been linked to AD.

- **Diabetes.** People with diabetes appear to have a higher risk for dementia, although the evidence for this association is modest. Poorly controlled diabetes, however, is a well-proven risk factor for stroke and cardiovascular disease-related events, which in turn increase the risk for vascular dementia.

- **Down syndrome.** Many people with Down syndrome develop early-onset AD, with signs of dementia by the time they reach middle age.

- **Genetics.** One's likelihood of developing a genetically linked form of dementia increases when more than one family member has the disorder. But in some cases, such as with CADASIL, having just one parent who carries a mutation increases the risk of inheriting the condition. In other instances, genetic mutations may underlie dementias in specific populations. For example, a mutation of the gene *TREM2* has been found to be common among people with a form of very early onset frontotemporal dementia that runs in Turkish families.

- **Hypertension.** High blood pressure has been linked to cognitive decline, stroke, and types of dementia that affect the white matter regions of the brain.

- **Mental illness.** Depression has been associated with mild mental impairment and cognitive function decline.

- **Smoking.** Smokers are prone to diseases that slow or stop blood from getting to the brain.

Diagnosis of Dementia

Doctors first assess whether the individual has an underlying treatable condition such as depression, abnormal thyroid function, drug-induced encephalopathy, normal pressure hydrocephalus, or vitamin B12 deficiency. Early diagnosis is important, as some causes for symptoms can be treated. In many cases, the specific type of dementia that a person has may not be confirmed until after the person has died and the brain is examined.

An assessment generally includes:

- **Patient history.** Typical questions about a person's medical and family history might include asking about whether dementia runs in the family, how and when symptoms began, and if the person is taking certain medications that might cause or exacerbate symptoms.

- **Physical exam.** Measuring blood pressure and other vital signs may help physicians detect conditions that might cause or occur with dementia. Such conditions may be treatable.

- **Neurological evaluations.** Assessing balance, sensory function, reflexes, vision, eye movements, and other functions helps identify signs of conditions that may affect the diagnosis or are treatable with drugs. Doctors also might use an electroencephalogram, a test that records patterns of electrical activity in the brain, to check for abnormal electrical brain activity.

The following procedures also may be used when diagnosing dementia:

- **Brain scans.** These tests can identify strokes, tumors, and other problems that can cause dementia. Scans also identify changes in the brain's structure and function. The most common scans are computed tomographic (CT) scans and magnetic resonance imaging (MRI). CT scans use X-rays to produce images of the brain and other organs. MRI scans use a computer, magnetic fields, and radio waves to produce detailed images of body structures, including tissues, organs, bones, and nerves.

- Other types of scans let doctors watch the brain as it functions. Two of these tests are single photon-emission computed tomography, which can be used to measure blood flow to the brain, and positron emission tomography (PET), which uses radioactive isotopes to provide pictures of brain activity. These scans are used to look for patterns of altered brain activity that are common in dementia. Researchers also use PET imaging with compounds that bind to beta-amyloid to detect levels of the protein, a hallmark of AD, in the living brain.

- **Cognitive and neuropsychological tests.** These tests measure memory, language skills, math skills, and other abilities related to mental functioning. For example, people with AD often show impairment in problem- solving, memory, and the ability to perform once-automatic tasks.

- **Laboratory tests.** Many tests help rule out other conditions. They include measuring levels of sodium and other electrolytes in the blood, a complete blood count, a blood sugar test, urine analysis, a check of vitamin B12 levels, cerebrospinal fluid analysis, drug and alcohol tests, and an analysis of thyroid function.

- **Presymptomatic tests.** Some dementias are associated with a known gene defect. In these cases, a genetic test could help people know if they are at risk for dementia. People should talk with family members, their primary healthcare professional, and a genetic counselor before getting tested.

- **Psychiatric evaluation.** This will help determine if depression or another mental health condition is causing or contributing to a person's symptoms.

Treatment of Vascular Dementia

Some dementias are treatable. However, therapies to stop or slow common neurodegenerative diseases such as AD have largely been unsuccessful, though some drugs are available to manage certain symptoms.

Vascular dementia is often managed with drugs to prevent strokes. The aim is to reduce the risk of additional brain damage. Some studies suggest that drugs that improve memory in AD might benefit people with early vascular dementia. Most of the modifiable risk factors that influence development of vascular dementia and VCI are the same risk factors for cerebrovascular disease, such as hypertension, atrial fibrillation, diabetes, and high cholesterol. Interventions that address these risk factors may be incorporated into the management of vascular dementia.

Section 32.4

Multi-Infarct Dementia (MID)

This section includes text excerpted from documents published by two public domain sources. Text under headings marked 1 are excerpted from "Multi-Infarct Dementia Information Page," National Institute of Neurological Disorders and Stroke (NINDS), February 13, 2017; Text under headings marked 2 are excerpted from "Binswanger's Disease," Genetic and Rare Diseases Information Center (GARD), National Center for Advancing Translational Sciences (NCATS), October 8, 2015.

What is Multi-Infarct Dementia?[1]

Multi-infarct dementia (MID) is a common cause of memory loss in the elderly. MID is caused by multiple strokes (disruption of blood flow to the brain). Disruption of blood flow leads to damaged brain tissue. Some of these strokes may occur without noticeable clinical symptoms. Doctors refer to these as "silent strokes." An individual having a silent stroke may not even know it is happening, but over time, as more areas of the brain are damaged and more small blood vessels are blocked, the symptoms of MID begin to appear. MID can be diagnosed by an MRI or CT of the brain, along with a neurological examination.

Symptoms of Multi-Infarct Dementia[1]

Symptoms include confusion or problems with short-term memory; wandering, or getting lost in familiar places; walking with rapid, shuffling steps; losing bladder or bowel control; laughing or crying inappropriately; having difficulty following instructions; and having problems counting money and making monetary transactions. MID, which typically begins between the ages of 60 and 75, affects men more often than women. Because the symptoms of MID are so similar to Alzheimer disease, it can be difficult for a doctor to make a firm diagnosis. Since the diseases often occur together, making a single diagnosis of one or the other is even more problematic.

Causes of Multi-Infarct Dementia[2]

Multi-infarct dementia (also known as Binswanger disease) occurs when the blood vessels that supply the deep structures of the brain become obstructed (blocked). As the arteries become more and more narrowed, the blood supplied by those arteries decreases and brain tissue dies. This can be caused by atherosclerosis, thromboembolism (blood clots) and other diseases such as cerebral autosomal dominant arteriopathy with subcortical infarcts and leukoencephalopathy (CADASIL).

Risk factors for multi-infarct dementia include:

- hypertension
- smoking
- hypercholesterolemia
- heart disease
- diabetes mellitus

Diagnosis of Multi-Infarct Dementia[2]

A diagnosis of multi-infarct dementia is often suspected based on the presence of characteristic signs and symptoms. Additional testing can then be ordered to confirm the diagnosis. This generally consists of imaging studies of the brain (i.e., computerized tomography (CT) scan and/or magnetic resonance imaging (MRI) scan).

Treatment of Multi-Infarct Dementia[1]

There is no treatment available to reverse brain damage that has been caused by a stroke. Treatment focuses on preventing future strokes by controlling or avoiding the diseases and medical conditions that put people at high risk for stroke: high blood pressure, diabetes, high cholesterol, and cardiovascular disease. The best treatment for MID is prevention early in life—eating a healthy diet, exercising, not smoking, moderately using alcohol, and maintaining a healthy weight.

Prognosis of Multi-Infarct Dementia[1]

The prognosis for individuals with MID is generally poor. The symptoms of the disorder may begin suddenly, often in a stepwise pattern after each small stroke. Some people with MID may even appear to improve for short periods of time, then decline after having more silent strokes. The disorder generally takes a downward course with intermittent periods of rapid deterioration. Death may occur from stroke, heart disease, pneumonia, or other infection.

Chapter 33

Communication Problems after Stroke

What Is Aphasia?

Aphasia is a disorder that results from damage to portions of the brain that are responsible for language. For most people, these areas are on the left side of the brain. Aphasia usually occurs suddenly, often following a stroke or head injury, but it may also develop slowly, as the result of a brain tumor or a progressive neurological disease. The disorder impairs the expression and understanding of language as well as reading and writing. Aphasia may co-occur with speech disorders, such as dysarthria or apraxia of speech, which also result from brain damage.

Who Can Acquire Aphasia?

Most people who have aphasia are middle-aged or older, but anyone can acquire it, including young children. About 1 million people in the

This chapter contains text excerpted from the following sources: Text beginning with the heading "What Is Aphasia?" is excerpted from "Aphasia," National Institute on Deafness and Other Communication Disorders (NIDCD), December 2015; Text under the heading "Brain Mapping of Language Impairments" is excerpted from "Brain Mapping of Language Impairments," National Institutes of Health (NIH), April 27, 2015; Text under the heading "Other Communication Problems after Stroke" is excerpted from "Speech and Communication (Aphasia, Dysarthria and Apraxia)," U.S. Department of Veterans Affairs (VA), December 27, 2013. Reviewed April 2017.

United States currently have aphasia, and nearly 180,000 Americans acquire it each year, according to the National Aphasia Association (NAA).

What Causes Aphasia?

Aphasia is caused by damage to one or more of the language areas of the brain. Most often, the cause of the brain injury is a stroke. A stroke occurs when a blood clot or a leaking or burst vessel cuts off blood flow to part of the brain. Brain cells die when they do not receive their normal supply of blood, which carries oxygen and important nutrients. Other causes of brain injury are severe blows to the head, brain tumors, gunshot wounds, brain infections, and progressive neurological disorders, such as Alzheimer disease.

What Types of Aphasia Are There?

There are two broad categories of aphasia: fluent and nonfluent, and there are several types within these groups.

Damage to the temporal lobe of the brain may result in **Wernicke aphasia**, the most common type of fluent aphasia. People with Wernicke aphasia may speak in long, complete sentences that have no meaning, adding unnecessary words and even creating made-up words.

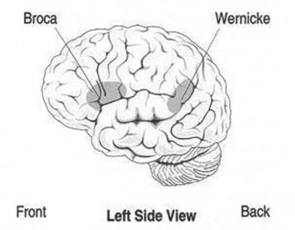

Figure 33.1. *Areas of the Brain Affected by Broca's and Wernicke's Aphasia*

For example, someone with Wernicke aphasia may say, "You know that smoodle pinkered and that I want to get him round and take care of him like you want before."

As a result, it is often difficult to follow what the person is trying to say. People with Wernicke aphasia are often unaware of their spoken mistakes. Another hallmark of this type of aphasia is difficulty understanding speech.

The most common type of nonfluent aphasia is **Broca aphasia**. People with Broca aphasia have damage that primarily affects the frontal lobe of the brain. They often have right-sided weakness or paralysis of the arm and leg because the frontal lobe is also important for motor movements. People with Broca aphasia may understand speech and know what they want to say, but they frequently speak in short phrases that are produced with great effort. They often omit small words, such as "is," "and" and "the."

For example, a person with Broca aphasia may say, "Walk dog," meaning, "I will take the dog for a walk," or "book book two table," for "There are two books on the table." People with Broca aphasia typically understand the speech of others fairly well. Because of this, they are often aware of their difficulties and can become easily frustrated.

Another type of aphasia, global aphasia, results from damage to extensive portions of the language areas of the brain. Individuals with global aphasia have severe communication difficulties and may be extremely limited in their ability to speak or comprehend language. They may be unable to say even a few words or may repeat the same words or phrases over and over again. They may have trouble understanding even simple words and sentences.

There are other types of aphasia, each of which results from damage to different language areas in the brain. Some people may have difficulty repeating words and sentences even though they understand them and can speak fluently (conduction aphasia). Others may have difficulty naming objects even though they know what the object is and what it may be used for (anomic aphasia).

Sometimes, blood flow to the brain is temporarily interrupted and quickly restored. When this type of injury occurs, which is called a transient ischemic attack, language abilities may return in a few hours or days.

How Is Aphasia Diagnosed?

Aphasia is usually first recognized by the physician who treats the person for his or her brain injury. Most individuals will undergo a magnetic resonance imaging (MRI) or computed tomography (CT) scan to confirm the presence of a brain injury and to identify its precise location. The physician also typically tests the person's ability to understand and produce language, such as following commands, answering questions, naming objects, and carrying on a conversation.

If the physician suspects aphasia, the patient is usually referred to a speech-language pathologist, who performs a comprehensive examination of the person's communication abilities. The person's ability to speak, express ideas, converse socially, understand language, and read and write are all assessed in detail.

How Is Aphasia Treated?

Following a brain injury, tremendous changes occur in the brain, which help it to recover. As a result, people with aphasia often see dramatic improvements in their language and communication abilities in the first few months, even without treatment. But in many cases, some aphasia remains following this initial recovery period. In these instances, speech-language therapy is used to help patients regain their ability to communicate.

Research has shown that language and communication abilities can continue to improve for many years and are sometimes accompanied by new activity in brain tissue near the damaged area. Some of the factors that may influence the amount of improvement include the cause of the brain injury, the area of the brain that was damaged and its extent, and the age and health of the individual.

Aphasia therapy aims to improve a person's ability to communicate by helping him or her to use remaining language abilities, restore language abilities as much as possible, and learn other ways of communicating, such as gestures, pictures, or use of electronic devices. Individual therapy focuses on the specific needs of the person, while group therapy offers the opportunity to use new communication skills in a small-group setting.

Technologies have provided new tools for people with aphasia. "Virtual" speech pathologists provide patients with the flexibility and convenience of getting therapy in their homes through a computer. The use of speech-generating applications on mobile devices like tablets can also provide an alternative way to communicate for people who have difficulty using spoken language.

Increasingly, patients with aphasia participate in activities, such as book clubs, technology groups, and art and drama clubs. Such experiences help patients regain their confidence and social self-esteem, in addition to improving their communication skills. Stroke clubs, regional support groups formed by people who have had a stroke, are available in most major cities. These clubs can help a person and his or her family adjust to the life changes that accompany stroke and aphasia.

Family involvement is often a crucial component of aphasia treatment because it enables family members to learn the best way to communicate with their loved one.

Family members are encouraged to:

- Participate in therapy sessions, if possible.

- Simplify language by using short, uncomplicated sentences.

- Repeat the content words or write down keywords to clarify meaning as needed.

- Maintain a natural conversational manner appropriate for an adult.

- Minimize distractions, such as a loud radio or TV, whenever possible.

- Include the person with aphasia in conversations.

- Ask for and value the opinion of the person with aphasia, especially regarding family matters.

- Encourage any type of communication, whether it is speech, gesture, pointing, or drawing.

- Avoid correcting the person's speech.

- Allow the person plenty of time to talk.

- Help the person become involved outside the home. Seek out support groups, such as stroke clubs.

Brain Mapping of Language Impairments

Through language—which includes sounds, gestures, and signs— we communicate our knowledge and beliefs. Between 6 million and 8 million people in the United States have some form of language impairment. In aphasia, portions of the brain that are responsible for expressing and understanding language are damaged. Aphasia usually occurs suddenly, often as the result of a stroke or head injury. It may also develop slowly, as in the case of a brain tumor, an infection, or dementia.

A team led by Dr. Daniel Mirman at Drexel University and Dr. Myrna F. Schwartz at the Moss Rehabilitation Research Institute set out to better understand the basis of language by studying people with aphasia using both neuroimaging and behavioral assessment. The research was funded by National Institutes of Health's (NIH) National Institute on Deafness and Other Communication Disorders (NIDCD).

The group studied 99 volunteers who had aphasia resulting from a stroke to the left side (hemisphere) of the brain. The participants averaged 58 years of age and used English as their native language.

The researchers asked the participants to complete a series of 17 language and cognitive measures that examined a wide range of language functions. These included the ability to perceive speech and process words both verbally and nonverbally (pictures), as well as short-term memory. For example, participants were asked whether 2 spoken words rhymed, to name items shown in pictures, to indicate whether spoken words were real English words or not, and to repeat lists of one-syllable words.

The scientists identified 2 major divisions in the way the language system is organized, resulting in 4 factors: the meaning versus the form of words, and speech recognition versus production. They next examined high-resolution MRI or CT brain scans of the participants to map the location of their lesions with their symptoms.

The researchers found that the 4 factors were associated with various lesion areas. For example, speech production and speech recognition were associated with damage to adjacent regions. Whereas some factors were linked to distinct brain regions, others converged, suggesting that certain areas might have broader functional significance.

"By studying language in people with aphasia, we can try to accomplish 2 goals at once: we can improve our clinical understanding of aphasia and get new insights into how language is organized in the mind and brain," Mirman says.

"A major challenge facing speech-language pathologists is the wide diversity of symptoms that one sees in stroke aphasia," Schwartz adds. "With this study, we took a major step towards explaining the symptom diversity in relation to a few primary underlying processes and their mosaic-like representation in the brain. These can serve as targets for new diagnostic assessments and treatment interventions."

Other Communication Problems after Stroke

Dysarthria

Dysarthria results from damage to the part of the brain that produces speech. As a result, speech may sound slurred. People with dysarthria may have problems saying sounds correctly.

Apraxia

Apraxia is a problem finding the "right" sounds to use when speaking. The speech may sound "flat." The person's tone may not change. He or she may only say one syllable at a time. Aphasia and apraxia of speech almost always occur at the same time.

Chapter 34

Swallowing Problems (Dysphagia) after Stroke

What Is Dysphagia?

The parts of the mouth and neck involved in swallowing are the tongue, pharynx or throat, larynx or voice box, esophagus or food channel, and trachea or windpipe.

People with dysphagia have difficulty swallowing and may even experience pain while swallowing (odynophagia). Some people may be completely unable to swallow or may have trouble safely swallowing liquids, foods, or saliva. When that happens, eating becomes a challenge. Often, dysphagia makes it difficult to take in enough calories and fluids to nourish the body and can lead to additional serious medical problems.

How Do We Swallow?

Swallowing is a complex process. Some 50 pairs of muscles and many nerves work to receive food into the mouth, prepare it, and move it from the mouth to the stomach. This happens in three stages. During the first stage, called the oral phase, the tongue collects the food or liquid, making it ready for swallowing. The tongue and jaw move

This chapter includes text excerpted from "Dysphagia," National Institute on Deafness and Other Communication Disorders (NIDCD), March 6, 2017.

solid food around in the mouth so it can be chewed. Chewing makes solid food the right size and texture to swallow by mixing the food with saliva. Saliva softens and moistens the food to make swallowing easier. Normally, the only solid we swallow without chewing is in the form of a pill or caplet. Everything else that we swallow is in the form of a liquid, a puree, or a chewed solid.

The second stage begins when the tongue pushes the food or liquid to the back of the mouth. This triggers a swallowing response that passes the food through the pharynx, or throat. During this phase, called the pharyngeal phase, the larynx (voice box) closes tightly and breathing stops to prevent food or liquid from entering the airway and lungs.

The third stage begins when food or liquid enters the esophagus, the tube that carries food and liquid to the stomach. The passage through the esophagus, called the esophageal phase, usually occurs in about three seconds, depending on the texture or consistency of the food, but can take slightly longer in some cases, such as when swallowing a pill.

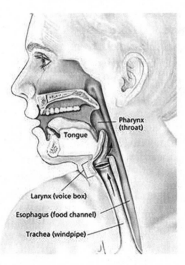

Figure 34.1. *Parts of the Mouth and Neck Involved in Swallowing*

How Does Dysphagia Occur?

Dysphagia occurs when there is a problem with the neural control or the structures involved in any part of the swallowing process. Weak tongue or cheek muscles may make it hard to move food around in the mouth for chewing. A stroke or other nervous system disorder may make it difficult to start the swallowing response, a stimulus that allows food and liquids to move safely through the throat. Another difficulty can occur when weak throat muscles, such as after cancer surgery, cannot move all of the food toward the stomach. Dysphagia may also result from disorders of the esophagus.

What Are Some Problems Caused by Dysphagia?

Dysphagia can be serious. Someone who cannot swallow safely may not be able to eat enough of the right foods to stay healthy or maintain an ideal weight.

Food pieces that are too large for swallowing may enter the throat and block the passage of air. In addition, when foods or liquids enter the airway of someone who has dysphagia, coughing or throat clearing sometimes cannot remove it. Food or liquid that stays in the airway may enter the lungs and allow harmful bacteria to grow, resulting in a lung infection called aspiration pneumonia.

Swallowing disorders may also include the development of a pocket outside the esophagus caused by weakness in the esophageal wall. This abnormal pocket traps some food being swallowed. While lying down or sleeping, someone with this problem may draw undigested food into the throat. The esophagus may also be too narrow, causing food to stick. This food may prevent other food or even liquids from entering the stomach.

How Is Dysphagia Treated?

There are different treatments for various types of dysphagia. Medical doctors and speech-language pathologists who evaluate and treat swallowing disorders use a variety of tests that allow them to look at the stages of the swallowing process. One test, the Flexible Endoscopic Evaluation of Swallowing with Sensory Testing (FEESST), uses a lighted fiber-optic tube, or endoscope, to view the mouth and throat while examining how the swallowing mechanism responds to such stimuli as a puff of air, food, or liquids.

A videofluoroscopic swallow study (VFSS) is a test in which a clinician takes a videotaped X-ray of the entire swallowing process by having you consume several foods or liquids along with the mineral barium to improve visibility of the digestive tract. Such images help identify where in the swallowing process you are experiencing problems. Speech-language pathologists use this method to explore what changes can be made to offer a safe strategy when swallowing. The changes may be in food texture, size, head and neck posture, or behavioral maneuvers, such as "chin tuck," a strategy in which you tuck your chin so that food and other substances do not enter the trachea when swallowing. If you are unable to swallow safely despite rehabilitation strategies, then medical or surgical intervention may be necessary for the short-term as you recover. In progressive conditions such as amyotrophic lateral sclerosis (ALS, or Lou Gehrig disease), a feeding tube in the stomach may be necessary for the long-term.

For some people, treatment may involve muscle exercises to strengthen weak facial muscles or to improve coordination. For others, treatment may involve learning to eat in a special way. For example, some people may have to eat with their head turned to one side or looking straight ahead. Preparing food in a certain way or avoiding certain foods may help in some situations. For instance, people who cannot swallow thin liquids may need to add special thickeners to their drinks. Other people may have to avoid hot or cold foods or drinks.

For some, however, consuming enough foods and liquids by mouth may no longer be possible. These individuals must use other methods to nourish their bodies. Usually this involves a feeding system, such as a feeding tube, that bypasses or supplements the part of the swallowing mechanism that is not working normally.

What Research Is Being Done on Dysphagia?

Scientists are conducting research that will improve the ability of physicians and speech-language pathologists to evaluate and treat swallowing disorders. Every aspect of the swallowing process is being studied in people of all ages, including those who do not have dysphagia, to give researchers a better understanding of how normal and disordered processes compare.

Research has also led to new, safe ways to study tongue and throat movements during the swallowing process. These methods will help physicians and speech-language pathologists safely evaluate a patient's progress during treatment.

Studies of treatment methods are helping scientists discover why some forms of treatment work with some people and not with others. This knowledge will help some people avoid serious lung infections and help others avoid tube feedings.

Where Can I Get Help?

If you have a sudden or gradual change in your ability to swallow, you should consult with your physician. He or she may refer you to an otolaryngologist—a doctor who specializes in diseases of the ear, nose, throat, head, and neck—and a speech-language pathologist. You may be referred to a neurologist if a stroke or other neurologic disorder is the cause of the swallowing problem.

Chapter 35

Muscle Spasticity and Weakness after Stroke

Chapter Contents

Section 35.1—Overview of Spasticity 410

Section 35.2—Foot Drop 413

Section 35.3—Constraint-Induced Movement
Therapy 414

Section 35.1

Overview of Spasticity

This section contains text excerpted from the following sources:
Text in this section begins with excerpts from "Spasticity
Information Page," National Institute of Neurological Disorders
and Stroke (NINDS), December 22, 2016; Text under the heading
"How Do You Manage Spasticity?" is excerpted from "How Do You
Manage Spasticity?" U.S. Department of Veterans Affairs (VA),
September 2009. Reviewed April 2017.

Spasticity is a condition in which there is an abnormal increase in
muscle tone or stiffness of muscle, which might interfere with movement, speech, or be associated with discomfort or pain. Spasticity
is usually caused by damage to nerve pathways within the brain or
spinal cord that control muscle movement. It may occur in association with spinal cord injury, multiple sclerosis, cerebral palsy, stroke,
brain or head trauma, amyotrophic lateral sclerosis, hereditary spastic
paraplegias, and metabolic diseases such as adrenoleukodystrophy,
phenylketonuria, and Krabbe disease.

Symptoms of Spasticity

Symptoms may include hypertonicity (increased muscle tone), clo-
nus (a series of rapid muscle contractions), exaggerated deep tendon
reflexes, muscle spasms, scissoring (involuntary crossing of the legs),
and fixed joints (contractures). The degree of spasticity varies from
mild muscle stiffness to severe, painful, and uncontrollable muscle
spasms. Spasticity can interfere with rehabilitation in patients with
certain disorders, and often interferes with daily activities.

Treatment of Spasticity

Treatment may include such medications as baclofen, diazepam,
tizanidine, or clonazepam. Physical therapy regimens may include
muscle stretching and range of motion exercises to help prevent
shrinkage or shortening of muscles and to reduce the severity of symptoms. Targeted injection of botulinum toxin into muscles with the most

410

time can help to selectively weaken these muscles to improve range of motion and function. Surgery may be recommended for tendon release or to sever the nerve-muscle pathway.

Prognosis of Spasticity

The prognosis for those with spasticity depends on the severity of the spasticity and the associated disorder(s).

How Do You Manage Spasticity?

Management of spasticity involves five key strategies, not just pharmacologic options.

- **Treat problems that increase the spasticity.** Evaluate for infections, fatigue, stress, and pain and address those that are modifiable. Develop a specific exercise program for patients. Referral to physiatrists and physical and occupational therapists not only can benefit spasticity management but also can address conserving energy that will lessen fatigue.

- **Develop a specific program for stiffness.** The most effective and simplest way to reduce spasticity is passive stretching. This is accomplished by stretching the affected joint slowly and moving it into a position that stretches the spastic muscles. After each muscle reaches its stretched position, it is held there for approximately one minute to allow it to slowly relax and release the undesired tension. This stretching program should begin at the ankle to stretch the calf muscle and then proceed upward to the muscles in the back of the thigh, the buttocks, the groin, and, after turning from the back to the stomach, the muscles in the front of the thigh. Although range of motion is important, holding the stretch is very important and patience is essential when doing the stretches. Exercising in a pool may also be extremely beneficial because the buoyancy of the water allows body movements with less energy expenditure and more efficient use of many muscles. The optimal pool temperature should be 85 degrees. Warmer temperatures will produce muscle fatigue and colder temperatures can actually cause spasticity.

- **Use specific mechanical devices.** These should be use to counteract spasticity and prevent contractures. Specific devices, such as finger or toe spreaders, are used to relax tightness in the feet and hands and aid immobility. Orthoses for the wrist, foot, and hand are used to maintain a natural position and to prevent limitations on movement and the development of spasticity.

- **Use pharmacologic approaches.** Baclofen is the most commonly used antispasmodic medication used in MS treatment. While a common medication, dosing is very patient-specific due to the narrow therapeutic window between effectiveness and inability to maintain functional ability. Tizandine is effective in decreasing stiffness and muscle spasms with less effect on strength than many other drugs. Because it can cause drowsiness, it is especially useful for nighttime stiffness and spasticity and can be used with baclofen for greater effectiveness. Dantrolene is a direct-acting muscle relaxant; however, it also has a narrow window between effectiveness and weakness, much like baclofen. Diazepam is often useful for spasms that occur at night. Because of its sedative effect, it also helps to induce sleep, but, as a barbiturate, it also has addictive potential, which may make it inappropriate for some patients. Clonazepam also can be used to promote significant relaxation but must be used with caution for the same reasons as diazepam. Cyproheptadine is an antihistamine that has antispasmodic properties and can be a good add-on. It can cause sedation, but at a dose of 4mg daily, it is useful for MS patients. Cyclobenzaprine is commonly used for back spasms. This drug can relieve limb spasms and works well in combination with other antispasmodics. Gabapentin is approved for seizures but also has antispasmodic properties. When taken in doses of more than 1g per day, it can ease problematic spasms. It can also be effective for pain caused by spasticity.

- **Use surgical interventions like a motor point block or a baclofen pump when necessary.** Patients with MS that have intractable spasticity and do not respond to oral medication, surgical intervention may be necessary. A motor point block, done by injecting phenol into specific groups of muscles, is useful for severe spasms that do not respond to drug therapy. This older surgical procedure may produce flaccidity in muscles. However, does not usually increase functional mobility and is not commonly used because newer techniques are available. At present, botulinum toxin is more commonly used to cause a temporary blockade of neuromuscular transmission. It is practical for treating small group muscle spasms, especially the muscles of the eye or face, but can also be useful for larger muscle groups depending on the dosage necessary to control spasticity.

412

A more invasive approach to controlling spasticity is the use of a baclofen pump that delivers baclofen directly into the spinal canal. Programming can require sometime, but this method is very effective for severe spasticity. This procedure requires test dosing before actual pump implantation. Finally, there are several more invasive, nonreversible procedures, such as tenotomy, neurectomy, and rhizotomy, which can be considered. In some circumstances, these may be effective strategies.

Section 35.2

Foot Drop

This section includes text excerpted from "Foot Drop Information Page," National Institute of Neurological Disorders and Stroke (NINDS), September 21, 2016.

Foot drop describes the inability to raise the front part of the foot due to weakness or paralysis of the muscles that lift the foot. As a result, individuals with foot drop scuff their toes along the ground or bend their knees to lift their foot higher than usual to avoid the scuffing, which causes what is called a "steppage" gait. Foot drop can be unilateral (affecting one foot) or bilateral (affecting both feet). Foot drop is a symptom of an underlying problem and is either temporary or permanent, depending on the cause.

Causes of Foot Drop

Causes include: neurodegenerative disorders of the brain that cause muscular problems, such as stroke, multiple sclerosis, and cerebral palsy; motor neuron disorders such as polio, some forms of spinal muscular atrophy and amyotrophic lateral sclerosis (commonly known as Lou Gehrig disease); injury to the nerve roots, such as in spinal stenosis; peripheral nerve disorders such as Charcot-Marie-Tooth disease or acquired peripheral neuropathy; local compression or damage to the peroneal nerve as it passes across the fibular bone below the knee; and muscle disorders, such as muscular dystrophy or myositis.

Treatment of Foot Drop

Treatment depends on the specific cause of foot drop. The most common treatment is to support the foot with lightweight leg braces and shoe inserts, called ankle-foot orthotics. Exercise therapy to strengthen the muscles and maintain joint motion also helps to improve gait. Devices that electrically stimulate the peroneal nerve during footfall are appropriate for a small number of individuals with foot drop. In cases with permanent loss of movement, surgery that fuses the foot and ankle joint or that transfers tendons from stronger leg muscles is occasionally performed.

Prognosis of Foot Drop

The prognosis for foot drop depends on the cause. Foot drop caused by trauma or nerve damage usually shows partial or even complete recovery. For progressive neurological disorders, foot drop will be a symptom that is likely to continue as a lifelong disability, but it will not shorten life expectancy.

Section 35.3

Constraint-Induced Movement Therapy

Constraint-Induced Movement Therapy, or CIMT, is a rehabilitative technique designed to help patients regain the use of an arm or hand that has experienced lost or reduced function after a stroke. Generally, when one limb or one half of the body is weakened or numbed, the natural tendency is for the patient to rely on the unaffected body part, a pattern known as "learned non-use," which has been shown to hinder recovery. In CIMT, the unaffected limb is restrained with a sling, bandage, or mitt, so the patient is forced to use and exercise the affected limb as much as possible. In this way, not only is the affected body part strengthened, but the brain actually rewires itself, repairing neural pathways and effecting recovery.

Some forms of CIMT experimentation have been around since at least the early twentieth century, but the technique really gained acceptance in the latter half of the century when it started being used more widely with good results. There are two forms of CIMT, each of which has its proponents.

Traditional Constraint-Induced Movement Therapy

Although each physical therapist and rehabilitation facility has a unique methodology, traditional, or original, CIMT is characterized by very long periods of time during which the patient is constrained. This is generally comprised of three components:

- Constraining the unaffected limb with intense use of the affected limb for up to six hours per day for ten days over a period of 14 days.

- Constraining the unaffected limb to promote the use of the affected limb during 90 percent of waking hours.

- Transferring rehabilitation gains to the patient's normal environment.

Traditional CIMT requires the patient to perform structured exercises and tasks under the one-on-one supervision of a trained therapist. This has led to occasional criticism of the technique involving concerns about patient safety from intense repetitive motion and the ability of patients to commit to the demanding regimen. In addition, some insurance companies balked at covering the high cost of the long supervised sessions. As a result, some practitioners have developed modified CIMT methodology.

Modified Constraint-Induced Movement Therapy

Modified CIMT, sometimes called MCIMT, relies on the same basic therapeutic techniques as the traditional version. There are numerous variations on the protocol, but MCIMT is generally characterized by less time with the unaffected limb constrained, less time spent in therapy sessions, and a more lenient and unsupervised transfer plan but a lengthier total rehabilitation period. For example, the regimen might include:

- Constraining the unaffected limb three days per week for several weeks.

- Supervised treatment sessions of as little as 30 minutes at a time.

- Two to seven sessions per week for two to twelve weeks.

- The goal of using the affected limb for 90 percent of waking hours but with specific targets and interim goals decided on an individual basis.

Proponents of MCIMT cite evidence that it is as effective as traditional CIMT in restoring or partially restoring the use of affected limbs following a stroke. In addition, they say, the regimen is less expensive than the original version and may be more readily accepted by insurance companies.

Whichever methodology is used, CIMT is intended to prevent or reverse learned non-use through exercises that mimic tasks that an individual performs in everyday life. But before participating in CIMT, patients need to be evaluated by a physician and occupational therapist, since not every individual is a candidate for this therapy. Some stroke impairments are too severe to be improved by this type of treatment, and MCIMT, in particular, may require that the patient have at least a minimum amount of strength and range of movement in the affected limb in order to participate.

References

1. "Constraint-Induced Movement Therapy," Flint Rehabilitation Devices, July 15, 2015.

2. "Constraint-Induced Movement Therapy (CIMT)," Northeastrehab.com, n.d.

3. "Constraint-Induced Movement Therapy After Stroke," Saebo. com, February 13, 2017.

4. Grotta, James C., MD, et al. "Constraint-Induced Movement Therapy," *Stroke*, October 28, 2004.

5. Kwakkel, Gert, PhD, et al. "Constraint-Induced Movement Therapy After Stroke," *Lancet Neurology*, February 14, 2015.

6. McDermott, Annabel, OT. "Constraint-Induced Movement Therapy—Upper Extremity," Canadian Partnership for Stroke Recovery, September 22, 2016.

Chapter 36

Balance Problems after Stroke

Problems with balance are extremely common after a stroke, with about 40 percent of stroke patients experiencing a fall within a year. Balance is a surprisingly complex function, involving three separate systems of the body: vision, somatosensory, and vestibular. Your eyes allow you to sense motion and determine where your head and body are located in relation to your surroundings. The somatosensory system uses sensors in your muscles, joints, and tendons to help your brain know how your feet, legs, and head are positioned. And the vestibular system employs structures in your inner ear to monitor head movements in relation to the pull of gravity to help you know if you're moving and in what direction you're oriented. Your brain processes all this information and then sends signals to your eyes, muscles, and other body parts to help keep you upright.

Common Balance Problems after Stroke

A stroke can affect each or all of the systems that control balance. It can influence the way the systems interact with each other or the way the brain sends signals to muscles through the nerves. Some of the most common balance problems include:

- **Weakness.** Most stroke patients experience some degree of muscle weakness, often on one side of the body. And this can result in difficulty sitting upright, standing, or walking.

- **Loss of sensation.** Some patients lose feeling in limbs, particularly legs. As a result, they sometimes can't feel the ground, making it difficult to walk and easy to lose balance.

- **Muscle stiffness.** Muscle and joint stiffness, or rigidity, can result in loss of coordination, making it difficult to walk and maintain balance.

- **Drop foot.** This is the term for difficulty lifting the front part of the foot. As a result, your toes can catch on the ground when you walk, and balance becomes affected.

- **Vision problems.** Some stroke patients have problems focusing, experience double vision, or have blind spots, all of which can cause balance issues.

- **Lack of energy.** It's not uncommon for stroke patients to tire easily. As a result, they can lose coordination and have difficulty controlling movement.

- **Dizziness.** Dizziness, or a spinning feeling, affects many stroke patients, especially those who experienced a brainstem stroke. This feeling of motion makes it particularly hard to maintain balance.

- **Ataxia.** This is a lack of muscle control that most often occurs with strokes that damage the back part of the brain. The reduced coordination makes it easy to lose balance.

- **Lack of concentration.** Trying to regain function and maintain balance after a stroke requires a significant amount of concentration, and many patients tire and lose focus.

- **Medication.** The side effects from some medications prescribed after a stroke can cause weakness, dizziness, and other problems that can cause loss of balance.

Treatment for Poststroke Balance Problems

Most patients with balance problems after a stroke see improvement within a few weeks to a few months. Generally, the sooner you begin to move, the more rapid your progress will be. A thorough mobility assessment by a physical therapist will tell you what type of movements and exercises will help you the most. These will be progressively more difficult as you progress, and depending on your specific balance issues, they can include:

- **Bed exercises.** Initial exercises might include such simple movements as sitting upright, lying back down, rolling over, and sitting on the edge of the bed with feet on the floor.

- **Seated exercises.** Many balance exercises can be performed in a sitting position on a bench or the side of a bed, such as shifting weight from side to side, leaning on each elbow, and standing up and sitting back down.

- **Simple standing exercises.** These include doing heel raises while holding onto something for support, stepping side to side with support, and reaching for objects.

- **Moderate standing exercises.** As progress is made, heel raises and side-stepping can be done without support, and slow heel-to-toe walking can be added, with support from a therapist, a walker, or a cane.

- **Advanced standing exercises.** When you're ready, you can move on to such activities as walking unaided, treadmill training, walking backwards, walking on soft or uneven surfaces, standing on one leg, side leg raises, and doing squats with a gym ball against a wall.

- **Yoga.** Many stroke patients find that simple yoga poses, using a chair for support at first, help improve strength and regain balance.

- **Vision exercises.** Patients with vision problems can work on their own or with a therapist on exercises that might include following an object moved from side to side and up and down, focusing on an object moved near and far, reading, and playing computer games. Some therapy centers also have specialized vision training equipment.

- **Dizziness training.** If you're experiencing dizziness or vertigo, one exercise that might help is focusing on a fixed object while moving your head in different directions. Although this might increase dizziness at first, with practice you should see improvement.

- **Constraint-induced movement therapy.** Some patients have difficulty maintaining balance because of weakness or numbness on one side of their bodies. In such cases, a physical therapist might use this technique, in which the stronger side of the body is restrained so the weaker side gets more exercise.

- **Functional electrical stimulation (FES).** Most commonly used for patients with drop foot, FES employs small electrical pulses to stimulate the peroneal nerve, which controls movement in the leg, ankle, and foot. This causes muscles to contract allowing the patient to lift his or her foot.

Ways to Help Avoid a Fall

Loss of balance after a stroke can be disorienting and confusing, but the biggest danger is the possibility of falling and causing further injury. Some ways to help avoid losing balance include:

- Exercise to improve balance.
- Eat a healthy diet to reduce dizziness.
- Be careful in the bathroom—that's where most falls take place.
- Walk slowly until you regain balance.
- Pause for a few seconds when changing positions (e.g., sitting to standing).
- Wear comfortable shoes or slippers that fit snugly.
- Remove throw rugs that can cause tripping.
- Be sure all areas of the house are well lighted.
- Store frequently used items low enough that you don't have to reach.
- Talk to your doctor to makes sure your medication isn't causing imbalance.

References

1. "Balance Changes after a Stroke," Wexner Medical Center, Ohio State University, August 13, 2012.

2. "Balance Problems after Stroke," Stroke Association (UK), April 2012.

3. "Common Problems after Stroke," Stroke Association (UK), February 2015.

4. "Keeping Your Balance after Stroke," American Stroke Association, March 5, 2015.

5. Marchione, Victor, MD. "Stroke and Balance Problems: Causes and Exercises to Regain Balance after Stroke," Bel Marra Health, November 16, 2016.

6. "Movement and Exercise after Stroke Fact Sheet," Stroke Foundation (Australia), n.d.

Chapter 37

Pain and Fatigue after Stroke

Chapter Contents

Section 37.1—Pain after Stroke 424

Section 37.2—Fatigue after Stroke 429

Section 37.1

Pain after Stroke

This section includes text excerpted from documents published
by two public domain sources. Text under headings marked 1 are
excerpted from "Pain after Stroke," U.S. Department of Veterans
Affairs (VA), December 27, 2013. Reviewed April 2017; Text under
heading marked 2 is excerpted from "Central Post-Stroke Pain,"
Genetic and Rare Diseases Information Center (GARD), National
Center for Advancing Translational Sciences (NCATS), May 25, 2011.
Reviewed April 2017.

What Do You Need to Know?[1]

Pain is common after a stroke. Pain means that the body is hurt
or something is wrong. Every stroke survivor's pain is different. The
pain may be mild or severe. It may last for a short time or be constant.

Pain after a stroke is caused by many things. Your loved one can
have one or more types of pain. The key is to find the cause of the pain
so it can be treated.

Local Pain

Local pain results from physical problems. After a part of the body
is paralyzed (unable to move) or weakened, the muscles may become
tight and stiff. These changes in the muscles can cause pain. This pain
is often felt in the joints, most often in the shoulders. Your loved one
may also have sore muscles from learning new ways to walk or move.
Pain may be caused by lying or sitting in one place too long. Other
common causes are pressure sores or painful leg cramps at night.

Central Pain

Central pain is a direct result of damage to the brain from the
stroke. Sensations like light touch are felt as pain when they should not
be painful. This pain is described as burning or aching. The pain is usually on the side of the body affected by the stroke. It is often constant
and may get worse over time. Changes in cold and hot temperatures
may increase the pain. Movement or touching may increase the pain.

Why Is It Important to Get Help?[1]

Talk to the healthcare team about your loved one's pain. Pain often leads to other problems. For instance, pain can cause depression and loss of sleep. Your loved one may stop moving a painful part of the body. Over time, the joint of this body part may "lock up" and your loved one will lose movement.

Central Poststroke Pain[2]

What Are the Signs and Symptoms of Central Poststroke Pain?

Central poststroke pain (CPSP) often begins shortly after the injury or damage that caused it, but may be delayed by months or even years, especially if it is related to poststroke pain. The character of the pain associated with CPSP differs widely among individuals, partly because of the variety of potential causes. It may affect a large portion of the body or may be more restricted to specific areas, such as hands or feet. The extent of pain is usually related to the cause of the central nervous system (CNS) injury or damage. Pain is typically constant, may be moderate to severe in intensity, and is often made worse by touch, movement, emotions, and temperature changes (usually cold temperatures). Individuals experience one or more types of pain sensations, the most prominent being burning. Mingled with the burning may be sensations of "pins and needles;" pressing, lacerating, or aching pain; and brief, intolerable bursts of sharp pain similar to the pain caused by a dental probe on an exposed nerve. Individuals may have numbness in the areas affected by the pain. The burning and loss of touch sensations are usually most severe on the distant parts of the body, such as the feet or hands.

How Is Central Poststroke Pain Diagnosed?

In the journal *Lancet Neurology*, the authors discuss making a diagnosis of CPSP. They recognize that a definite diagnosis of CPSP may be difficult, mainly because of the variable signs and symptoms, the frequent concurrence of several pain types, and the lack of clear diagnostic criteria for CPSP. The diagnosis may be based on a combination of the history, a clinical and sensory examination, imaging of lesions (such as computerized tomography (CT) scan or magnetic resonance imaging (MRI)), and other examinations. The history of stroke may be confirmed by imaging (either CT or MRI) to visualize the cause

425

(type, location, and size) and to rule out other central causes of the pain. Details about the pain, including when and how the pain began; pain quality; and the presence of dysesthesia (impaired sensitivity) or allodynia (pain resulting from something that should not normally cause pain) are helpful in the diagnosis. Sometimes patients are asked to indicate the area of pain on a drawing of the body (a pain drawing). The clinical examination may include sensory testing to confirm and pinpoint the presence of sensory abnormalities, but also to rule out other causes of pain.

Experts have proposed that mandatory criteria for the diagnosis of CPSP include:

- Pain within an area of the body corresponding to the abnormality of the CNS

- History suggestive of a stroke and onset of pain at or after stroke onset

- Confirmation of a CNS lesion by imaging, or negative or positive sensory signs confined to the area of the body corresponding to the lesion

- Other causes of pain are excluded or considered highly unlikely

  Supportive criteria may include:

- No primary relation to movement, inflammation, or other local tissue damage

- Descriptions such as burning, painful cold, electric shocks, aching, pressing, stinging, and pins and needles, although all pain descriptions may apply

- Allodynia or dysesthesia to touch or cold

What Treatments Should You Discuss with Your Healthcare Team?[1]

Pain usually lessens with treatment. There are many treatments to ask about.

Pain Medicines

Pain medicines are one of the most important treatments. Use pain medicines that your healthcare team suggests. Follow the directions on the label of the medicine. Give pain medicines on a regular basis.

Do not wait until the pain gets bad to give pain medicines. Do not stop using medicines for fear of addiction. When pain medicines are used correctly, they do not cause addiction.

Over-the-counter (OTC) pain medicines, like Tylenol® or Advil® relieve mild pain. These OTC medicines may interact with other medicines your loved one takes. Check with your healthcare team before taking any OTC medicines. For more severe pain, stronger prescription pain medicines like narcotics are often needed.

Medicines used to treat depression, spasticity (tightness and stiffness of muscles) or seizures may relieve central pain. Shots or injections of cortisone (steroids) into joints like the shoulder may help.

Exercises

Exercises to strengthen muscles can help your loved one move better. For example, stretching exercises decrease the tightness and soreness of the muscles. Talk with a physical therapist about the best exercise plan.

Heat Therapy

Heat therapy like heating pads and warm baths may soothe sore muscles and stiff joints.

Transcutaneous Electrical Nerve Stimulation

Transcutaneous electrical nerve stimulation (often called TENS or TNS) improves the strength of the muscles and often reduces pain. Patches or electrodes are placed on the skin. A mild electrical current runs through these patches. This is not painful.

Complementary or Alternative Therapies

Complementary or alternative therapies like acupuncture, massage therapy, and yoga often relieve pain.

What If the Pain Continues?[1]

Everyone has the right to good pain control. Ask your healthcare team to try different treatments to relieve the pain. If the pain continues, ask about other types of care.

* Pain clinics are helpful for people whose pain is difficult to treat. Ask about pain clinics in your area.

- Psychologists help stroke survivors find ways to live with pain that cannot be completely relieved. Psychologists also help survivors who are sad or depressed due to living with pain.

How Can You Help Your Loved One Describe the Pain?[1]

Your healthcare team needs to know how your loved one feels. Ask your loved one to rate the pain. Use a pain scale of "0–10," with "0" being no pain and "10" being the worst pain your loved one has ever felt. If your loved one can't speak, use a pain scale.

Take note of where your loved one hurts. What things bring on the pain? What makes it worse? When does the pain occur? How does it feel? Report these symptoms to your healthcare team.

Remember that some stroke survivors have trouble speaking. Watch for signs of pain such as moaning or changes in behaviors. Some stroke survivors may not feel pain. They may not know when they are cut or burned by hot water. Watch for sores and other injuries.

Talk with Your Loved One about the Pain

- Pain almost always is a real problem. Believe your loved one's complaints.

- Allow time for your loved one to talk about the pain.

- Talk about feelings of sadness related to the pain. Watch for signs of depression. Report problems to your healthcare team.

Helpful Tips[1]

- Help your loved one remain active to keep muscles strong and reduce pain.

- Talk with your healthcare team about correct ways to exercise. Also ask about how best to position paralyzed or weak arms and legs. Splints or other devices may be helpful.

- Support a weak or paralyzed arm to reduce pain in the shoulder. Ask your healthcare team about using an arm sling. Provide support for the arm on a lapboard or raised armrest. Use pillows while lying in bed.

- Have your loved one wear loose, comfortable clothing.

- Help your loved one relax. Find an activity that your loved one enjoys such as playing with the dog or watching television.

Suggest activities like listening to music, reading a book, prayer, or meditation.

• Use warm baths, showers, warm washcloths, or heating pads. Be sure to check the temperature so as not to cause burns. Cool cloths and ice may also help. Talk with your healthcare team about the best plan.

Section 37.2

Fatigue after Stroke

This section includes text excerpted from "RESCUE Fact Sheet—Feeling Tired after Stroke," U.S. Department of Veterans Affairs (VA), December 27, 2013. Reviewed April 2017.

Fatigue is defined as loss of energy or strength. Around 30–70 percent of stroke survivors feel very tired or have fatigue.

What Do You Need to Know?

It is normal for your loved one to tire easily. After a stroke, simple tasks, like sitting up or standing, may be exhausting. With time, your loved one should get back strength and energy.

Health issues that decrease energy after a stroke include:

• Muscle weakness

• Paralysis

• Pain

• Poor nutrition and weight loss

• Sadness or depression

Why Is It Important to Get Help?

Fatigue can slow down your loved one's recovery. It is important for your healthcare team to learn the cause of fatigue. Sometimes

429

fatigue is due to medical problems that can be treated. At other times, fatigue is due to side effects of medicines. The good news is there are treatments and ways to decrease fatigue.

What Treatments Should You Discuss with Your Healthcare Team?

- Medicines often help if fatigue is due to pain or depression.

- A social worker, psychologist, or psychiatrist can help your loved one with depression.

- A physical therapist (PT) can teach exercises to build strength. A PT can show your loved one how to move and save energy.

- An occupational therapist (OT) can teach new ways to do everyday tasks to save energy. An OT can suggest changes to make in your home to help your loved one move around.

Helpful Tips

- Encourage your loved one to eat healthy foods like fruits and vegetables.

- Give your loved one plenty of water to drink. Decreased amounts of liquids can cause fatigue.

- Plan frequent rest periods.

- Help your loved one get a good night's sleep. Limit caffeine after lunch. Get up and go to bed at the same time each day.

- Help your loved one stay active. Too much bed rest can weaken muscles.

- Work with your healthcare team to develop an exercise plan.

Remember

- Fatigue is a common problem after stroke.

- Talk with your healthcare team about your loved one's fatigue.

- Frequent rest periods are important.

- Help your loved one exercise and stay active.

Chapter 38

Bowel Control Problems and Stroke

Did you know bowel control problems affect about 18 million U.S. adults—one out of every 12 people? If you have a bowel control problem, you are not alone.

What Is a Bowel Control Problem?

A bowel control problem, also called fecal incontinence, means you are unable to hold a bowel movement until you reach a toilet. You may also have a bowel control problem if you pass stool into your underwear without being aware of it happening.

Who Gets Bowel Control Problems?

Although people of any age can have bowel control problems, they are more common in older adults. If you have any of the following, you may be more likely to have a bowel control problem:

- **Muscle or nerve damage.** Stroke; possible sources of muscle or nerve damage are hemorrhoid or cancer surgery; a long-term habit of straining to pass stool; childbirth; diseases that affect nerves, such as diabetes or multiple sclerosis; and spinal cord injury.

This chapter includes text excerpted from "Bowel Control Problems," National Institute of Diabetes and Digestive and Kidney Diseases (NIDDK), June 2014.

- **Diarrhea.** Diarrhea is passing loose, watery stools three or more times a day. Loose stools fill the rectum quickly and are more difficult to hold than solid stools.

- **Urgency.** You feel you need to get to the toilet immediately.

- **Constipation.** Constipation is having fewer than three bowel movements a week, which can lead to large, hard stools that get stuck in the rectum. Watery stool builds up behind the hard stool and can leak out around the hard stool. Inactivity, such as sitting for many hours a day, can keep stool in the rectum and cause constipation related problems.

- **Poor overall health**. You may be more likely to have bowel control problems if you have chronic, or long lasting, illnesses.

- **Loss of stretch in the rectum.** Rectal surgery, radiation treatment, and inflammatory bowel disease can cause scarring that stiffens the rectal walls. The rectum then can't stretch as much to hold stool, increasing the risk of bowel control problems.

- **Hemorrhoids.** Hemorrhoids can prevent the anus from closing completely.

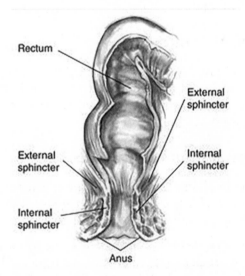

Figure 38.1. *Sphincter Muscles Involved in Bowel Control*

(Source: "Bowel Control Problems (Fecal Incontinence)," National Institute of Diabetes and Digestive and Kidney Diseases (NIDDK).)

What Can I Do about Bowel Control Problems?

Although you may be embarrassed to talk about your bowel control problem, your doctor will not be shocked or surprised. Your doctor will take your medical history, perform a physical exam, may suggest one or more medical tests, and may refer you to a specialist. Treatment may include changes to your diet, medicines to soften your stool or control diarrhea, exercises to strengthen your bowel control muscles, training to have bowel movements at certain times during the day, and possibly surgery.

Eating, Diet, and Nutrition

Changes in diet, such as eating the right amount of fiber and drinking plenty of water, may improve your bowel control. Keeping a food diary can help you identify foods that cause bowel control problems.

Chapter 39

Bladder Control Problems and Stroke

For the urinary system to do its job, muscles and nerves must work together to hold urine in the bladder and then release it at the right time. Nerves carry messages from the bladder to the brain to let it know when the bladder is full. They also carry messages from the brain to the bladder, telling muscles either to tighten or release. A nerve problem might affect your bladder control if the nerves that are supposed to carry messages between the brain and the bladder do not work properly.

What Bladder Control Problems Does Nerve Damage Cause?

Nerves that work poorly can lead to three different kinds of bladder control problems.

Overactive bladder. Damaged nerves may send signals to the bladder at the wrong time, causing its muscles to squeeze without warning. The symptoms of overactive bladder include

- urinary frequency—defined as urination eight or more times a day or two or more times at night

---

This chapter includes text excerpted from "Urologic Diseases—Bladder Control Problems and Nerve Disease," National Institute of Diabetes and Digestive and Kidney Diseases (NIDDK), June 2012. Reviewed April 2017.

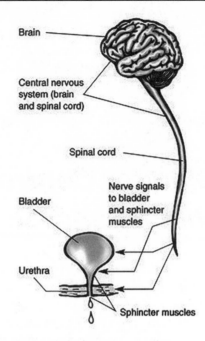

Figure 39.1. *Bladder Control Problems*

Nerves carry signals from the brain to the bladder and sphincter.

- urinary urgency—the sudden, strong need to urinate immediately

- urge incontinence—leakage of urine that follows a sudden, strong urge to urinate

Poor control of sphincter muscles. Sphincter muscles surround the urethra and keep it closed to hold urine in the bladder. If the nerves to the sphincter muscles are damaged, the muscles may become loose and allow leakage or stay tight when you are trying to release urine.

Urine retention. For some people, nerve damage means their bladder muscles do not get the message that it is time to release urine or are too weak to completely empty the bladder. If the bladder becomes too full, urine may back up and the increasing pressure may damage the kidneys. Or urine that stays too long may lead to an infection in the kidneys or bladder. Urine retention may also lead to overflow incontinence.

What Causes Nerve Damage?

Many events or conditions can damage nerves and nerve pathways. Some of the most common causes are:

- stroke
- vaginal childbirth
- infections of the brain or spinal cord
- diabetes
- accidents that injure the brain or spinal cord
- multiple sclerosis
- heavy metal poisoning

In addition, some children are born with nerve problems that can keep the bladder from releasing urine, leading to urinary infections or kidney damage.

How Will the Doctor Test for Nerve Damage and Bladder Control Problems?

Any evaluation for a health problem begins with a medical history and a general physical examination. Your doctor can use this information to narrow down the possible causes for your bladder problem.

If nerve damage is suspected, the doctor may need to test both the bladder itself and the nervous system, including the brain. Three different kinds of tests might be used:

- **Urodynamics.** These tests involve measuring pressure in the bladder while it is being filled to see how much it can hold and then checking to see whether the bladder empties completely and efficiently.

- **Imaging.** The doctor may use different types of equipment—X-rays, magnetic resonance imaging (MRI), and computerized tomography (CT) scans—to take pictures of the urinary tract and nervous system, including the brain.

- **EEG and EMG.** An electroencephalograph (EEG) is a test in which wires with pads are placed on the forehead to sense any dysfunction in the brain. The doctor may also use an electromyograph (EMG), which uses wires with pads placed on the lower abdomen to test the nerves and muscles of the bladder.

What Are the Treatments for Overactive Bladder?

The treatment for a bladder control problem depends on the cause of the nerve damage and the type of voiding dysfunction that results.

In the case of overactive bladder, your doctor may suggest a number of strategies, including bladder training, electrical stimulation, drug therapy, and, in severe cases where all other treatments have failed, surgery.

Bladder training. Your doctor may ask you to keep a bladder diary—a record of your fluid intake, trips to the bathroom, and episodes of urine leakage. This record may indicate a pattern and suggest ways to avoid accidents by making a point of using the bathroom at certain times of the day—a practice called timed voiding. As you gain control, you can extend the time between trips to the bathroom. Bladder training also includes Kegel exercises to strengthen the muscles that hold in urine.

Electrical stimulation. Mild electrical pulses can be used to stimulate the nerves that control the bladder and sphincter muscles. Depending on which nerves the doctor plans to treat, these pulses can be given through the vagina or anus, or by using patches on the skin. Another method is a minor surgical procedure to place the electric wire near the tailbone. This procedure involves two steps. First, the

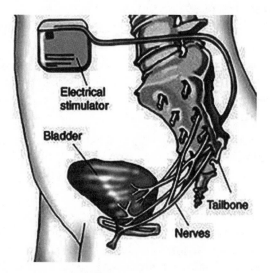

Figure 39.2. *Electrical Stimulation*

wire is placed under the skin and connected to a temporary stimulator, which you carry with you for several days. If your condition improves during this trial period, then the wire is placed next to the tailbone and attached to a permanent stimulator under your skin. The Food and Drug Administration (FDA) has approved this device, marketed as the InterStim system, to treat urge incontinence, urgency-frequency syndrome, and urinary retention in patients for whom other treatments have not worked.

Drug therapy. Different drugs can affect the nerves and muscles of the urinary tract in different ways.

- Drugs that relax bladder muscles and prevent bladder spasms include oxybutynin chloride (Ditropan), tolterodine (Detrol), hyoscyamine (Levsin), and propantheline bromide (Pro-Banthine), which belong to the class of drugs called anticholinergics. Their most common side effect is dry mouth, although large doses may cause blurred vision, constipation, a faster heartbeat, and flushing. A patch delivery system for oxybutynin (Oxytrol) may decrease side effects. Ditropan XL and Detrol LA are timed-release formulations that deliver a low level of the drug continuously in the body. These drugs have the advantage of once-a-day administration. In 2004, the FDA approved trospium chloride (Sanctura), darifenacin (Enablex), and solifenacin succinate (VESIcare) for the treatment of overactive bladder.

- Drugs for depression that also relax bladder muscles include imipramine hydrochloride (Tofranil), a tricyclic antidepressant. Side effects may include fatigue, dry mouth, dizziness, blurred vision, nausea, and insomnia.

Additional drugs are being evaluated for the treatment of overactive bladder and may soon receive FDA approval.

Surgery. In extreme cases, when incontinence is severe and other treatments have failed, surgery may be considered. The bladder may be made larger through an operation known as augmentation cystoplasty, in which a part of the diseased bladder is replaced with a section taken from the patient's bowel. This operation may improve the ability to store urine but may make the bladder more difficult to empty, making regular catheterization necessary. Additional risks of surgery include the bladder breaking open and leaking urine into the body, bladder stones, mucus in the bladder, and infection.

How Do You Do Kegel Exercises?

Kegel exercises strengthen the muscles that hold up the bladder and keep it closed.

The first step in doing Kegel exercises is to find the right muscles. Imagine you are trying to stop yourself from passing gas. Squeeze the muscles you would use. If you sense a "pulling" feeling, those are the right muscles for pelvic exercises.

Try not to squeeze other muscles at the same time. Be careful not to tighten your stomach, legs, or buttocks. Squeezing the wrong muscles can put more pressure on your bladder control muscles. Just squeeze the pelvic muscles. Don't hold your breath.

At first, find a quiet spot to practice—your bathroom or bedroom—so you can concentrate. Pull in the pelvic muscles and hold for a count of 3. Then relax for a count of 3. Repeat, but don't overdo it. Work up to 3 sets of 10 repeats. Start doing your pelvic muscle exercises lying down. This position is the easiest because the muscles do not need to work against gravity. When your muscles get stronger, do your exercises sitting or standing. Working against gravity is like adding more weight.

Be patient. Don't give up. It takes just 5 minutes a day. You may not feel your bladder control improve for 3 to 6 weeks. Still, most people do notice an improvement after a few weeks.

Some people with nerve damage cannot tell whether they are doing Kegel exercises correctly. If you are not sure, ask your doctor or nurse to examine you while you try to do them. If you are not squeezing the right muscles, you can still learn proper Kegel exercises by doing special training with biofeedback, electrical stimulation, or both.

What Are the Treatments for Lack of Coordination between the Bladder and Urethra?

The job of the sphincter muscles is to hold urine in the bladder by squeezing the urethra shut. If the urethral sphincter fails to stay closed, urine may leak out of the bladder. When nerve signals are coordinated properly, the sphincter muscles relax to allow urine to pass through the urethra as the bladder contracts to push out urine. If the signals are not coordinated, the bladder and the sphincter may contract at the same time, so urine cannot pass easily.

Drug therapy for an uncoordinated bladder and urethra. Scientists have not yet found a drug that works selectively on the urethral sphincter muscles, but drugs used to reduce muscle spasms or tremors are sometimes used to help the sphincter relax. Baclofen (Lioresal) is prescribed for muscle spasms or cramping in patients with multiple sclerosis and spinal injuries. Diazepam (Valium) can be taken as a muscle relaxant or to reduce anxiety. Drugs called alpha-adrenergic blockers can also be used to relax the sphincter. Examples of these drugs are alfuzosin (UroXatral), tamsulosin (Flomax), terazosin (Hytrin), and doxazosin (Cardura). The main side effects are low blood pressure, dizziness, fainting, and nasal congestion. All of these drugs have been used to relax the urethral sphincter in people whose sphincter does not relax well on its own.

Botox injection. Botulinum toxin type A (Botox) is best known as a cosmetic treatment for facial wrinkles. Doctors have also found that botulinum toxin is useful in blocking spasms like eye ticks or relaxing muscles in patients with multiple sclerosis. Urologists have found that injecting botulinum toxin into the tissue surrounding the sphincter can help it to relax. Although the FDA has approved botulinum toxin only for facial cosmetic purposes, researchers are studying the safety and effectiveness of botulinum toxin injection into the sphincter for possible FDA approval in the future.

What Are the Treatments for Urine Retention?

Urine retention may occur either because the bladder wall muscles cannot contract or because the sphincter muscles cannot relax.

Catheter. A catheter is a thin tube that can be inserted through the urethra into the bladder to allow urine to flow into a collection bag. If you are able to place the catheter yourself, you can learn to carry out the procedure at regular intervals, a practice called clean intermittent catheterization. Some patients cannot place their own catheters because nerve damage affects their hand coordination as well as their voiding function. These patients need to have a caregiver place the catheter for them at regular intervals. If regular catheter placement is not feasible, the patients may need to have an indwelling catheter that can be changed less often. Indwelling catheters have several risks, including infection, bladder stones, and bladder tumors. However, if the bladder cannot be emptied any other way, then the catheter is the only way to stop the buildup of urine in the bladder that can damage the kidneys.

Urethral stent. Stents are small tube-like devices inserted into the urethra and allowed to expand, like a spring, widening the opening for urine to flow out. Stents can help prevent urine backup when the bladder wall and sphincter contract at the same time because of improper nerve signals. However, stents can cause problems if they move or lead to infection.

Surgery. Men may consider a surgery that removes the external sphincter (a sphincterotomy) or a piece of it (a sphincter resection) to prevent urinary retention. The surgeon will pass a thin instrument through the urethra to deliver electrical or laser energy that burns away sphincter tissue. Possible complications include bleeding that requires a transfusion and, rarely, problems with erections. This procedure causes loss of urine control and requires the patient to collect urine by wearing an external catheter that fits over the penis like a condom. No external collection device is available for women.

Urinary diversion. If other treatments fail and urine regularly backs up and damages the kidneys, the doctor may recommend a urinary diversion, a procedure that may require an outside collection bag attached to a stoma, a surgically created opening where urine passes out of the body. Another form of urinary diversion replaces the bladder with a continent urinary reservoir, an internal pouch made from sections of the bowel or other tissue. This method allows the person to store urine inside the body until a catheter is used to empty it through a stoma.

Chapter 40

Vision Problems after Stroke

Vision problems are very common after stroke, with up to two-thirds of patients experiencing at least some degree of vision impairment. These issues occur most often in cases in which the right side of the brain is affected, but they can result from other types of stroke damage, as well. Sight involves not just the eyes but also the optic nerves, which travel the entire length of the brain. And although the occipital lobe at the back of the brain is the primary area that processes visual information, almost all areas of the brain receive input from vision, so there are many ways that a stroke can affect the way a patient sees. Like other effects of stroke, vision problems can be permanent, but in most cases they can improve over time, especially with proper treatment.

Common Vision Problems after Stroke

There is a wide variety of visual impairment that can occur following a stroke, but some of the most common problems include:

- **Visual field loss.** The visual field is the portion of a person's surroundings that can be seen at any given time. Visual field loss, called hemianopia, results in patients only being able to see either the right or left side of what they're looking at.

- **Central field loss.** With this condition, the center part of the vision field is affected. The patient might only be able to see objects at the very edges of the field but not in the middle.

- **Double vision.** Known as diplopia, double vision is most often the result of stroke damage to the brainstem. Here, the patient might see two of the same object, lose depth perception, and become disoriented.

- **Visual neglect.** Visual neglect, or inattention, usually results from damage to the parietal lobe of the brain, where spatial information is processed. With this condition, patients may not be aware of objects on one side. For example, they might only eat food on half of their plates, being unaware that the other half exists.

- **Eye movement issues.** Vision requires the coordinated movement of both eyes, and stroke can affect the way the brain controls these movements. This could result in such problems as difficulty focusing on objects or continuous jerky movement of the eyes.

- **Visual agnosia.** With this unusual disorder, the patient is able to see objects or people but is unable to identify them because of damage to the visual processing area of the brain. However, the patient may be able to recognize objects by touch or smell.

Other problems caused by vision problems resulting from stroke can include difficulty identifying colors, inability to calculate distance to objects, dizziness, and hallucinations.

Treatment for Vision Problems after Stroke

Because there are so many different types of visual impairment following a stroke, treatment can vary considerably. Depending on the condition, an ophthalmologist (eye doctor), optometrist (eye care professional), orthoptist (eye muscle specialist), and optician (eyeglasses and contact lens dispenser) can all be involved in a designing and carrying out a treatment plan. Some possible treatments include:

- **Optical therapy.** Also called vision field relocation, this treatment uses prisms or mirror—usually mounted on glasses—to shift images from the impaired side to the side with better vision, sometimes increasing the visual field by 20 percent.

- **Visual restoration therapy.** Here, flashing lights and images on a computer screen are used to stimulate neural cells and improve vision in blind areas of the visual field. By performing a set of vigorous exercises every day for several months, partially blind stroke patients can often improve vision significantly.

- **Eye movement therapy.** This type of treatment helps train a patient's eyes to scan objects within his or her post-stroke visual field. Exercises focus on strengthening and retraining eye muscles for improved control and stamina.

- **Surgery.** In some cases, surgical repair of eye muscles can correct double vision and movement disorders.

Vision Aids

Most patients who experience visual impairment after stroke improve at least to some degree with treatment. But in cases in which the problems persist (or while therapy continues), there are various devices that can help patients cope with vision issues. These include:

- **Eye patches.** While eye patches may not permanently correct conditions like double vision, they can be a simple, inexpensive means of coping with certain perception issues.

- **Magnifiers.** All types of magnifiers are available to help make reading easier. These range from simple pocket-sized magnifying glasses to large, lighted table-top models.

- **Typoscope.** This is a dark piece of nonreflective black cardboard with a rectangular slot in the center. When placed over reading material, it eliminates glare from the surrounding white spaces and makes it easier to focus on a line of text.

- **Reading stands.** A stand can not only position reading material closer and hold it steady, it can also prevent stooping to read, reducing neck strain and headaches.

- **Proper lighting.** Adequate lighting is important for individuals experiencing vision problems following a stroke. Adjustable lamps focus light on reading material or objects, keeping it out of the person's eyes. And if vision is better in one eye, an adjustable lamp can be positioned over the shoulder of the unaffected eye.

- **Binoculars or telescopes.** A small telescope or set of binoculars can be helpful for reading street signs or viewing distant objects. Some binoculars can be mounted on eyeglasses for added convenience.

- **Sunglasses.** Tinted glasses can not only protect the eyes from glare, they're also helpful in improving distance vision and depth perception.

References

1. "Common Problems after Stroke," Stroke Association (UK), February 2015.

2. Gupta, Mrinali Patel, MD. "Stroke/Hemianopsia," Vision-aware.org, n.d.

3. Lazarony, Lucy. "Overcome Post-Stroke Vision Challenges," Strokesmart.org, June 17, 2014.

4. "Stroke Related Eye Conditions," Royal National Institute of Blind People (UK), 2016.

5. "Vision," National Stroke Association," n.d.

6. "Vision Disturbances after Stroke," American Stroke Association, November 15, 2016.

Chapter 41

Poststroke Rehabilitation Facilities

Chapter Contents

Section 41.1—Overview of Poststroke Rehabilitation
         and Types of Poststroke Therapies 448

Section 41.2—How to Choose a Rehabilitation
         Facility 458

Section 41.3—Tips for Choosing a Rehabilitation
         Facility 461

447

Section 41.1

Overview of Poststroke Rehabilitation and Types of Poststroke Therapies

This section includes text excerpted from "Post-Stroke Rehabilitation," *Know Stroke*, National Institute of Neurological Disorders and Stroke (NINDS), September 2014.

In the United States more than 700,000 people suffer a stroke each year, and approximately two-thirds of these individuals survive and require rehabilitation. The goals of rehabilitation are to help survivors become as independent as possible and to attain the best possible quality of life. Even though rehabilitation does not "cure" the effects of stroke in that it does not reverse brain damage, rehabilitation can substantially help people achieve the best possible long-term outcome.

What Is Poststroke Rehabilitation?

Rehabilitation helps stroke survivors relearn skills that are lost when part of the brain is damaged. For example, these skills can include coordinating leg movements in order to walk or carrying out the steps involved in any complex activity. Rehabilitation also teaches survivors new ways of performing tasks to circumvent or compensate for any residual disabilities. Individuals may need to learn how to bathe and dress using only one hand, or how to communicate effectively when their ability to use language has been compromised. There is a strong consensus among rehabilitation experts that the most important element in any rehabilitation program is carefully directed, well-focused, repetitive practice—the same kind of practice used by all people when they learn a new skill, such as playing the piano or pitching a baseball.

Rehabilitative therapy begins in the acute-care hospital after the person's overall condition has been stabilized, often within 24 to 48 hours after the stroke. The first steps involve promoting independent movement because many individuals are paralyzed or seriously weakened. Patients are prompted to change positions frequently while lying in bed and to engage in passive or active range of motion exercises to

448

strengthen their stroke-impaired limbs. ("Passive" range-of-motion exercises are those in which the therapist actively helps the patient move a limb repeatedly, whereas "active" exercises are performed by the patient with no physical assistance from the therapist.) Depending on many factors—including the extent of the initial injury—patients may progress from sitting up and being moved between the bed and a chair to standing, bearing their own weight, and walking, with or without assistance. Rehabilitation nurses and therapists help patients who are able to perform progressively more complex and demanding tasks, such as bathing, dressing, and using a toilet, and they encourage patients to begin using their stroke-impaired limbs while engaging in those tasks. Beginning to reacquire the ability to carry out these basic activities of daily living represents the first stage in a stroke survivor's return to independence.

For some stroke survivors, rehabilitation will be an ongoing process to maintain and refine skills and could involve working with specialists for months or years after the stroke.

What Disabilities Can Result from a Stroke?

The types and degrees of disability that follow a stroke depend upon which area of the brain is damaged. Generally, stroke can cause five types of disabilities:

- paralysis or problems controlling movement;
- sensory disturbances including pain;
- problems using or understanding language;
- problems with thinking and memory; and
- emotional disturbances.

Paralysis or Problems Controlling Movement (Motor Control)

Paralysis is one of the most common disabilities resulting from stroke. The paralysis is usually on the side of the body opposite the side of the brain damaged by stroke, and may affect the face, an arm, a leg, or the entire side of the body. This one-sided paralysis is called hemiplegia (one-sided weakness is called hemiparesis). Stroke patients with hemiparesis or hemiplegia may have difficulty with everyday activities such as walking or grasping objects. Some stroke patients have problems with swallowing, called dysphagia, due to damage to the part of the brain that controls the muscles for swallowing. Damage to a lower part of the brain, the cerebellum, can affect the body's ability to coordinate movement, a disability called ataxia, leading to problems with body posture, walking, and balance.

Sensory Disturbances including Pain

Stroke patients may lose the ability to feel touch, pain, temperature, or position. Sensory deficits also may hinder the ability to recognize objects that patients are holding and can even be severe enough to cause loss of recognition of one's own limb. Some stroke patients experience pain, numbness or odd sensations of tingling or prickling in paralyzed or weakened limbs, a symptom known as paresthesias.

The loss of urinary continence is fairly common immediately after a stroke and often results from a combination of sensory and motor deficits. Stroke survivors may lose the ability to sense the need to urinate or the ability to control bladder muscles. Some may lack enough mobility to reach a toilet in time. Loss of bowel control or constipation also may occur. Permanent incontinence after a stroke is uncommon, but even a temporary loss of bowel or bladder control can be emotionally difficult for stroke survivors.

Stroke survivors frequently have a variety of chronic pain syndromes resulting from stroke-induced damage to the nervous system (neuropathic pain). In some stroke patients, pathways for sensation in the brain are damaged, causing the transmission of false signals that result in the sensation of pain in a limb or side of the body that has the sensory deficit. The most common of these pain syndromes is called "thalamic pain syndrome" (caused by a stroke to the thalamus, which processes sensory information from the body to the brain), which can be difficult to treat even with medications. Finally, some pain that occurs after stroke is not due to nervous system damage, but rather to mechanical problems caused by the weakness from the stroke. Patients who have a seriously weakened or paralyzed arm commonly experience moderate to severe pain that radiates outward from the shoulder. Most often, the pain results from lack of movement in a joint that has been immobilized for a prolonged period of time (such as having your arm or shoulder in a cast for weeks) and the tendons and ligaments around the joint become fixed in one position. This is commonly called a "frozen" joint; "passive" movement (the joint is gently moved or flexed by a therapist or caregiver rather than by the individual) at the joint in a paralyzed limb is essential to prevent painful "freezing" and to allow easy movement if and when voluntary motor strength returns.

Problems Using or Understanding Language (Aphasia)

At least one-fourth of all stroke survivors experience language impairments, involving the ability to speak, write, and understand spoken and written language. A stroke-induced injury to any of the brain's language-control centers can severely impair verbal communication. The dominant centers for language are in the left side of the brain for right-handed individuals and many left-handers as well. Damage to a language center located on the dominant side of the brain, known as Broca's area, causes expressive aphasia. People with this type of aphasia have difficulty conveying their thoughts through words or writing. They lose the ability to speak the words they are thinking and to put words together in coherent, grammatically correct sentences. In contrast, damage to a language center located in a rear portion of the brain, called Wernicke's area, results in receptive aphasia. People with this condition have difficulty understanding spoken or written language and often have incoherent speech. Although they can form grammatically correct sentences, their utterances are often devoid of meaning. The most severe form of aphasia, global aphasia, is caused by extensive damage to several areas of the brain involved in language function. People with global aphasia lose nearly all their linguistic abilities; they cannot understand language or use it to convey thought.

Problems with Thinking and Memory

Stroke can cause damage to parts of the brain responsible for memory, learning, and awareness. Stroke survivors may have dramatically shortened attention spans or may experience deficits in short-term memory. Individuals also may lose their ability to make plans, comprehend meaning, learn new tasks, or engage in other complex mental activities. Two fairly common deficits resulting from stroke are anosognosia, an inability to acknowledge the reality of the physical impairments resulting from stroke, and neglect, the loss of the ability to respond to objects or sensory stimuli located on the stroke-impaired side. Stroke survivors who develop apraxia (loss of ability to carry out a learned purposeful movement) cannot plan the steps involved in a complex task and act on them in the proper sequence. Stroke survivors with apraxia also may have problems following a set of instructions.

451

Apraxia appears to be caused by a disruption of the subtle connections that exist between thought and action.

Emotional Disturbances

Many people who survive a stroke feel fear, anxiety, frustration, anger, sadness, and a sense of grief for their physical and mental losses. These feelings are a natural response to the psychological trauma of stroke. Some emotional disturbances and personality changes are caused by the physical effects of brain damage. Clinical depression, which is a sense of hopelessness that disrupts an individual's ability to function, appears to be the emotional disorder most commonly experienced by stroke survivors. Signs of clinical depression include sleep disturbances, a radical change in eating patterns that may lead to sudden weight loss or gain, lethargy, social withdrawal, irritability, fatigue, self-loathing, and suicidal thoughts. Post-stroke depression can be treated with antidepressant medications and psychological counseling.

What Medical Professionals Specialize in Poststroke Rehabilitation?

Poststroke rehabilitation involves physicians; rehabilitation nurses; physical, occupational, recreational, speech-language, and vocational therapists; and mental health professionals.

Physicians

Physicians have the primary responsibility for managing and coordinating the long-term care of stroke survivors, including recommending which rehabilitation programs will best address individual needs. Physicians also are responsible for caring for the stroke survivor's general health and providing guidance aimed at preventing a second stroke, such as controlling high blood pressure or diabetes and eliminating risk factors such as cigarette smoking, excessive weight, a high-cholesterol diet, and high alcohol consumption.

Neurologists usually lead acute-care stroke teams and direct patient care during hospitalization. They sometimes participate on the long-term rehabilitation team. Other subspecialists often lead the rehabilitation stage of care, especially physiatrists, who specialize in physical medicine and rehabilitation.

Rehabilitation Nurses

Nurses specializing in rehabilitation help survivors relearn how to carry out the basic activities of daily living. They also educate survivors about routine healthcare, such as how to follow a medication schedule, how to care for the skin, how to move out of a bed and into a wheelchair, and special needs for people with diabetes. Rehabilitation nurses also work with survivors to reduce risk factors that may lead to a second stroke, and provide training for caregivers.

Nurses are closely involved in helping stroke survivors manage personal care issues, such as bathing and controlling incontinence. Most stroke survivors regain their ability to maintain continence, often with the help of strategies learned during rehabilitation. These strategies include strengthening pelvic muscles through special exercises and following a timed voiding schedule. If problems with incontinence continue, nurses can help caregivers learn to insert and manage catheters and to take special hygienic measures to prevent other incontinence-related health problems from developing.

Physical Therapists

Physical therapists specialize in treating disabilities related to motor and sensory impairments. They are trained in all aspects of anatomy and physiology related to normal function, with an emphasis on movement. They assess the stroke survivor's strength, endurance, range of motion, gait abnormalities, and sensory deficits to design individualized rehabilitation programs aimed at regaining control over motor functions.

Physical therapists help survivors regain the use of stroke-impaired limbs, teach compensatory strategies to reduce the effect of remaining deficits, and establish ongoing exercise programs to help people retain their newly learned skills. Disabled people tend to avoid using impaired limbs, a behavior called learned non-use. However, the repetitive use of impaired limbs encourages brain plasticity** and helps reduce disabilities.

Strategies used by physical therapists to encourage the use of impaired limbs include selective sensory stimulation such as tapping or stroking, active and passive range-of-motion exercises, and temporary restraint of healthy limbs while practicing motor tasks.

In general, physical therapy emphasizes practicing isolated movements, repeatedly changing from one kind of movement to another, and rehearsing complex movements that require a great deal of coordination and balance, such as walking up or down stairs or moving safely between obstacles. People too weak to bear their own weight can still practice repetitive movements during hydrotherapy (in which water provides sensory stimulation as well as weight support) or while being partially supported by a harness. A recent trend in physical therapy emphasizes the effectiveness of engaging in goal-directed activities, such as playing games, to promote coordination. Physical therapists frequently employ selective sensory stimulation to encourage use of impaired limbs and to help survivors with neglect regain awareness of stimuli on the neglected side of the body.

Occupational and Recreational Therapists

Like physical therapists, occupational therapists are concerned with improving motor and sensory abilities, and ensuring patient safety in the post-stroke period. They help survivors relearn skills needed for performing self-directed activities (also called occupations) such as personal grooming, preparing meals, and housecleaning. Therapists can teach some survivors how to adapt to driving and provide on-road training. They often teach people to divide a complex activity into its component parts, practice each part, and then perform the whole sequence of actions. This strategy can improve coordination and may help people with apraxia relearn how to carry out planned actions.

Occupational therapists also teach people how to develop compensatory strategies and change elements of their environment that limit activities of daily living. For example, people with the use of only one hand can substitute hook and loop fasteners (such as Velcro) for buttons on clothing. Occupational therapists also help people make changes in their homes to increase safety, remove barriers, and facilitate physical functioning, such as installing grab bars in bathrooms.

Recreational therapists help people with a variety of disabilities to develop and use their leisure time to enhance their health, independence, and quality of life.

Speech-Language Pathologists

Speech-language pathologists help stroke survivors with aphasia relearn how to use language or develop alternative means of communication. They also help people improve their ability to swallow, and they work with patients to develop problem-solving and social skills needed to cope with the after-effects of a stroke.

Many specialized therapeutic techniques have been developed to assist people with aphasia. Some forms of short-term therapy can improve comprehension rapidly. Intensive exercises such as repeating the therapist's words, practicing following directions, and doing reading or writing exercises form the cornerstone of language rehabilitation. Conversational coaching and rehearsal, as well as the development of prompts or cues to help people remember specific words, are sometimes beneficial. Speech-language pathologists also help stroke survivors develop strategies for circumventing language disabilities. These strategies can include the use of symbol boards or sign language. Recent advances in computer technology have spurred the development of new types of equipment to enhance communication.

Speech-language pathologists use special types of imaging techniques to study swallowing patterns of stroke survivors and identify the exact source of their impairment. Difficulties with swallowing have many possible causes, including a delayed swallowing reflex, an inability to manipulate food with the tongue, or an inability to detect food remaining lodged in the cheeks after swallowing. When the cause has been pinpointed, speech-language pathologists work with the individual to devise strategies to overcome or minimize the deficit. Sometimes, simply changing body position and improving posture during eating can bring about improvement. The texture of foods can be modified to make swallowing easier; for example, thin liquids, which often cause choking, can be thickened. Changing eating habits by taking small bites and chewing slowly can also help alleviate dysphagia.

Vocational Therapists

Approximately one-fourth of all strokes occur in people between the ages of 45 and 65. For most people in this age group, returning to work is a major concern. Vocational therapists perform many of the same functions that ordinary career counselors do. They can help people with residual disabilities identify vocational strengths and develop résumés that highlight those strengths. They also can help identify potential employers, assist in specific job searches, and provide referrals to stroke vocational rehabilitation agencies.

Most important, vocational therapists educate disabled individuals about their rights and protections as defined by the Americans with Disabilities Act of 1990. This law requires employers to make "reasonable accommodations" for disabled employees. Vocational therapists frequently act as mediators between employers and employees to negotiate the provision of reasonable accommodations in the workplace.

Nurses specializing in rehabilitation help survivors relearn how to carry out the basic activities of daily living. They also educate survivors about routine healthcare, such as how to follow a medication schedule, how to care for the skin, how to move out of a bed and into a wheelchair, and special needs for people with diabetes. Rehabilitation nurses also work with survivors to reduce risk factors that may lead to a second stroke, and provide training for caregivers.

Nurses are closely involved in helping stroke survivors manage personal care issues, such as bathing and controlling incontinence. Most stroke survivors regain their ability to maintain continence, often with the help of strategies learned during rehabilitation. These strategies include strengthening pelvic muscles through special exercises and following a timed voiding schedule. If problems with incontinence continue, nurses can help caregivers learn to insert and manage catheters and to take special hygienic measures to prevent other incontinence-related health problems from developing.

When Can a Stroke Patient Begin Rehabilitation?

Rehabilitation should begin as soon as a stroke patient is stable, sometimes within 24 to 48 hours after a stroke. This first stage of rehabilitation can occur within an acute-care hospital; however, it is very dependent on the unique circumstances of the individual patient.

Recently, in the largest stroke rehabilitation study in the United States, researchers compared two common techniques to help stroke patients improve their walking. Both methods—training on a body-weight supported treadmill or working on strength and balance exercises at home with a physical therapist—resulted in equal improvements in the individual's ability to walk by the end of one year. Researchers found that functional improvements could be seen as late as one year after the stroke, which goes against the conventional wisdom that most recovery is complete by 6 months. The trial showed that 52 percent of the participants made significant improvements in walking, everyday function and quality of life, regardless of how severe their impairment was, or whether they started the training at 2 or 6 months after the stroke.

Where Can a Stroke Patient Get Rehabilitation?

At the time of discharge from the hospital, the stroke patient and family coordinate with hospital social workers to locate a suitable living arrangement. Many stroke survivors return home, but some move into some type of medical facility.

Inpatient Rehabilitation Units

Inpatient facilities may be freestanding or part of larger hospital complexes. Patients stay in the facility, usually for 2 to 3 weeks, and engage in a coordinated, intensive program of rehabilitation. Such programs often involve at least 3 hours of active therapy a day, 5 or 6 days a week. Inpatient facilities offer a comprehensive range of medical services, including full-time physician supervision and access to the full range of therapists specializing in post-stroke rehabilitation.

Outpatient Units

Outpatient facilities are often part of a larger hospital complex and provide access to physicians and the full range of therapists specializing in stroke rehabilitation. Patients typically spend several hours, often 3 days each week, at the facility taking part in coordinated therapy sessions and return home at night. Comprehensive outpatient facilities frequently offer treatment programs as intense as those of inpatient facilities, but they also can offer less demanding regimens, depending on the patient's physical capacity.

Nursing Facilities

Rehabilitative services available at nursing facilities are more variable than are those at inpatient and outpatient units. Skilled nursing facilities usually place a greater emphasis on rehabilitation, whereas traditional nursing homes emphasize residential care. In addition, fewer hours of therapy are offered compared to outpatient and inpatient rehabilitation units.

Home-Based Rehabilitation Programs

Home rehabilitation allows for great flexibility so that patients can tailor their program of rehabilitation and follow individual schedules. Stroke survivors may participate in an intensive level of therapy several hours per week or follow a less demanding regimen. These arrangements are often best suited for people who require treatment by only one type of rehabilitation therapist. Patients dependent on Medicare coverage for their rehabilitation must meet Medicare's "homebound" requirements to qualify for such services; at this time lack of transportation is not a valid reason for home therapy. The major disadvantage of home-based rehabilitation programs is the lack of specialized equipment. However, undergoing treatment at home gives people the advantage of practicing skills and developing compensatory strategies in the context of their own living environment. In the recent stroke rehabilitation trial, intensive balance and strength rehabilitation in the home was equivalent to treadmill training at a rehabilitation facility in improving walking.

Section 41.2

How to Choose a Rehabilitation Facility

"How to Choose a Rehabilitation Facility,"
© 2017 Omnigraphics. Reviewed April 2017.

Stroke rehabilitation, often called rehab, is a crucial part of recovering from a stroke. Proper rehabilitation techniques can help patients increase strength and flexibility, re-learn basic skills like talking, eating, and walking, regain independence, and improve their overall quality of life. Effective rehab frequently requires a team of healthcare professionals from a variety of fields, such as neurology, nursing, physical therapy, occupational therapy, psychiatry, psychology, speech therapy, nutrition, and social work. Of course stroke patients and their families want the best rehab program available. But since each patient is different, both in terms of specific condition and individual preferences, finding the right rehab facility can be a challenging task.

Types of Rehabilitation Settings

Depending on the severity of the stroke, personal preference, insurance coverage, and other factors, rehabilitation can take place in a number of different locations, including:

- **Acute care facility.** This is often a special unit of a hospital, to which a patient is transferred after he or she is stabilized, usually a few days after the stroke. Here, for four to seven days, the patient receives ongoing medical care and testing while spending several hours per day going through progressively more complex basic tasks, such as moving limbs, sitting up, standing, bathing, and dressing.

- **Sub-acute care facility.** Sub-acute care can take place at a special hospital unit or a separate dedicated facility, such as a nursing home or skilled nursing center. This therapy is less intense than acute care, but it generally continues for a longer period of time. The patient continues to see a neurologist or other physician while receiving care by the nursing staff and undergoing a combination, physical, occupational, and speech therapy and appropriate counseling.

- **Outpatient facility.** Once stroke patients return home, they usually continue rehabilitation on an outpatient basis, which can take place at a doctor's office, a clinic, part of a hospital, or a rehab center. Here, the therapy is more intense than the patient could perform on his or her own, with the goal of regaining as much function as possible through a variety of exercises and tests.

- **Home care.** No one wants to stay in a hospital or residential facility longer than necessary, and research shows that stroke patients who are able to continue rehabilitation at home earlier generally do better. Home care is best for patients who require treatment by just one or two specialists, who can visit and supervise therapy on a regular basis. Although home care may lack the specialized equipment available at a dedicated facility, it has the advantage of allowing the patient to perform exercises and practice skills in his or her own environment.

Factors to Consider When Choosing a Rehabilitation Facility

Because of the different effects of a stroke, patient needs can vary considerably, as can the types of appropriate care facilities. But here are some factors to take into account:

- **Accreditation.** Quality standards for rehabilitation facilities are established by the Commission on Accreditation of Rehab Facilities (CARF) and the Joint Commission on Accreditation of Healthcare Organizations (JCAHO), as well as by Medicare. Ask how the facility meets these standards.

- **Specialized programs.** One of the most important factors is to be sure the facility offers programs and equipment that meet the specific needs of the patient. Ask about details of the program: what therapy is planned, how often it will be done, and who will be involved.

- **Trained staff.** Rehab staff must be trained and experienced in providing the particular type of therapy required by the patient. Those who require ongoing medical care, for example, will require on-site physicians and skilled nursing staff, while patients who are having difficulty walking will need a physical therapist.

- **Workload.** The number of patients served by the facility and the number seen by each medical professional or therapist will have an effect on the patient's successful rehabilitation. Ask questions to ensure that staff members are not overloaded.

- **Treatment plan.** Ask about the patient's specific treatment plan, what team members were involved in developing it, and how often it will be updated.

- **Progress evaluation.** It's important to try and quantify the patient's rehabilitation to get an accurate picture of his or her progress. Ask about the facility's process for formal evaluations, how often they're done, and who is involved.

- **Additional services.** Some rehab facilities offer supplemental services, including art, music, relaxation, and pet therapy, as well as a variety of games, coordination exercises, and support groups. Some of these may appeal to certain patients and could be very beneficial to their rehabilitation.

- **Family participation.** Ask if family members are involved in developing treatment plans and participating in therapy sessions. Family support can provide important information, help improve patient morale, and also prepare family members to assist with home care at some point.

- **Transition and ongoing therapy.** Once residential therapy is completed, it's important that the facility has a process for preparing the patient for discharge with appropriate instructions for home care. In addition, some facilities are equipped to provide ongoing in-home therapy with their own trained staff.

- **Insurance.** Don't forget to ask about insurance coverage. Be sure the facility, its staff, and the anticipated therapy are covered by the patient's insurance plan before committing to a facility.

References

1. "10 Tips for Choosing a Rehab Facility," Cleveland Clinic, December 20, 2013.

2. "Choosing the Right Stroke Rehab Facility," American Stroke Association, n.d.

3. Gerber, Charlotte. "10 Questions to Ask When Choosing a Rehabilitation Facility," Verwell.com, August 12, 2016.

4. "Home Is the Best Place for Stroke Rehabilitation," Medscape. com, May 5, 2000.

5. "National Stroke Association's Guide to Choosing Stroke Rehabilitation Services," National Stroke Association, 2006.

6. "Rehab Facilities," Stroke-rehab.com, n.d.

Section 41.3

Tips for Choosing a Rehabilitation Facility

Finding the right rehabilitation facility can be challenging because there are many factors to consider, says Yana Shumyatcher, MD, a Physical Medicine and Rehabilitation specialist at Cleveland Clinic Rehabilitation Hospital at Euclid Hospital. "Asking the right questions can help," she says.

Below, find ten questions to ask when choosing a rehab facility:

1. Does it offer programs specific to your needs?

You should check if physicians at the facility prescribe therapies for specific services. These can include rehabilitation after stroke, brain injury, Parkinson disease, amputation, orthopaedic surgery, cardiac rehabilitation and organ transplantation.

2. **Is 24-hour care provided and how qualified is the staff?**

   Check if around-the-clock physician coverage is provided. Also, check if the nursing staff includes registered nurses certified in rehabilitation nursing and if they are experienced in acute care.

3. **How are treatment plans developed?**

   Find out how treatment plans are developed at any facility you are considering. Physicians and nurses may work with physical, occupational, speech/language and recreational therapists, psychologists and social workers to develop patient treatment plans.

4. **How often is therapy provided?**

   Patients should receive at least three hours of therapy daily, five days a week, as required for licensed rehabilitation facilities.

5. **What supplemental services are offered?**

   Find out what other services the facilities offer, which could include programming in horticulture, art, music, relaxation, cooking, pet therapy, balance/coordination and stroke exercise. They may also have support groups.

6. **Do caregivers assist with discharge and insurance questions?**

   You might ask if patients are assigned to social workers or case managers, who can help coordinate services needed at home and who can also help verify insurance benefits.

7. **Is family participation encouraged?**

   A partnership involving the patient, family, and medical providers is essential to maximizing every opportunity for recovery. Find out how involved family members may be and if they are encouraged to observe therapy, participate in key meetings and learn how to assist in the care of the patient

8. **Are outpatient physician and therapy services offered?**

   Ask if there will be comprehensive services, including outpatient therapy and home care, available through rehabilitation professionals in your area.

9. **Is access to patient electronic medical records provided?**

   Find out if each patient's rehabilitation team can access his or her medical history, medication lists, radiology and laboratory results, and treatment status electronically.

10. **Do patients have on-site access to other specialists?**

    Find out if medical and surgical subspecialists, therapists and physiatrists are also available.

Part Six

Life after Stroke

Chapter 42

Recovering from Stroke

Recovery time after a stroke is different for everyone—it can take weeks, months, or even years. Some people recover fully, but others have long-term or lifelong disabilities.

What to Expect after a Stroke

If you have had a stroke, you can make great progress in regaining your independence. However, some problems may continue:

- Paralysis (inability to move some parts of the body), weakness, or both on one side of the body.

- Trouble with thinking, awareness, attention, learning, judgment, and memory.

- Problems understanding or forming speech.

- Trouble controlling or expressing emotions.

- Numbness or strange sensations.

- Pain in the hands and feet that worsens with movement and temperature changes.

This chapter contains text excerpted from the following sources: Text in this chapter begins with excerpts from "Stroke—Recovering from Stroke," Centers for Disease Control and Prevention (CDC), January 17, 2017; Text under the heading "Intensive Physical Therapy Boosts Stroke Recovery" is excerpted from "Intensive Physical Therapy Boosts Stroke Recovery," U.S. Department of Veterans Affairs (VA), June 2, 2015.

- Trouble with chewing and swallowing.

- Problems with bladder and bowel control.

- Depression.

Stroke Rehabilitation

Rehab can include working with speech, physical, and occupational therapists.

- **Speech therapy** helps people who have problems producing or understanding speech.

- **Physical therapy** uses exercises to help you relearn movement and coordination skills you may have lost because of the stroke.

- **Occupational therapy** focuses on improving daily activities, such as eating, drinking, dressing, bathing, reading, and writing.

Therapy and medicine may help with depression or other mental health conditions following a stroke. Joining a patient support group may help you adjust to life after a stroke. Talk with your healthcare team about local support groups, or check with an area medical center.

Support from family and friends can also help relieve fear and anxiety following a stroke. Let your loved ones know how you feel and what they can do to help you.

Preventing Another Stroke

If you have had a stroke, you are at high risk for another stroke:

- One in four strokes each year are recurrent.

- The chance of stroke within 90 days of a transient ischemic attack (TIA) may be as high as 17 percent, with the greatest risk during the first week.

That's why it's important to treat the causes of stroke, including heart disease, high blood pressure, atrial fibrillation (fast, irregular heartbeat), high cholesterol, and diabetes. Your doctor may prescribe you medicine or tell you to change your diet, exercise, or adopt other healthy lifestyle habits. Surgery may also be helpful in some cases.

Intensive Physical Therapy Boosts Stroke Recovery

After a stroke, the brain and body can start recovering immediately, and can show improvement up to six months afterwards. However, a U.S. Department of Veterans Affairs (VA) study has found that for those with persistent disability even after completing standard rehabilitation therapy, intensive physical therapy can provide additional recovery even the therapy begins a year or more after the stroke.

The study, covered by the Daily Caller and other media outlets, was led by Dr. Janis Daly, director of the Brain Rehabilitation Research Center of Excellence at the Gainesville (FL) VA Medical Center and a researcher at the University of Florida.

The average change in function for patients who had been severely affected by their stroke was clinically significant for arm movements and for performing complex tasks. For example, a man who had been unable to lift a spoon to his mouth is now able to feed himself.

To help the 39 participants regain movements of their shoulders, arms, and hands, the study team delivered an intensive physical therapy program that included five hours of rehabilitation per day, five days per week, for 12 weeks. They tested three different modes of rehabilitation, including motor-learning rehabilitation, which involves the repetitive practicing of tasks as deliberately as possible; electrical stimulation rehabilitation, in which electrodes stimulated forearm muscles to cause the hand to lift; and robotics-assisted rehabilitation, in which robots provided support to help the patients make reaching movements on their own, gradually lessening the support as the patients regained function.

The motor-learning group received five full hours of this therapy daily. Those using the other two modes received motor learning most of the time, but either electrical stimulation or robotics therapy for the remaining time. Each of the groups improved significantly, on average doubling or nearly doubling their scores on a scale that assesses coordination. Recovery for all three groups was equal, with no statistically significant difference between the groups.

"The magnitude of recovery we observed in our study is higher than any other studies that have been published so far, which supports the promise of longer treatment and more intensive treatment after stroke, even for those who are more severely impaired," said Daly in a University of Florida news release.

Chapter 43

Making the Home Safer for Stroke Survivors

After a stroke, your loved one may fall or have trouble moving around. You can make changes to improve home safety. These types of changes are called "home modification."

What Do You Need to Know?

Some changes are easy and you can do them yourself. For bigger changes, you may need professional help. The changes you make depend on the needs of your loved one.

What Can You Do?

Look around and find ways to make your home safe. Watch your loved one walk in the home to find areas that are unsafe.

Bathroom

- Buy non-slip bath mats, tub or shower benches and toilet chairs.

- Install handrails beside the toilet and in the tub or shower.

This chapter includes text excerpted from "Ways to Make the Home Safer (Home Modification)," U.S. Department of Veterans Affairs (VA), December 27, 2013. Reviewed April 2017.

- Install a hand-held shower head so your loved one can sit during a shower.

Kitchen

- Buy a stove with controls in the front. Your loved one will be able to reach the controls when cooking.
- Lower counters to make them easier to reach while sitting.
- Keep oven mitts and heat-proof mats close to the stove. Leave areas near the stove clear to place hot dishes.
- Place a fire extinguisher in easy reach.

Bedroom

- Put bedrails on the bed for safety.
- Place a commode beside the bed so your loved one won't need to walk to the bathroom. This can prevent falls at night.

What Changes Can Be Made for Stroke Survivors Who Use Wheelchairs?

Remove the cabinet under the stove or sink so your loved one can roll under. Use heat-proof covering (insulation) on pipes in roll-under sinks and stoves to prevent burns.

Stroke survivors may have trouble moving wheelchairs on heavy carpet. Use nonslip flooring if you remove the carpet. Widen doorways to help stroke survivors get in and out of the home. Outdoor and indoor ramps can also be built.

What Are Some General Home Changes?

Place pads on soft furniture to help with toileting accidents—Cover the pads so that other people will not notice.

Remove throw rugs—Use double-sided tape to hold down carpets.

Keep floors clear—Place large furniture far apart to help your loved one move around. Make sure furniture does not move if leaned on. Cover sharp corners of furniture.

Place handrails on both sides of stairs for safety—Elevators or lifts for the home can help stroke survivors who cannot climb stairs.

Replace door knobs and faucet knobs with lever handles— This will help stroke survivors who have trouble using their hands and arms.

What Are Some Other Safety Changes?

- Place a phone in each room or give your loved one a cell phone to call for help. Large-button phones are helpful for people who have trouble seeing.

- A medical alert system that the stroke survivor can carry may help.

- Lighting should be bright (use high wattage light bulbs) to prevent falls. Install overhead lights or nightlights in doorways, hallways and bathrooms.

- Install and regularly check smoke detectors and carbon monoxide detectors.

- Move all cords out of the way. Make sure cords are in good repair to prevent shock or fires.

Helpful Tips

- If possible, have your loved one visit the home before the last day in the hospital. Some hospitals and rehabilitation centers will let patients take weekend trips to visit family. This will help you learn how to make the house safe before your loved one comes home.

- Occupational therapists, visiting nurses and physical therapists can come to your house and help you make changes.

- Purchase items for home safety at medical equipment stores and through catalogs.

How Can You Pay for Home Modification?

Insurance and Medicaid

Some changes to the home may be covered by insurance. Talk to private insurance companies to see what can be covered. Medicaid may pay for some needed medical items.

Government Funding

The U.S. Department of Veterans Affairs (VA) has some funding through its Home Loans program, benefits.va.gov/homeloans. Contact other government resources, such as the U.S. Department of Housing and Urban Development (HUD) and the Social Security Administration (SSA) to help with funding. You may also get information from Eldercare Locator.

Private Funding

Nonprofit and volunteer groups may pay for some home changes. Contact groups like Rebuilding Together (rebuildingtogether.org) and NeighborWorks Network (www.neighborworks.org).

Chapter 44

Rehabilitative and Assistive Technology

What Is Rehabilitative and Assistive Technology?

Rehabilitative and assistive technology refers to tools, equipment, or products that can help a person with a disability to function successfully at school, home, work, and in the community.

Assistive technology can be as simple as a magnifying glass or as complex as a computerized communication system. An assistive device can be as large as an automated wheelchair lift for a van or as small as a handheld hook to assist with buttoning a shirt.

The term "rehabilitative technology" is sometimes used to refer to aids used to help people recover their functioning after injury or illness. But the term often is used interchangeably with the term "assistive technology."

The *Eunice Kennedy Shriver* National Institute of Child Health and Human Development (NICHD) supports research for developing technologies, devices, computerized and robotic devices, and other aids aimed at helping people with disabilities achieve their full potential.

Rehabilitative engineering involves the application of engineering and scientific principles to study how people with disabilities function

This chapter includes text excerpted from "Rehabilitative and Assistive Technology," *Eunice Kennedy Shriver* National Institute of Child Health and Human Development (NICHD), December 5, 2012. Reviewed April 2017.

in society. It includes studying barriers to optimal function and designing solutions so that people with disabilities can interact successfully in their environments.

How Many People Use Assistive Devices?

The Centers for Disease Control and Prevention (CDC) estimated that:

- One in five Americans—about 53 million people—has a disability of some kind.

- 33 million Americans have a disability that makes it difficult for them to carry out daily activities; some have challenges with everyday activities, such as attending school or going to work, and may need help with their daily care.

- 2.2 million people in the United States depend on a wheelchair for day-to-day tasks and mobility.

- 6.5 million people use a cane, a walker, or crutches to assist with their mobility.

What Are Some Types of Assistive Devices and How Are They Used?

Some examples of assistive technologies are:

- People with physical disabilities that affect movement can use mobility aids, such as wheelchairs, scooters, walkers, canes, crutches, prosthetic devices, and orthotic devices, to enhance their mobility.

- Hearing aids can improve hearing ability in persons with hearing problems.

- Cognitive assistance, including computer or electrical assistive devices, can help people function following brain injury.

- Computer software and hardware, such as voice recognition programs, screen readers, and screen enlargement applications, help people with mobility and sensory impairments use computer technology.

- In the classroom and elsewhere, assistive devices, such as automatic page-turners, book holders, and adapted pencil grips, allow learners with disabilities to participate in educational activities.

- Closed captioning allows people with hearing impairments to enjoy movies and television programs.

- Barriers in community buildings, businesses, and workplaces can be removed or modified to improve accessibility. Such modifications include ramps, automatic door openers, grab bars, and wider doorways.

- Lightweight, high-performance wheelchairs have been designed for organized sports, such as basketball, tennis, and racing.

- Adaptive switches make it possible for a child with limited motor skills to play with toys and games.

- Many types of devices help people with disabilities perform such tasks as cooking, dressing, and grooming. Kitchen implements are available with large, cushioned grips to help people with weakness or arthritis in their hands. Medication dispensers with alarms can help people remember to take their medicine on time. People who use wheelchairs for mobility can use extendable reaching devices to reach items on shelves.

What Are Some Types of Rehabilitative Technologies?

Rehabilitative technologies are any technologies that help people recover function after injury or illness. Just a few examples include the following:

- **Robotics.** Specialized robots help people regain function in arms or legs after a stroke.

- **Virtual reality.** People who are recovering from injury can retrain themselves to perform motions within a virtual environment.

- **Musculoskeletal modeling and simulations.** These computer simulations of the human body can pinpoint the underlying mechanical problems in a person with a movement-related disability. This can help design better assistive aids or physical therapies.

- **Transcranial magnetic stimulation (TMS).** TMS sends magnetic impulses through the skull to stimulate the brain. This system can help people who have had a stroke recover movement and brain function.

- **Transcranial direct current stimulation (tDCS).** In tDCS, a mild electrical current travels through the skull and stimulates the brain of patients recovering from stroke. This can help recover movement.

- **Motion analysis.** Motion analysis captures video of human motion with specialized computer software that analyzes the motion in detail. The technology gives healthcare providers a detailed picture of a person's specific movement challenges to be used as a guide for proper therapy.

For What Conditions Are Assistive Devices Used?

Some disabilities are quite visible, and others are "hidden." Most disabilities can be grouped into four major categories:

- **Cognitive disability:** intellectual and learning disabilities/disorder, distractibility, reading disorders, inability to remember or focus on large amounts of information

- **Hearing disability:** hearing loss or impaired hearing

- **Physical disability:** paralysis, difficulties with walking or other movement, inability to use a computer mouse, slow response time, limited fine or gross motor control

- **Visual disability:** blindness, low vision, color blindness

Mental illness, including anxiety disorders, mood disorders, eating disorders, and psychosis, for example, is also a disability.

Hidden disabilities can include some people with visual impairments and those with dexterity difficulties, such as repetitive strain injury. People who are hard of hearing or have mental health difficulties also may be included in this category.

Some people have disabling medical conditions that may be regarded as hidden disabilities—for example, epilepsy; diabetes; sickle cell conditions; human immunodeficiency virus / acquired immune deficiency syndrome (HIV/AIDS); cystic fibrosis; cancer; and heart, liver or kidney problems. The conditions may be short term or long term, stable or progressive, constant or unpredictable and fluctuating, controlled by medication or another treatment, or untreatable. Many people with hidden disabilities can benefit from assistive technologies for certain activities or during certain stages of their diseases or conditions.

People who have spinal cord injuries, traumatic brain injury, cerebral palsy, muscular dystrophy, spina bifida, osteogenesis imperfecta, multiple sclerosis, demyelinating diseases, myelopathy, progressive muscular atrophy, amputations, or paralysis often benefit from complex rehabilitative technology. This means that the assistive devices these people use are individually configured to help each person with his or her own unique disability.

How Does Rehabilitative and Assistive Technology Benefit People with Disabilities?

Deciding which type of rehabilitative or assistive technology would be most helpful for a person with a disability is usually made by the disabled person and his or her family and caregivers, along with a team of professionals and consultants. The team is trained to match particular assistive technologies to specific needs to help the person function more independently. The team may include family doctors, regular and special education teachers, speech-language pathologists, rehabilitation engineers, occupational therapists, and other specialists, including representatives from companies that manufacture assistive technology.

Assistive technology enables students with disabilities to compensate for the impairments they experience. This specialized technology promotes independence and decreases the need for other educational support.

Appropriate assistive technology helps people with disabilities overcome or compensate, at least in part, for their limitations. Rehabilitative technology can help restore function in people who have developed a disability due to disease, injury, or aging. Rehabilitative and assistive technology can enable individuals to:

- Care for themselves and their families

- Work

- Learn in schools and other educational institutions

- Access information through computers and reading

- Enjoy music, sports, travel, and the arts

- Participate fully in community life

Assistive technology also benefits employers, teachers, family members, and everyone who interacts with users of the technology. Increasing opportunities for participation benefits everyone.

As assistive technologies are becoming more commonplace, people without disabilities are benefiting from them. For example, people who are poor readers or for whom English is a second language are taking advantage of screen readers. The aging population is making use of screen enlargers and magnifiers.

Chapter 45

Driving after Stroke

You have been a safe driver for years. For you, driving means freedom and control. As you get older, changes in your physical and mental health can affect how safely you drive.

Driving is a major concern after you have a stroke. A stroke is a "brain attack" that occurs when the blood flow to the brain is interrupted. A stroke makes brain cells die and damages the brain. Brain injury may change the way you do things, especially your ability to drive safely.

How Can a Stroke Affect the Way I Drive?

At first, you may not realize all the effects of the stroke. So it is crucial that you talk with your family and work closely with your healthcare provider before you start driving again after you have a stroke.

Below are some ways a stroke may affect the way you drive:

- You may not be able to speak, to think or see clearly, or to control your body.

- You may have temporary or permanent weakness or paralysis on one side of your body.

- You may be forgetful, careless, or irritable.

- You may get frustrated easily and be confused while driving.

- You may drift across lane markings, into other lanes.

This chapter includes text excerpted from "Driving after You Have a Stroke," National Highway Traffic Safety Administration (NHTSA), February 23, 2015.

Can I Still Drive after a Stroke?

You may be able to drive after a stroke. It depends on where the stroke took place in your brain and how much damage it caused. Many people recover after a stroke and are able to drive safely. But many others will have some type of disability afterward.

Your healthcare provider will tell you how the stroke affected you, and when and if you can drive. It is important to note that in many areas, it is dangerous and even illegal to drive after a stroke without your doctor's consent.

What Can I Do When a Stroke Affects My Driving Safety?

You may not realize how a stroke has changed your ability to drive safely. After initial treatment, your healthcare provider can tell you about warning signs and symptoms of stroke. Warning signs tend to come on suddenly and may include:

- Numbness or weakness of the face, arm, or leg, especially on one side of the body.
- Confusion, trouble speaking or understanding.
- Trouble seeing in one or both eyes.
- Trouble walking, dizziness, loss of balance or coordination.
- Severe headache with no known cause.

Your healthcare provider can give you information about rehabilitation after the stroke. He or she also may suggest that you see a driver rehabilitation specialist to help you adjust to any changes caused by the stroke. A driver rehabilitation specialist can test how well you drive on and off the road. This specialist also may help you improve your driving skills by training you to use special equipment that can be fitted on your car to make it easier for you to drive safely.

To find a driver rehabilitation specialist, go to www.aota.org/older-driver. Under "Driving and Community Mobility," click the button in the center of the page marked "Search for a Driver Rehabilitation Specialist." This will link you to a national database. There you can search for names and addresses of local driver rehabilitation specialists.

What Can I Do If I Have to Limit or Stop Driving?

With proper treatment and support, you may be able to drive safely after a stroke. Even if you have to limit or give up driving, you can stay active and do the things you like to do.

First, plan ahead. Talk with family and friends about how you can shift from driver to passenger. Below are some ways to get where you want to go and see the people you want to see:

- Rides with family and friends.

- Taxis.

- Shuttle buses or vans.

- Public buses, trains, and subways.

- Walking.

- Paratransit services (special transportation services for people with disabilities; some offer door-to-door service).

Take someone with you. You may want to have a family member or friend go with you when you use public transportation or when you walk. Having someone with you can help you get where you want to go without confusion.

Find out about transportation services in your area. Many community-based volunteer programs offer free or low-cost transportation.

Where Can I Get Help with Transportation?

To find transportation services in your area, visit www.eldercare. gov or call the national ElderCare Locator at 800-677-1116, and ask for your local Office on Aging.

If you have a disability, check out Easter Seals Project ACTION (Accessible Community Transportation In Our Nation) at www.projectaction.org or call 800-659-6428. This project works with the transportation industry and the disability community to give people with disabilities more ways to get around.

Chapter 46

Nutrition and Exercise Tips for Poststroke Patients

Chapter Contents

Section 46.1—Advice for People with Swallowing
        Difficulties 486

Section 46.2—Nutrition and Exercise after Stroke................... 488

Section 46.1

Advice for People with Swallowing Difficulties

This section contains text excerpted from the following sources: Text in this section begins with excerpts from "Dysphagia," National Institute on Deafness and Other Communication Disorders (NIDCD), March 6, 2017; Text beginning with the heading "Tips for Safe Swallowing" is excerpted from "Safe Swallowing," U.S. Department of Veterans Affairs (VA), May 2013. Reviewed April 2017.

People with dysphagia have difficulty swallowing and may even experience pain while swallowing (odynophagia). Some people may be completely unable to swallow or may have trouble safely swallowing liquids, foods, or saliva. When that happens, eating becomes a challenge. Often, dysphagia makes it difficult to take in enough calories and fluids to nourish the body and can lead to additional serious medical problems.

What Causes Dysphagia?

Dysphagia has many possible causes and happens most frequently in older adults. Any condition that weakens or damages the muscles and nerves used for swallowing may cause dysphagia. For example, people with diseases of the nervous system, such as cerebral palsy or Parkinson disease, often have problems swallowing. Additionally, stroke or head injury may weaken or affect the coordination of the swallowing muscles or limit sensation in the mouth and throat.

People born with abnormalities of the swallowing mechanism may not be able to swallow normally. Infants who are born with an opening in the roof of the mouth (cleft palate) are unable to suck properly, which complicates nursing and drinking from a regular baby bottle.

In addition, cancer of the head, neck, or esophagus may cause swallowing problems. Sometimes the treatment for these types of cancers can cause dysphagia. Injuries of the head, neck, and chest may also create swallowing problems. An infection or irritation can cause narrowing of the esophagus. Finally, for people with dementia, memory loss and cognitive decline may make it difficult to chew and swallow.

Where Can I Get Help?

If you have a sudden or gradual change in your ability to swallow, you should consult with your physician. He or she may refer you to an otolaryngologist—a doctor who specializes in diseases of the ear, nose, throat, head, and neck—and a speech-language pathologist. You may be referred to a neurologist if a stroke or other neurologic disorder is the cause of the swallowing problem.

Tips for Safe Swallowing

* Eat while sitting in an upright position.
* Avoid distractions—focus on eating!
* Eat and drink slowly; take small bites.
* Chew thoroughly and swallow completely.
* Sit upright for 30 minutes after eating.

Diet Level and Food Consistency

Your healthcare provider, dietitian or speech-language pathologist will recommend the right diet level and liquid consistency for you.

* **Dysphagia Pureed:** Foods on this diet are pureed to a pudding-like consistency.

* **Dysphagia Mechanically-Altered:** Foods on this diet are soft textured, moist and easy to chew. Meats must be ground or minced into pieces no larger than 1/4-inch. Vegetables must smaller than 1/2-inch pieces, thoroughly cooked and mashed with a fork. Foods from the Dysphagia Pureed diet can also be eaten on this diet.

* **Dysphagia Advanced:** Foods must be moist and cut into bite-sized pieces. No sticky, chewy, hard, or stringy foods are allowed. Foods from the dysphagia pureed and mechanically-altered diets can also be eaten on this diet.

Liquid Consistency

- **Nectar Thick:** Nectar thick liquids are thickened to the consistency of peach or pear nectar. Liquids must stay this thickness at room and body temperature. Nectar thick liquids will coat a spoon lightly.

- **Honey Thick:** Honey thick liquids are thicker than nectar thick liquids but not as thick as pudding. Liquids should pour slowly off a spoon and coat the spoon like honey. The liquid should not run off like a thin liquid or plop like pudding. Liquids must remain at this consistency at room or body temperature.

Thickeners are available to thicken thin liquids to the desired consistency; they come in powder or gel form. Follow the manufacturer's instructions for mixing. Pre-thickened beverages are also available.

Section 46.2

Nutrition and Exercise after Stroke

This section contains text excerpted from the following sources:
Text in this section begins with excerpts from "RESCUE Fact
Sheet—Healthy Eating," U.S. Department of Veterans Affairs
(VA), December 27, 2013. Reviewed April 2017; Text beginning
with the heading "Exercise after Stroke" is excerpted from
"Exercise after Stroke," U.S. Department of Veterans Affairs (VA),
December 27, 2013. Reviewed April 2017.

Good nutrition or healthy eating is a key to stroke recovery. Healthy eating can help to keep your blood pressure, blood sugar, and weight under control. Healthy eating may even help prevent another stroke.

What Do You Need to Know?

Grains

Include grains in your diet every day. Grains have fiber, vitamins, and minerals. Fiber lowers the chance of having another stroke. Wheat, rice, oats, and barley are common grains. Whole grains are best. Whole grain cereals, brown rice, whole wheat pasta and whole wheat breads are good choices. Make half of your grains "whole."

Vegetables

Vegetables are another good source of fiber, vitamins, and minerals. Choose dark green, leafy vegetables like spinach, broccoli, and collard greens. Orange vegetables like sweet potatoes and carrots are good choices too. Vary your vegetables.

Fruits

Fruits are also good sources of fiber, vitamins, and minerals. Choose different fresh, dried, canned, or frozen fruits. It's best to choose whole fruits rather than juices. Juices have more sugar and less fiber than whole fruits.

Milk, Yogurt, and Cheese

Dairy products contain calcium and vitamin D. They help keep bones strong. Choose low-fat (1%) or fat-free milk (skim) products. If you can't have milk products, there are other choices. For instance, some cereals and juices are fortified or have extra calcium and vitamin D.

Meats, Beans, and Other Protein Sources

Proteins are found in meat, fish, beans, eggs, and nuts. Proteins help with muscle, bone, and skin health. Pinto beans, kidney beans, chickpeas, and split peas are also high in protein. It is important to limit red meat, which is high in saturated fat. Fish and poultry are better choices. Avoid processed foods, as they have a lot of salt. Stay away from frying. Instead, boil, bake, or grill meats. Be sure to remove the skin and extra fat before cooking.

Fats, Oils, and Sweets

A healthy diet includes some fats. The key is to choose healthy fats. Vegetable fats like olive, corn, and soybean oils are better for the heart than animal fats like butter and lard. Trans fats are man-made fats. Trans fats are unhealthy and increase the chances of heart attacks and strokes. Trans fats are found in baked goods and some restaurant food. Soft, low-fat tub margarine is better to use than stick margarine. Snacking on nuts is a healthy choice.

Drink Plenty of Liquids

Drinking liquids helps prevent constipation (trouble having a bowel movement). Drinking water is one of the best ways to get the right amount of liquids. To improve flavor, add a lemon or lime slice. Unsweetened tea, low-fat or fat-free milk and 100 percent fruit juice are good choices, too. Liquids are also found in foods like fruits and vegetables.

What about Salt?

Too much salt can raise your blood pressure. Cut back on salty snacks and processed food. Remember that you should have only 2/3 of a teaspoon of table salt each day. This includes everything you eat or drink, not just what is added when cooking or eating. Remember that canned foods and many canned soups have added salt.

Nutrition Tips

- Cook several extra meals at one time. Date and freeze the extra meals to eat later.

- Read the food labels or "nutrition facts" on packaged or processed foods. Many of these products are high in fat and salt.

- Add more salads, vegetables, and fruits to you diet.

- Season foods with lemon juice, herbs, and spices instead of salt or butter.

Exercise after Stroke

Physical activity or exercise can be any activity that gets the body moving. This includes things like walking and dancing. It can even include household chores like sweeping.

Why Is Exercise Important?

Exercise is good for both the mind and body. It can help your loved one get back strength that was lost due to stroke. It can make muscles more flexible. This will help improve how your loved one moves.

Physical exercise is important in reducing the risk of your loved one having another stroke. Stroke guidelines suggest that the survivor gets 20 to 60 minutes of aerobic exercise three to seven days per week. To make it easier, the exercise can be broken into smaller times. Walking for 10–15 minutes several times a day is a good way to get aerobic exercise.

Physical Benefits of Exercise

- Lowers chance of another stroke.
- Improves energy level.
- Makes bones and muscles stronger.
- Lowers blood pressure.
- Helps improve sleep.
- Improves flexibility.
- Reduces risk of falls.

Mental Benefits of Exercise

- Reduces stress.
- Lowers feelings of depression and anxiety.
- Improves self-worth.
- Promotes independence.

What Do You Need to Know?

Stroke can reduce your loved one's ability to exercise. If they are depressed, the motivation to exercise may be lowered. With decreased physical activity, muscles become weaker. The chances of another stroke or other health problem will increase.

It is important for your loved one to get regular exercise. Most survivors are able to do some form of exercise after their stroke. The type of exercise your loved one can do depends on the disability. The key is to stay as physically active as possible. Talk to your healthcare team before your loved one starts an exercise program.

What Are the Different Types of Exercise?

Aerobic Exercise

- Includes walking, dancing or riding a bike.
- Helps to lower blood pressure and maintain a healthy body weight.
- Low-impact exercises like swimming help protect the joints.

Do 30 minutes of moderate exercise 5 days a week or 20 minutes of intense exercise 3 days a week.

Strengthening Exercise

- Includes conditioning exercises, like sit-ups and push-ups.

- Includes using balance balls and weights.

- Helps to make muscles stronger.

Do muscle strengthening exercises at least two times a week.

Flexibility Exercise

- Includes stretching and yoga.

- Helps to keep joints flexible.

- Lowers chance of injury.

Do exercises that increase flexibility at least 2 times a week.

How Do You Get Your Loved One to Exercise?

- Help your loved one choose activities they enjoy doing. Walking the dog or gardening can be a fun way to get exercise.

- Join in on the exercise. You can improve your health together.

- Be a cheerleader for your loved one. Even small progress deserves praise.

- Keep an activity journal. Seeing the progress made can help motivate your loved one to continue.

- Look into adaptive recreation if your loved one has a disability. Adaptive recreation allows people with disabilities to get involved in sports or other fitness activities.

Exercise Tips

- Have your loved one start slowly. Don't overdo it.

- Remember to have them warm up and cool down when exercising.

- Make sure your loved one drinks plenty of water before, during and after exercise.

Chapter 47

Skin Care after Stroke

Skin is an important part of the body that works in many ways to maintain health.

- Protects the body from outside injury, illness, and germs

- Prevents loss of fluids and nutrients

- Helps to control body temperature in hot and cold weather

Skin includes several layers of tissue. Some tissues are filled with tiny blood vessels that move oxygen and nutrients to the skin. The skin also has nerves which send messages from different parts of the body to the brain. These create awareness of touch, pain, and temperature. Other nerves provide information about where body parts (arms, legs) are positioned in space and whether you are lying on an object.

After experiencing a stroke, patients may be at risk for skin problems due to decreased movement and feeling. Several types of skin problems can occur:

- Sores, blisters, rashes or skin color changes may develop if someone remains sitting or lying in one spot for long periods of time.

- Loss of feeling may affect ability to notice contact with something sharp or hot.

Text in this chapter is from "Skin Care after a Stroke," © 2017 Nursing Practice Council, Shirley Ryan AbilityLab (formerly Rehabilitation Institute of Chicago). Used by Permission: Betts LIFE Center, Shirley Ryan AbilityLab (formerly Rehabilitation Institute of Chicago).

- Bladder or bowel accidents are special concerns because they can cause the skin to become irritated.

- Older people tend to have greater skin problems after a stroke because skin becomes less elastic with age.

Keeping Skin Healthy

Healthy skin is intact, well lubricated with natural oils and nourished by a good blood supply. Skin stays healthy with a balanced diet, good hygiene, regular skin checks and pressure relief. Relieving pressure and checking skin ensures a good blood supply. Skin problems can often be prevented. The following tips will help.

Hygiene

- Keep skin clean and dry. Urine, sweat or stool can cause skin breakdown. Bathing every day in a tub or shower may not be necessary and may also wash away natural oils that lubricate the skin. A daily sponge bath, however, is good for exfoliation of dry skin and overall personal hygiene. Always try to keep palm side of affected hand and underarm clean.

- Dry well after bathing, but avoid hard rubbing with a towel—it can hurt the skin.

- Back rubs can be very relaxing, but should be done with lotion or oil, not alcohol, which is very drying to the skin.

- Trim nails regularly and avoid sharp edges or hangnails.

- Individuals with diabetes should do self foot care examinations and see a podiatrist regularly.

Nutrition

- Eat a healthy diet. Protein, vitamins and iron are especially important. Consult with a nutrition professional for help planning a diet that will meet your needs.

- Drink six to eight cups of fluid every day.

- Tube feedings are chosen to provide all necessary nutrients.

- Pureeing or chopping foods does not change the nutritional value.

Skin Inspection

- Check skin regularly to spot injuries when they are just starting.

- Inspect entire body, especially bony areas.

- Check at least twice a day—morning and evening—when you change position. Check more often if increasing sitting or turning times.

- Check skin every hour when using new equipment.

- Do not depend on others to tell you how your skin looks. If you need help, however, clearly explain what warning signs to look for.

- Use a long handled mirror to help with hard to see areas.

- Be alert to areas that have been injured and healed. Scar tissue breaks down very easily.

- Look for red areas, blisters, openings in the skin or rashes. In red areas, use the back of your stronger hand to feel for heat.

- Do not forget to check groin area. Men who wear an external catheter should check genital area for sores or other problems.

Chapter 48

Sleep after Stroke

Sleep problems are common after a stroke. The good news is there are ways to improve your loved one's sleep.

What Do You Need to Know?

Both old and young adults need about 7–9 hours of sleep. Poor sleep is not a normal part of getting older. But, after a stroke, your loved one may have more sleep problems. Sleep is important for good health. Everyone should expect to get a good night's sleep.

What Might Be Causing Your Loved One's Sleep Problems?

More than half of stroke survivors have one of the following sleep problems:

Sleep Apnea

This is a serious condition. Sleep apnea increases the risk of having a second stroke. It is caused by abnormal breathing patterns. Loud snoring, choking and gasping sounds during sleep may mean that your loved one has sleep apnea. Tell your healthcare team about these symptoms. There are good treatments.

This chapter includes text excerpted from "Sleeping Problems," U.S. Department of Veterans Affairs (VA), December 27, 2013. Reviewed April 2017.

Change in Sleep-Wake Cycles

After a stroke, some survivors do not get sleepy at night. It may be difficult to wake the stroke survivor in the morning. This happens when the sleep-wake schedule is no longer affected by sunlight and the darkness of night. Talk with your healthcare team. Bright light therapy may help.

What Are Some Other Common Sleep Problems?

Here is a list of other reasons your loved one may have trouble sleeping:

- frequently waking to use the bathroom—often due to prostate or bladder problems
- pain or discomfort
- stress, anxiety and depression
- conditions such as asthma, arthritis or heart failure
- medicines and certain foods or drinks

Why Is It Important to Get Help?

Poor sleep can slow your loved one's recovery. Sleep problems can lead to depression, memory problems and night-time falls.

Your healthcare team can help resolve your loved one's sleep problems. Discuss the following sleep complaints with your healthcare team:

- Waking up many times a night.
- Trouble falling asleep and staying asleep.
- Feeling tired during the day. Taking frequent naps.
- Discomfort and tingling feelings in the legs at night. These are symptoms of restless leg syndrome.
- Jerking or kicking the legs during sleep. These are symptoms of periodic limb movement disorder.

Signs of a Serious Problem

Contact your healthcare team right away if your loved one has the following symptoms:

- Wakes suddenly and is confused or acts strangely

- Has shortness of breath or chest pain

Be Careful What Your Loved One Eats and Drinks

Certain foods and drinks can lead to sleep problems.

- Provide food and drinks that are caffeine-free. Avoid coffee, tea, certain soft drinks and chocolate after the late afternoon.

- Plan to eat the dinner meal three hours before your loved one goes to bed.

- Make sure your loved one is full or not hungry before bedtime. But, avoid heavy meals that can cause poor sleep.

- Talk about limiting drinks two hours before bedtime. Drinking fluids at night can lead to frequent trips to the bathroom.

- Discuss avoiding alcoholic drinks at night. Alcohol helps people fall asleep, but their sleep is often restless.

Watch the Medicines Your Loved One Takes

Check to see if medicines could affect your loved one's sleep. Cold and allergy medicines that you buy over-the-counter (OTC) often cause sleep problems. Check with your healthcare team before taking OTC medicines.

Try to improve sleep before taking sleeping pills. Never give your loved one sleeping pills you buy over-the-counter. These pills may cause confusion and memory problems.

Your healthcare team may prescribe your loved one sleeping pills. These pills should only be taken for two or three nights in a row.

How Can You Help Your Loved One Relax at Nighttime?

- Give your loved one a massage or backrub before going to bed.

- Suggest drinking a glass of warm milk at bedtime.

- Suggest ways to relax. Take slow, deep breaths in bed. Count the breaths. Block other thoughts that come to mind. Think of peaceful scenes, such as the beach.

What Are Some Bedtime Tips to Teach Your Loved One?

- Follow a regular sleep schedule. Go to bed and wake up the same time every day.

- Have a bedtime routine. For example, take a warm bath before bedtime. Listen to calm music or read a book.

- Use the bedroom only for sleep or sex. Do not eat food or watch TV in bed.

- Keep the bedroom quiet, dark and at a comfortable temperature.

- Get out of bed if not asleep in 15 to 30 minutes. Read or listen to soothing music. Go back to bed only when sleepy.

Helpful Tips

- Get plenty of exercise every day. Stop exercising at least three hours before bedtime.

- Try to get some natural light each afternoon.

- Nap for only 15 to 30 minutes or avoid napping. For some people, napping may cause sleep problems.

- Go to a sleep specialist or find a sleep clinic if problems continue.

Remember

- Talk with your healthcare team about your loved one's sleep problems. Be alert if your loved one has loud snoring, gasping breaths and jerking, painful legs.

- Watch the medicines your loved one takes. Never use over-the-counter sleeping pills. Take prescribed sleeping medicines for no more than two to three days in a row.

- Help your loved one follow a regular sleep schedule. Go to bed and wake up the same time every day.

Chapter 49

Sexuality after Stroke

Stroke brings about many unexpected waves of change that are difficult to adjust to and may even be embarrassing to talk about, such as sex after stroke. Resuming a healthy intimate life is important, but it can also be a challenging part of the recovery process for the stroke survivor. It is important for the stroke survivor and their partner to be informed and equipped to face the changes in sexual activity and function that may follow a stroke.

The changes that affect how stroke survivors feel about sex and intimacy are emotional, physical and mental. Stroke survivors may experience difficulty having sex because of erectile dysfunction or vaginal dryness, immobility, incontinence, fatigue, side-effects of medicines, fear of another stroke, decreased libido, or depression.

Partners of stroke survivors are also faced with adapting to the changes in sex and intimacy. It is common for stroke survivor's partners to experience fear of causing relapse, lack of excitation, anguish, and even disgust towards sex. They may be uncomfortable with the change in physical appearance of the stroke survivor or have difficulty seeing their loved one as they did prior to the stroke.

Open communication about the changes between stroke survivor and their partner is important to reconnecting and rekindling the feelings of closeness. Even if a stroke survivor is unable to have intercourse, it is still possible to enjoy other sexual activities and intimacy.

This chapter includes text excerpted from "Sex after Stroke," U.S. Department of Veterans Affairs (VA), April 2009. Reviewed April 2017.

Open discussion about sex after a stroke between the stroke survivor, their partner, and the healthcare provider is an important part of a safe and healthy stroke recovery.

Common Questions Caregivers Have about Sex after Stroke

Can My Husband / Wife and I Still Have Sex?

Yes. There may be difficulties and adjustments that might need to be made, but sexual relations can usually continue after having a stroke. It is an important component for a healthy relationship.

Why Has My Partner's Desire for Sex Decreased since the Stroke?

In many instances, changes in sexual activity is linked to changes in role function of the stroke survivor and their partner. Immobility, cognitive impairment, and side effects from medication sometimes lead to a reduction in libido, arousal, or even orgasm in both men and women. Men may experience erectile dysfunction (ED) and concerns about sexual performance can also greatly reduce sexual interest.

Can I Induce Another Stroke While Having Sex with My Partner?

Though there is no strong evidence that engaging in sexual activity is likely to cause a stroke (it is very rare), a common fear among stroke survivors and their loved ones is that the exertion and excitement of sex may cause harm, or even induce another stroke. It may take a simple "Go ahead, you'll be fine" from the provider to eliminate the fear for both the stroke survivor and their partner.

What Are the Sexual Consequences of Stroke?

There are several issues following a stroke that may affect your partner, including: changes in self-perception (sexual attractiveness), diminished self-image and/or low self-esteem, fear of being rejected or abandoned, concerns about sexual failure, decreased libido, decreased coital frequency, decreased satisfaction with sexual life.

What Can I Do to Adjust?

Understand that the stroke survivor will experience physical, mental and emotional changes following the stroke, and that it will take some time to adjust. Counseling is highly recommended to deal with these changes. Explore the many alternative ways to share closeness and intimacy. Your healthcare team may be able to suggest some treatments and other ways to improve your sexual relationship.

Chapter 50

Dealing with Depression after Stroke

After a stroke, your loved one may have many negative feelings. Your loved one may think that things will never get better. This is not true—help is available!

Almost half of all stroke survivors have depression. Depression is a normal response to the losses that occur from a stroke.

What Are the Signs and Symptoms of Depression?

Here is a list of the signs and symptoms of depression. Five or more of these signs or symptoms that last more than two weeks are warning signals for depression.

- Sadness or an "empty" mood

- Feeling guilty, worthless or helpless

- Problems concentrating, remembering or making decisions

- Appetite and/or weight changes

- Feeling hopeless

- Lack of energy or feeling tired and "slowed down"

This chapter includes text excerpted from "Depression after Stroke," U.S. Department of Veterans Affairs (VA), December 27, 2013. Reviewed April 2017.

- Problems with sleep, such as trouble getting to sleep, staying asleep or sleeping too much

- Feeling restless or irritable

- Loss of interest or pleasure in hobbies and activities, including sex, that were once enjoyed

What Do You Need to Know?

Depression is real—People need help when they have depression.

Physical and emotional changes are common after a stroke—Accept your loved one's changes.

Expect improvements over time—Things often get better.

Why Is It Important to Get Help?

Treatment of depression will help the stroke survivor recover faster. It will make your job as a caregiver easier. For instance, treating depression helps with:

- Thinking skills and memory

- Physical recovery and rehabilitation

- Language and speech

- Emotions and motivation

What Treatments Should You Discuss with Your Healthcare Team?

Get help from your healthcare team quickly. The stroke survivor and family members may explain away the person's depression. Make sure that the stroke survivor receives treatment.

- Medicines, such as antidepressants, improve symptoms.

- Psychotherapy (talk therapy) is used along with medicines. Talk therapy gives your loved one a safe place to talk about feelings.

- Support groups provide help from other stroke survivors and caregivers. They know what you and your loved one are going through. There are support groups for stroke survivors and caregivers like you.

Helpful Tips

- Know the warning signals of depression. Watch for the signs and symptoms of depression. Get help quickly.

- Be patient with your loved one. After a stroke, it will take time for your loved one to understand the changes.

- Help your loved one exercise and take part in fun activities.

- Encourage friends and your family to visit and talk with your loved one.

- Have a good attitude. Focus on how much your stroke survivor can do. Smile and relax about things you can't change.

Chapter 51

Caring for Someone with Memory Problems after Stroke

Most people have some memory problems after a stroke. The severity of the problems depends on how much brain damage occurred. Persons with less severe strokes naturally recover their memory over weeks or months. For others, there are medical treatments and things you can do to help.

Why Is It Important to Get Help?

Discuss your loved one's memory problems with your healthcare team. They can do a physical exam and basic memory tests. Certain medicines and health problems can worsen memory loss. For some people, there are helpful treatments.

How Can You Find Help for Your Loved One?

Talk with a social worker or your healthcare team. Ask about a referral to a memory clinic or for other services. Below is a list of healthcare providers who can help:

- Neurologists or cognitive neurologists diagnose and treat memory problems.

This chapter includes text excerpted from "Memory Problems," U.S. Department of Veterans Affairs (VA), December 27, 2013. Reviewed April 2017.

- Neuropsychologists conduct tests and work with neurologists to treat problems.

- Occupational therapists and specialist memory nurses suggest practical tips. They provide care in the office or the patient's home.

Your local stroke associations can provide information.

What Do You Need to Know?

Strokes affect people in different ways. Many stroke survivors remember things more slowly. They often forget to do tasks like taking their medicines. Persons with strokes often have trouble with short-term memory or recalling things that just happened. Learning new names and telephone numbers is often hard. Most stroke survivors retain their long-term memory. For example, they remember events that occurred in the past.

What Are the Common Types of Memory Problems after Stroke?

The type of memory loss depends on the part of the brain that was damaged.

People whose stroke affected the right side of the body often have problems with verbal memory. Verbal memory includes remembering names, stories or information related to language or words.

Visual memory is often impaired in people whose stroke affected the left side of the body. Visual memory includes remembering faces, shapes or things you see.

How Can You Use Memory Aids to Help Your Loved One?

- Place an easy-to-read digital clock on a bedside table.

- Hang a big calendar on the wall.

- Post emergency and important phone numbers in large letters near the phone.

- Place a notepad in a handy place to jot down things to remember.

- Use a pill box to sort the pills that need to be taken each day.

How Can You Support Your Loved One?

- Make a memory book of favorite photos of people and places.

- Talk about the past. Share memories.

- Allow your loved one time to find the right words.

- Work at being understanding. It's normal to get frustrated. Keep in mind this is not your loved one's fault.

- Join a stroke support group. Other stroke caregivers can give you ideas for dealing with memory loss.

How Can You Help Your Loved One Stay Mentally Active?

The following activities may help improve memory:

- Crossword puzzles and word games

- Cards, dominoes and board games

- Computer games that are made to improve memory

Helpful Tips

- Help your loved one focus on one thing at a time. Avoid noise and lots of people.

- Keep information simple. Break down activities into small steps.

- Have a daily routine. Do tasks at the same time each day.

- Label drawers with pictures or words to describe their contents.

- Leave reminder notes around the house. For example, leave a note to turn off the stove or lock the door.

Remember

- Problems with memory are common after stroke. They affect each stroke survivor in different ways.

- There are things you can do to help your loved one. Examples include reminder notes and making a memory book.

- Support your loved one. Remember that memory problems are not your loved one's fault.

Chapter 52

Tips for Caregivers of Stroke Patients

Caregivers care for someone with an illness, injury, or disability. Caregiving can be rewarding, but it can also be challenging. Stress from caregiving is common. Women especially are at risk for the harmful health effects of caregiver stress. These health problems may include depression or anxiety. There are ways to manage caregiver stress.

What Is a Caregiver?

A caregiver is anyone who provides care for another person in need, such as a child, an aging parent, a husband or wife, a relative, friend, or neighbor. A caregiver also may be a paid professional who provides care in the home or at a place that is not the person's home.

People who are not paid to give care are called informal caregivers or family caregivers. This fact sheet focuses on family caregivers who provide care on a regular basis for a loved one with an injury, an illness such as dementia, or a disability. The family caregiver

This chapter contains text excerpted from the following sources: Text in this chapter begins with excerpts from "Caregiver Stress" Office on Women's Health (OWH), U.S. Department of Health and Human Services (HHS), January 25, 2015; Text beginning with the heading "What Treatments Should I Discuss with My Healthcare Team?" is excerpted from "Caregiver Stress and Depression," U.S. Department of Veterans Affairs (VA), December 27, 2013. Reviewed April 2017.

often has to manage the person's daily life. This can include helping with daily tasks like bathing, eating, or taking medicine. It can also include arranging activities and making health and financial decisions.

Who Are Caregivers?

Most Americans will be informal caregivers at some point during their lives. A 2012 survey found that 36 percent of Americans provided unpaid care to another adult with an illness or disability in the past year. That percentage is expected to go up as the proportion of people in the United States who are elderly increases. Also, changes in healthcare mean family caregivers now provide more home-based medical care. Nearly half of family caregivers in the survey said they give injections or manage medicines daily.

Also, most caregivers are women. And nearly three in five family caregivers have paid jobs in addition to their caregiving.

What Is Caregiver Stress?

Caregiver stress is due to the emotional and physical strain of caregiving. Caregivers report much higher levels of stress than people who are not caregivers. Many caregivers are providing help or are "on call" almost all day. Sometimes, this means there is little time for work or other family members or friends. Some caregivers may feel overwhelmed by the amount of care their aging, sick or disabled family member needs.

Although caregiving can be very challenging, it also has its rewards. It feels good to be able to care for a loved one. Spending time together can give new meaning to your relationship.

Remember that you need to take care of yourself to be able to care for your loved one.

Who Gets Caregiver Stress?

Anyone can get caregiver stress, but more women caregivers say they have stress and other health problems than men caregivers. And some women have a higher risk for health problems from caregiver stress, including those who:

- **Care for a loved one who needs constant medical care and supervision.** Caregivers of people with Alzheimer disease or dementia are more likely to have health problems and to be depressed than caregivers of people with conditions that do not require constant care.

- **Care for a spouse.** Women who are caregivers of spouses are more likely to have high blood pressure, diabetes, and high cholesterol and are twice as likely to have heart disease as women who provide care for others, such as parents or children.

Women caregivers also may be less likely to get regular screenings, and they may not get enough sleep or regular physical activity.

What Are the Signs and Symptoms of Caregiver Stress?

Caregiver stress can take many forms. For instance, you may feel frustrated and angry one minute and helpless the next. You may make mistakes when giving medicines. Or you may turn to unhealthy behaviors like smoking or drinking too much alcohol.

Other signs and symptoms include:

- Feeling overwhelmed
- Feeling alone, isolated, or deserted by others
- Sleeping too much or too little
- Gaining or losing a lot of weight
- Feeling tired most of the time
- Losing interest in activities you used to enjoy
- Becoming easily irritated or angered
- Feeling worried or sad often
- Having headaches or body aches often

Talk to your doctor about your symptoms and ways to relieve stress. Also, let others give you a break. Reach out to family, friends, or a local resource.

How Does Caregiver Stress Affect My Health?

Some stress can be good for you, as it helps you cope and respond to a change or challenge. But long-term stress of any kind, including caregiver stress, can lead to serious health problems.

Some of the ways stress affects caregivers include:

- **Depression and anxiety.** Women who are caregivers are more likely than men to develop symptoms of anxiety and depression.

Anxiety and depression also raise your risk for other health problems, such as heart disease and stroke.

- **Weak immune system.** Stressed caregivers may have weaker immune systems than noncaregivers and spend more days sick with the cold or flu. A weak immune system can also make vaccines such as flu shots less effective. Also, it may take longer to recover from surgery.

- **Obesity.** Stress causes weight gain in more women than men. Obesity raises your risk for other health problems, including heart disease, stroke, and diabetes.

- **Higher risk for chronic diseases.** High levels of stress, especially when combined with depression, can raise your risk for health problems, such as heart disease, cancer, diabetes, or arthritis.

- **Problems with short-term memory or paying attention.** Caregivers of spouses with Alzheimer's disease are at higher risk for problems with short-term memory and focusing.

Caregivers also report symptoms of stress more often than people who are not caregivers.

What Can I Do to Prevent or Relieve Caregiver Stress?

Taking steps to relieve caregiver stress helps prevent health problems. Also, taking care of yourself helps you take better care of your loved one and enjoy the rewards of caregiving.

Here are some tips to help you prevent or manage caregiver stress:

- **Learn ways to better help your loved one.** Some hospitals offer classes that can teach you how to care for someone with an injury or illness. To find these classes, ask your doctor or call your local Area Agency on Aging (AOA).

- **Find caregiving resources in your community to help you.** Many communities have adult daycare services or respite services to give primary caregivers a break from their caregiving duties.

- **Ask for and accept help.** Make a list of ways others can help you. Let helpers choose what they would like to do. For instance, someone might sit with the person you care for while you do an errand. Someone else might pick up groceries for you.

- **Join a support group for caregivers.** You can find a general caregiver support group or a group with caregivers who care for someone with the same illness or disability as your loved one. You can share stories, pick up caregiving tips, and get support from others who face the same challenges as you do.

- **Get organized.** Make to-do lists, and set a daily routine.

- **Take time for yourself.** Stay in touch with family and friends, and do things you enjoy with your loved ones.

- **Take care of your health.** Find time to be physically active on most days of the week, choose healthy foods, and get enough sleep.

- **See your doctor for regular checkups.** Make sure to tell your doctor or nurse you are a caregiver. Also, tell her about any symptoms of depression or sickness you may have.

If you work outside the home and are feeling overwhelmed, consider taking a break from your job. Under the federal Family and Medical Leave Act (FMLA), eligible employees can take up to 12 weeks of unpaid leave per year to care for relatives. Ask your human resources office about your options.

What Treatments Should I Discuss with My Healthcare Team?

Ignoring the stress of caregiving is the number one cause of "caregiver burn-out." Be honest with yourself about what you are feeling. Do not pretend that everything is okay. Proper treatment helps most people with depression. Ask your healthcare team about the best treatment for you.

- Medicines, such as antidepressants are almost always helpful.

- Psychotherapy (talk therapy) is used along with medicines. Talk therapy gives you a safe place to talk about your feelings.

- Support groups provide a place to share your feelings with other caregivers.

- Other caregivers understand what you are going through. They can help you find solutions to your problems.

How Can You Take Better Care of Yourself?

Taking care of yourself will make you a better caregiver.

- **Put taking care of yourself at the top of your list**—Have regular medical check-ups. Eat right and exercise.

- **Ask for help**—Take on only what you can manage. Don't try to do everything by yourself. Be prepared with a mental list of ways other people can help.

- **Find time for yourself**—You need breaks from caregiving. Do things you enjoy. Go for walks or visit your friends. Take yoga or relaxation classes. Get a massage. Treat yourself to special outings on a regular basis.

- **Laugh and have fun**—Joke with your loved one. Laugh out loud. Read a funny book. Watch a funny movie or a comedy on TV.

Helpful Tips

- **Accept your feelings**—Feelings of anger and sadness are normal from time to time. Be patient with yourself.

- **Remember that caregiving has rewards**—About half of all caregivers report positive feelings about caregiving. Caregiving often leads to stronger relationships with loved ones. Many stroke survivors do not show their true feelings. But, know that your loved one needs and appreciates your care.

- **Don't take things personally**—Your loved one may say or do hurtful things. Remember that these behaviors are due to their illness.

- **Practice getting rid of negative thoughts**—Replace negative thoughts with positive thinking or memories. Practice this every day. Focus on the things you can do. Relax about those things that you cannot. Forget and forgive your mistakes. We all make them.

- **Get information**—Learn about strokes. Learn about resources and ways to provide good care. This will help you plan for the future.

Chapter 53

Stroke Support Group

Stroke support groups help survivors and families cope with life after stroke. Support group members share experiences and encourage one another.

Why Are They Important?

Life after a stroke is often difficult. Talking to others who have been through stroke and recovery may help. Support groups focus on your strengths and successes. Some support groups invite guest speakers who are healthcare providers. Support groups are a good place to make friends.

They can help you and your loved one:

- Solve problems and get tips on caregiving

- Find local resources

- Get information on ways to improve health

- Learn about strokes and recovery

- Try new things, such as bowling or taking a dance class

What Do You Need to Know?

Stroke support groups are often run by hospitals, the U.S. Department of Veterans Affairs (VA) or stroke-related volunteer groups.

This chapter includes text excerpted from "Stroke Support Group," U.S. Department of Veterans Affairs (VA), December 27, 2013. Reviewed April 2017.

Many groups include members trained to answer your questions. There are different types of stroke support groups. Some groups include people with other medical conditions. To some, this makes the group more interesting. There are also support groups for caregivers only. Groups meet at days and times convenient for members.

How Do You Find a Stroke Support Group?

If you are looking for a stroke support group in your area, consider the following resources.

- Talk with your local VA social worker. Other healthcare professionals such as nurses, psychologists and physical therapists can help.

- Search the National Stroke Association's Stroke Group Registry.

- Call the American Stroke Association's "Warmline." It connects families with other stroke support groups.

- Check your local newspaper for announcements about stroke support groups.

How Do You Find Stroke Support Groups Online?

You may prefer an online support group. Online support groups are often helpful if you lack time or can't leave the house.

You can find online support groups through these websites:

- The Stroke Network (www.strokenetwork.org)

- The American Stroke Association (www.strokeassociation.org)

Helpful Tips

- You may have to visit several support groups to find the right one.

- Support groups do not take the place of medical care. Your healthcare provider knows what's best for you and your loved one.

- You can even start a stroke support group.

Remember

- It's hard to adjust to the changes after stroke. Stroke support groups offer help and encouragement. They can help people get back into social activities.

- Different kinds of stroke support groups are available. Your loved one and you may go to a local group. You also may use an online group.

- Stroke support groups do not take the place of medical care.

Chapter 54

Health Insurance and Disability Concerns after Stroke

Chapter Contents

Section 54.1—Affordable Care Act (ACA)..................................... 524

Section 54.2—Health Insurance Information for
           Stroke Patients.. 526

Section 54.3—Social Security Disability Benefits..................... 529

523

Section 54.1

Affordable Care Act (ACA)

This section includes text excerpted from "Affordable Care Act (ACA)," HealthCare.gov, Centers for Medicare and Medicaid Services (CMS), July 3, 2016.

The comprehensive healthcare reform law enacted in March 2010 (sometimes known as ACA, PPACA, or "Obamacare").

The law has three primary goals:

- Make affordable health insurance available to more people. The law provides consumers with subsidies ("premium tax credits") that lower costs for households with incomes between 100% and 400% of the federal poverty level.

- Expand the Medicaid program to cover all adults with income below 138% of the federal poverty level. (Not all states have expanded their Medicaid programs.)

- Support innovative medical care delivery methods designed to lower the costs of healthcare generally.

Rights and Protections

The healthcare law offers rights and protections that make coverage more fair and easy to understand. Some rights and protections apply to plans in the Health Insurance Marketplace or other individual insurance, some apply to job-based plans, and some apply to all health coverage. The protections outlined below may not apply to grandfathered health insurance plans.

How the Healthcare Law Protects You

- Requires insurance plans to cover people with pre-existing health conditions, including pregnancy, without charging more

- Provides free preventive care

- Gives young adults more coverage options

- Ends lifetime and yearly dollar limits on coverage of essential health benefits
- Helps you understand the coverage you're getting
- Holds insurance companies accountable for rate increases
- Makes it illegal for health insurance companies to cancel your health insurance just because you get sick
- Protects your choice of doctors
- Protects you from employer retaliation

Ending Lifetime and Yearly Limits

The healthcare law stops insurance companies from limiting yearly or lifetime coverage expenses for essential health benefits.

Lifetime Limits

Insurance companies can't set a dollar limit on what they spend on essential health benefits for your care during the entire time you're enrolled in that plan.

Yearly Limits

Insurance companies can't set a yearly dollar limit on what they spend for your coverage.

Does This Apply to My Plan?

Protections against lifetime limits on coverage apply to all individual and job-based health plans, including grandfathered plans.

Protections against annual limits apply to most health plans, but they don't apply to grandfathered individual health plans. Check your plan's materials to find out if your health plan is grandfathered.

Are There Any Exceptions I Should Know About?

Insurance companies can still put yearly or lifetime dollar limits on spending for healthcare services that aren't considered essential health benefits.

Section 54.2

Health Insurance Information for Stroke Patients

This section contains text excerpted from the following sources: Text under the heading "Buying Long-Term Care Insurance" is excerpted from "Buying Long-Term Care Insurance," Administration for Community Living (ACL), February 22, 2017; Text under the heading "State Medicaid Programs" is excerpted from "State Medicaid Programs," Administration for Community Living (ACL), February 22, 2017.

Buying Long-Term Care Insurance

People with certain conditions may not qualify for long-term care insurance. Since standards vary between different insurance companies, if one company denies you, it is possible that another company will accept you. Common reasons why you might not be able to buy long-term care insurance include:

- You had a **stroke within the past year to two years** or a history of strokes

- You currently use long-term care services

- You **already need help** with Activities of Daily Living (ADL)

- You have **acquired immune deficiency syndrome (AIDS)** or AIDS-Related Complex (ARC)

- You have **Alzheimer Disease** or any form of **dementia** or cognitive dysfunction

- You have a **progressive neurological condition** such as multiple sclerosis or Parkinson Disease

- You have **metastatic cancer** (cancer that has spread beyond its original site)

Insurance companies also consider other health conditions when determining your eligibility. If you buy your long-term care insurance before you develop one of the health conditions listed above, then your policy will cover the care you need for that condition.

Before You Buy

You should consider a number of things before purchasing LTC insurance:

- **Don't buy more** insurance than you think you may need. You may have enough income to pay a portion of your care costs and you may only need a small policy for the remainder. You also may have **family members** willing and able to supplement your care needs.

- **Don't buy too little** insurance. That will only delay the use of your own assets or income to pay for care. Think about how you feel about having care costs that are not covered. **While you can usually decrease your coverage, it is more difficult to increase coverage,** especially if your health has declined.

- Look carefully at each policy. There is **no "one-size-fits-all"** policy.

- If you choose a policy that only pays for room and board in a facility, **plan for other expenses**, such as supplies, medications, linens, and other items and services that your policy may not cover.

- **It costs less to buy coverage when you are younger.** The average age of people buying long-term care insurance today is about 60. The average age of those purchasing policies offered at work is about 50.

- Make sure that you can **afford** the long-term care insurance policy over time, as your monthly income may change.

- Research and consider different options and talk with a **professional** before finalizing your decision.

- Don't feel pressured into making a decision.

State Medicaid Programs

Medicaid is a joint federal and state government program that helps people with **low income** and assets pay for some or all of their healthcare bills. **It covers medical care,** like doctor visits and hospital

527

costs, **long-term care services** in nursing homes, and long-term care services provided at home, such as visiting nurses and assistance with personal care. Unlike Medicare, Medicaid does pay for custodial care in nursing homes and at home.

Overall program rules for who can be eligible for Medicaid and what services are covered are based on federal requirements, but **states have considerable leeway** in how they operate their programs. States are required to cover certain groups of individuals, but have the option to cover additional groups. Similarly, states are required to cover certain services, but have the option of covering additional services if they wish to do so. As a result, **eligibility rules and services that are covered vary from state to state**.

To be eligible for Medicaid you must meet certain requirements, including having income and assets that do not exceed the levels used by your state.

Once your state determines that you are eligible for Medicaid, the state will make an additional determination of whether you qualify for long-term care services. When determining whether you qualify for long-term care services, most states use a specific number of personal care and other service needs to qualify for nursing home care or home and community-based services. There may be different eligibility requirements for different types of home and community-based services.

Your State Medical Assistance office is the best source for information about how to qualify for Medicaid in your state and if you qualify for long-term care services.

Section 54.3

Social Security Disability Benefits

This section contains text excerpted from the following sources:
Text in this section begins with excerpts from "Disability
Benefits," U.S. Social Security Administration (SSA), May 2015;
Text under the heading "Compassionate Allowances" is
excerpted from "Compassionate Allowances," U.S. Social
Security Administration (SSA), March 24, 2016.

Disability is something most people don't like to think about. But the chances that you'll become disabled probably are greater than you realize. Studies show that a 20-year old worker has a 1-in-4 chance of becoming disabled before reaching full retirement age. For specific information about your situation, you should speak with a Social Security representative. Social Security pays disability benefits through two programs: the Social Security disability insurance (SSDI) program and the Supplemental Security Income (SSI) program.

Frequently Asked Questions on Disability Benefits

Who Can Get Social Security Disability Benefits?

Social Security pays benefits to people who can't work because they have a medical condition that's expected to last at least one year or result in death. Federal law requires this very strict definition of disability. While some programs give money to people with partial disability or short-term disability, Social Security does not.

Certain family members of disabled workers can also receive money from Social Security.

How Do I Meet the Earnings Requirement for Disability Benefits?

In general, to get disability benefits, you must meet two different earnings tests:

1. A recent work test, based on your age at the time you became disabled; and

2. A duration of work test to show that you worked long enough under Social Security.

Certain blind workers have to meet only the duration of work test.

The following table shows the rules for how much work you need for the recent work test, based on your age when your disability began. The U.S. Social Security Administration (SSA) bases the rules in this table on the **calendar quarter** in which you turned or will turn a certain age.

The calendar quarters are:

First Quarter: January 1 through March 31

Second Quarter: April 1 through June 30

Third Quarter: July 1 through September 30

Fourth Quarter: October 1 through December 31

Table 54.1. Rules for Work Needed for the Recent Work Test

If You Become Disabled...	Then, You Generally Need:
In or before the quarter you turn age 24	Work during half the time for the period beginning with the quarter after you turned 21 and ending with the quarter you became disabled. Example: If you become disabled in the quarter you turned age 27, then you would need three years of work out of the six-year period ending with the quarter you became disabled.
In the quarter you turn age 31 or later	Work during five years out of the 10- year period ending with the quarter your disability began.

The following table shows examples of how much work you need to meet the duration of work test if you become disabled at various selected ages. For the duration of work test, your work doesn't have to fall within a certain period of time.

Note: This table doesn't cover all situations.

Table 54.2. Examples of Work Needed for the Duration of Work Test

If You Become Disabled...	Then, You Generally Need:
Before age 28	1.5 years of work
Age 30	2 years
Age 34	3 years

Table 54.2. Continued

If You Become Disabled...	Then, You Generally Need:
Age 42	5 years
Age 44	5.5 years
Age 46	6 years
Age 48	6.5 years
Age 50	7 years
Age 52	7.5 years
Age 54	8 years
Age 56	8.5 years
Age 58	9 years
Age 60	9.5 years

How Do I Apply for Disability Benefits?

There are two ways that you can apply for disability benefits. You can:

1. Apply online at www.socialsecurity.gov; or

2. Call the toll-free number, 800-772-1213, to make an appointment to file a disability claim at your local Social Security office or to set up an appointment for someone to take your claim over the telephone. The disability claims interview lasts about one hour. If you're deaf or hard of hearing, you may call the toll-free TTY number, 800-325-0778, between 7am and 7pm on business days. If you schedule an appointment, you'll be sent a Disability Starter Kit to help you get ready for your disability claims interview.

You have the right to representation by an attorney or other qualified person of your choice when you do business with Social Security.

When Should I Apply and What Information Do I Need?

You should apply for disability benefits as soon as you become disabled. Processing an application for disability benefits can take three to five months. To apply for disability benefits, you'll need to complete an application for Social Security benefits. You can apply online at www. socialsecurity.gov. The SSA may be able to process your application faster if you help by getting any other information they need.

531

The information needed includes:

- Your Social Security number;

- Your birth or baptismal certificate;

- Names, addresses and phone numbers of the doctors, caseworkers, hospitals and clinics that took care of you, and dates of your visits;

- Names and dosage of all the medicine you take;

- Medical records from your doctors, therapists, hospitals, clinics, and caseworkers that you already have in your possession;

- Laboratory and test results;

- A summary of where you worked and the kind of work you did; and

- A copy of your most recent W-2 Form (Wage and Tax Statement) or, if you're self-employed, your federal tax returns for the past year.

In addition to the basic application for disability benefits, you'll also need to fill out other forms. One form collects information about your medical condition and how it affects your ability to work. Other forms give doctors, hospitals, and other healthcare professionals who have treated you, permission to send SSA information about your medical condition.

Don't delay applying for benefits if you can't get all of this information together quickly. The SSA will help you get it.

Who Decides If I Am Disabled?

The SSA will review your application to make sure you meet some basic requirements for disability benefits. They'll check whether you worked enough years to qualify. Also, they'll evaluate any current work activities. If you meet these requirements, they'll process your application and forward your case to the Disability Determination Services office in your state.

This state agency completes the initial disability determination decision for SSA. Doctors and disability specialists in the state agency ask your doctors for information about your condition. They'll consider all the facts in your case. They'll use the medical evidence from your doctors, hospitals, clinics, or institutions where you've been treated and all other information. They'll ask your doctors about:

- Your medical condition(s);

- When your medical condition(s) began;

- How your medical condition(s) limit your activities;

- Medical tests results; and

- What treatment you've received.

They'll also ask the doctors for information about your ability to do work-related activities, such as walking, sitting, lifting, carrying, and remembering instructions. Your doctors don't decide if you're disabled.

The state agency staff may need more medical information before they can decide if you're disabled. If your medical sources can't provide needed information, the state agency may ask you to go for a special examination. The SSA prefers to ask your own doctor, but sometimes the exam may have to be done by someone else. Social Security will pay for the exam and for some of the related travel costs.

How SSA Makes the Decision

The SSA uses a five-step process to decide if you're disabled.

1. **Are you working?**

   If you're working and your earnings average more than a certain amount each month, generally you won't be considered to be disabled. The amount changes each year. If you're not working, or your monthly earnings average to the current amount or less, the state agency then looks at your medical condition.

2. **Is your medical condition "severe"?**

   For you to be considered to have a disability by Social Security's definition, your medical condition must significantly limit your ability to do basic work activities—such as lifting, standing, walking, sitting, and remembering—for at least 12 months. If your medical condition isn't severe SSA won't consider you to be disabled. If your condition is severe, the SSA proceeds to step three.

3. **Does your impairment(s) meet or medically equal a listing?**

SSA's list of impairments (the listings) describes medical conditions that they consider severe enough to prevent a person from completing substantial gainful activity, regardless of age, education, or work experience. If your medical condition (or combination of medical conditions) isn't on this list, the state agency looks to see if your condition is as severe as a condition on the list. If the severity of your medical condition meets or equals the severity of a listed impairment, the state agency will decide that you have a qualifying disability. If the severity of your condition doesn't meet or equal the severity level of a listed impairment, the state agency goes on to step four.

4. **Can you do the work you did before?**

   At this step, SSA decides if your medical impairment(s) prevents you from performing any of your past work. If it doesn't, they'll decide you don't have a qualifying disability. If it does, they'll proceed to step five.

5. **Can you do any other type of work?**

   If you can't do the work you did in the past, SSA look to see if there's other work you can do despite your impairment(s). They will consider your age, education, past work experience, and any skills you may have that could be used to do other work. If you can't do other work, They will decide that you're disabled. If you can do other work, they'll decide that you don't have a qualifying disability.

Special Rules for Blind People

There are special rules for people who are blind.

The Agency Will Tell You the Decision

When the state agency makes a determination on your case, they'll send a letter to you. If your application is approved, the letter will show the amount of your benefit, and when your payments start. If your application isn't approved, the letter will explain why and tell you how to appeal the determination if you don't agree with it.

What if I disagree?

If you disagree with a decision made on your claim, you can appeal it. The steps you can take are explained in The Appeals Process, which is available from Social Security.

How SSA will contact you?

Generally, the agency mail or call you when they want to contact you about your benefits, but sometimes, a Social Security representative may come to your home. The representative will show you identification before talking about your benefits. Calling the Social Security office to ask if someone was sent to see you is a good idea.

If you're blind or have low vision, you can choose to receive notices from SSA in one of the following ways:

- Standard print notice by first-class mail;

- Standard print notice by certified mail;

- Standard print notice by first-class mail and a follow-up telephone call;

- Braille notice and a standard print notice by first-class mail;

- Microsoft Word file on a data compact disc (CD) and a standard print notice by first-class mail;

- Audio CD and a standard print notice by first-class mail; or

- Large print (18-point size) notice and a standard print notice by first-class mail.

What Happens When My Claim Is Approved?

SSA will send a letter to you telling you your application is approved, the amount of your monthly benefit, and the effective date. Your monthly disability benefit is based on your average lifetime earnings. Your first Social Security disability benefits will be paid for the sixth full month after the date your disability began.

Here is an example: If the state agency decides your disability began on January 15, your first disability benefit will be paid for the month of July. Social Security benefits are paid in the month following the month for which they are due, so you'll receive your July benefit in August.

You'll also receive *What You Need To Know When You Get Disability Benefits*, which gives you important information about your benefits and tells you what changes you must report to SSA.

Can My Family Get Benefits?

Certain members of your family may qualify for benefits based on your work. They include:

- Your spouse, if he or she is age 62 or older;

- Your spouse at any age, if he or she is caring for a child of yours who is younger than age 16 or disabled;

- Your unmarried child, including an adopted child, or, in some cases, a stepchild or grandchild. The child must be younger than age 18 (or younger than 19 if still in high school);

- Your unmarried child, age 18 or older, if he or she has a disability that started before age 22. The child's disability must also meet the definition of disability for adults.

Note: In some situations, a divorced spouse may qualify for benefits based on your earnings, if he or she was married to you for at least 10 years, is not currently married, and is at least age 62. The money paid to a divorced spouse doesn't reduce your benefit or any benefits due to your current spouse or children.

How Do Other Payments Affect My Benefits?

If you're getting other government benefits, the amount of your Social Security disability benefits may be affected. For more information, you should see the following publications:

- How Workers' Compensation And Other Disability Payments May Affect Your Benefits (www.ssa.gov/pubs/EN-05-10018.pdf);

- Windfall Elimination Provision (www.ssa.gov/pubs/EN-05-10045.pdf); and

- Government Pension Offset (www.ssa.gov/pubs/EN-05-10007.pdf).

You can get these publications from the website (www.ssa.gov/pubs), or contact SSA to request them.

What Do I Need to Tell Social Security?

If You Have an Outstanding Warrant for Your Arrest

You must tell SSA if you have an outstanding arrest warrant for any of the following felony offenses:

- Flight to avoid prosecution or confinement;

- Escape from custody; and

- Flight-escape.

You can't receive regular disability benefits, or any underpayments you may be due, for any month in which there is an outstanding arrest warrant for any of these felony offenses.

If You're Convicted of a Crime

Tell Social Security right away if you're convicted of a crime. Regular disability benefits, or any underpayments, that may be due aren't paid for the months a person is confined for a crime, but any family members who are eligible for benefits based on that person's work may continue to receive benefits.

Monthly benefits, or any underpayments that may be due, are usually not paid to someone who commits a crime and is confined to an institution by court order and at public expense. This applies if the person has been found

- Not guilty by reason of insanity or similar factors (such as mental disease, mental defect, or mental incompetence); or

- Incompetent to stand trial.

If You Violate a Condition of Parole or Probation

You must tell SSA if you're violating a condition of your probation or parole imposed under federal or state law. You can't receive regular disability benefits or any underpayment that may be due for any month in which you violate a condition of your probation or parole.

When Do I Get Medicare?

You'll get Medicare coverage automatically after you've received disability benefits for two years.

What Do I Need to Know about Working?

After you start receiving Social Security disability benefits, you may want to try working again. Social Security has special rules called work incentives that allow you to test your ability to work and still receive monthly Social Security disability benefits. You can also get help with education, rehabilitation, and training you may need to work.

If you do take a job or become self-employed, tell SSA about it right away. They need to know when you start or stop work and if there are any changes in your job duties, hours of work, or rate of pay. You can call them toll-free at 800-772-1213. If you're deaf or hard of hearing, you may call the TTY number, 800-325-0778.

The Ticket to Work Program

Under this program, Social Security and SSI disability beneficiaries can get help with training and other services they need to go to work at no cost to them. Most disability beneficiaries are eligible to participate in the Ticket to Work program and can select an approved provider of their choice who can offer the kind of services they need.

Compassionate Allowances

Social Security has an obligation to provide benefits quickly to applicants whose medical conditions are so serious that their conditions obviously meet disability standards.

Compassionate Allowances (CAL) are a way of quickly identifying diseases and other medical conditions that invariably qualify under the Listing of Impairments based on minimal objective medical information. Compassionate Allowances allow Social Security to target the most obviously disabled individuals for allowances based on objective medical information that can be obtained quickly. Compassionate Allowances is not a separate program from the SSDI or SSI programs.

CAL conditions are selected using information received at public outreach hearings, comments received from the Social Security and Disability Determination Services communities, counsel of medical and scientific experts, and SSA's research with the National Institutes of Health (NIH). Also, they consider which conditions are most likely to meet their current definition of disability.

Social Security has held seven Compassionate Allowances public outreach hearings. The hearings were on stroke and traumatic brain injury, rare diseases, cancers, early-onset Alzheimer disease and related dementias, schizophrenia, cardiovascular disease and multiple organ transplants, and autoimmune diseases.

Chapter 55

Choosing Long-Term Care
for Those Disabled by Stroke

Chapter Contents

Section 55.1—Long-Term Care 540
Section 55.2—Assisted Living.. 555

Section 55.1

Long-Term Care

This section includes text excerpted from "Long-Term Care: What Is Long-Term Care?" NIHSeniorHealth, National Institute on Aging (NIA), May 2015.

What Is Long-Term Care?

Long-term care involves a variety of services designed to meet a person's health or personal care needs during a short or long period of time. These services help people live as independently and safely as possible when they can no longer perform everyday activities on their own.

Most Care Provided at Home

Long-term care is provided in different places by different caregivers, depending on a person's needs. Most long-term care is provided at home by unpaid family members and friends. It can also be given in a facility such as a nursing home or in the community, for example, in an adult day care center.

The most common type of long-term care is personal care—help with everyday activities, also called "activities of daily living." These activities include bathing, dressing, grooming, using the toilet, eating, and moving around—for example, getting out of bed and into a chair.

Long-term care also includes community services such as meals, adult day care, and transportation services. These services may be provided free or for a fee.

Health Drives the Need for Care

People often need long-term care when they have a serious, ongoing health condition or disability. The need for long-term care can arise suddenly, such as after a stroke or heart attack. Most often, however, it develops gradually, as people get older and frailer or as an illness or disability gets worse.

How Long Does Care Last?

Long-term care can last a short time or a long time. Short-term care lasts several weeks or a few months while someone is recovering from a sudden illness or injury. For example, a person may get short-term rehabilitation therapy at a nursing facility after hip surgery, then go home.

Long-term care can be ongoing, as with someone who is severely disabled from a stroke or who has Alzheimer disease. Many people can remain at home if they have help from family and friends or paid services. But some people move permanently to a nursing home or other type of facility if their needs can no longer be met at home.

About 70 percent of people over age 65 need some type of long-term care during their lifetime. More than 40 percent need care in a nursing home for some period of time.

Who Will Need Long-Term Care?

It is difficult to predict how much or what type of long-term care a person might need. Several things increase the risk of needing long-term care.

- Age—The risk generally increases as people get older.

- Gender—Women are at higher risk than men, primarily because they often live longer.

- Marital status—Single people are more likely than married people to need care from a paid provider.

- Lifestyle—Poor diet and exercise habits can increase a person's risk.

- Health and family history—These factors also affect risk.

Home-Based Services

Services from Unpaid Caregivers

Home-based long-term care includes health, personal, and support services to help people stay at home and live as independently as possible. Most long-term care is provided either in the home of the person receiving services or at a family member's home. In-home services may be short-term—for someone who is recovering from an operation, for example—or long-term, for people who need ongoing help.

Most home-based services involve personal care, such as help with bathing, dressing, and taking medications, and supervision to make sure a person is safe. Unpaid family members, partners, friends, and neighbors provide most of this type of care.

Family and friends can also help loved ones if they live far away.

Services from Paid Caregivers

Home-based long-term care services can also be provided by paid caregivers, including caregivers found informally, and healthcare professionals such as nurses, home healthcare aides, therapists, and homemakers, who are hired through home healthcare agencies. These services include:

- home healthcare
- homemaker services
- friendly visitor/companion services
- emergency response systems

Home Healthcare

Home healthcare involves part-time medical services ordered by a physician for a specific condition. These services may include nursing care to help a person recover from surgery, an accident, or illness. Home healthcare may also include physical, occupational, or speech therapy and temporary home health aide services. These services are provided by home healthcare agencies approved by Medicare, a government insurance program for people over age 65.

Homemaker Services

Home health agencies offer personal care and homemaker services that can be purchased without a physician's order. Personal care includes help with bathing and dressing. Homemaker services include help with meal preparation and household chores. Agencies do not have to be approved by Medicare to provide these kinds of services.

Friendly Visitor / Companion Services

Friendly visitor/companion services are usually staffed by volunteers who regularly pay short visits (less than 2 hours) to someone who is frail or living alone. You can also purchase these services from home health agencies.

Emergency Response Systems

Emergency response systems automatically respond to medical and other emergencies via electronic monitors. The user wears a necklace or bracelet with a button to push in an emergency. Pushing the button summons emergency help to the home. This type of service is especially useful for people who live alone or are at risk of falling. A monthly fee is charged.

To find home-based services, contact Eldercare Locator at 800-677-1116 or visit www.eldercare.gov. You can also call your local Area Agency on Aging (AAA), Aging and Disability Resource Center (ADRC), department of human services or aging, or a social service agency.

Community-Based Services

Helping People Live Independently

Like home-based services, community-based long-term care services help people—old and young—stay at home and live as independently as possible. These services can be given at home or at a location in the community. Some programs are limited to people with disabilities or low-income people, but many are open to all. Community-based services are often provided by a local government, social service agency, or private company.

Living in a Continuing Care Community

Community-based services may supplement other services provided at home. They can also give family members a break from caregiving. These services include:

- adult day service programs
- senior centers
- transportation services
- meals programs
- respite care

Adult Day Care

Adult day service programs provide health, social, and other services in a safe place, generally on weekdays. They are designed for adults with mental or physical impairments. They are also for adults who need time to socialize and a place to go when their family care-givers are at work. Some programs provide rides to and from their locations.

Senior Centers

Senior centers offer a variety of services, including meals, recreation, social services, and classes. Many of them also provide information and referrals to help people find the care and services they need. Generally, senior centers are for healthy older adults without cognitive problems.

Transportation Services

Transportation services help people get to and from medical appointments, shopping centers, and other places in the community. Some senior housing complexes and community groups offer transportation services. Many public transit agencies have services for people with disabilities. Some services are free. Others charge a fee.

Meal Programs

Community-based meals programs include services that deliver meals to homebound people ("Meals on Wheels"). Some programs offer group meals at senior centers, places of worship, and other locations.

Respite Care

Respite care temporarily relieves families of the responsibility of caring for family members who cannot care for themselves. It is provided in a variety of settings, including homes, adult day centers, and nursing homes.

"Villages"

One new type of service is the local "village," in which neighborhood residents band together to trade and buy services they need to live independently. Members typically pay an annual fee to obtain services such as home repair and rides to the doctor but not skilled nursing care.

How to Locate Services

It can be difficult to find the right kind of long-term care services. There are sources to turn to for help with this task. For example, geriatric care managers are professionals, usually nurses or social workers, who help people with their long-term care needs. They can assess a person's needs, develop a plan of care, and identify and coordinate whatever services are needed.

To find community-based services, contact Eldercare Locator at 800-677-1116 or visit www.eldercare.gov. You can also call your local Area AAA, ADRC, department of human services or aging, or a social service agency.

Facility-Based Services

Providing Full-Time Assistance

At some point, support from family, friends, and local programs may not be enough. People who require help full time might move to a residential facility that provides many or all of the long-term care services they need.

Facility-based long-term care services include:

- adult foster care
- board and care homes
- assisted living facilities
- nursing homes
- continuing care retirement communities

Some facilities have only housing and housekeeping, but many also provide personal care and medical services. Many facilities offer special programs for people with Alzheimer disease and other types of dementia.

Board and Care Homes

Board and care homes, also called residential care facilities or group homes, are small private facilities, usually with 20 or fewer residents. Rooms may be private or shared. Residents receive personal care and meals and have staff available around the clock. Nursing and medical care usually are not provided on site.

Assisted Living

Assisted living is for people who need help with daily care, but not as much help as a nursing home provides. Assisted living facilities range in size from as few as 25 residents to 120 or more. Typically, a few "levels of care" are offered, with residents paying more for higher levels of care.

Assisted living residents usually live in their own apartments or rooms and share common areas. They have access to many services, including up to three meals a day; assistance with personal care; help with medications, housekeeping, and laundry; 24-hour supervision, security, and onsite staff; and social and recreational activities. Exact arrangements vary from state to state.

Nursing Homes

Nursing homes, also called skilled nursing facilities, provide a wide range of health and personal care services. Their services focus on medical care more than most assisted living facilities. These services typically include nursing care, 24-hour supervision, three meals a day, and assistance with everyday activities. Rehabilitation services such as physical, occupational, and speech therapy are also available.

Some people stay at a nursing home for a short time after being in the hospital. After they recover, they go home. However, most nursing home residents live there permanently because they have ongoing physical or mental conditions that require constant care and supervision.

Continuing Care Retirement Communities (CCRCs)

Continuing care retirement communities (CCRCs), also called life care communities, offer different levels of service in one location. Many of them offer independent housing (houses or apartments), assisted living, and skilled nursing care all on one campus. Healthcare services and recreation programs are also provided.

In a CCRC, where you live depends on the level of service you need. People who can no longer live independently move to the assisted living facility or sometimes receive home care in their independent living unit. If necessary, they can enter the CCRC's nursing home.

For More Information

There are many sources of information about facility-based long-term care. A good place to start is the Eldercare Locator at 800-677-1116 or www.eldercare.gov. You can also call your local AAA, ADRC, department of human services or aging, or a social service agency.

Planning for Long-Term Care

You can never know for sure if you will need long-term care. Maybe you will never need it. But an unexpected accident, illness, or injury can change your needs, sometimes suddenly. The best time to think about long-term care is before you need it.

Planning for the possibility of long-term care gives you time to learn about services in your community and what they cost. It also allows you to make important decisions while you are still able. You will need to make:

- housing decisions

- health decisions

- legal decisions

- financial decisions

People with Alzheimer disease or other cognitive impairment should begin planning for long-term care as soon as possible.

Housing Decisions: Staying In Your Home

In thinking about long-term care, it is important to consider where you will live as you age and how your place of residence can best support your needs if you can no longer fully care for yourself.

Most people prefer to stay in their own home for as long as possible. When planning to receive long-term care in your home, there are many things to consider including:

- the condition of your home

- whether it can be modified, if necessary, to accommodate a wheelchair or other devices/equipment

- the availability of long-term care services in your area, such as adult day care or nearby medical facilities

- how "age-friendly" your community is. Does it offer public transportation, home delivered meals and other needed services?

- tax and legal issues

Housing Decisions: Housing with Services

If it becomes necessary, several types of housing come with support services. Primarily, these are:

- **Public Housing** for low-to-moderate income elderly and persons with disabilities. Typically assistance with services is provided by a staff person called a Service Coordinator.

- **Assisted Living or "board and care" homes** are group living settings that offer housing in addition to assistance with personal care and other services, such as meals. Generally, they do not provide medical care.

- **CCRCs** provide a range of housing options, including independent living units, assisted living and nursing homes, all on the same campus. Nursing facilities, or nursing homes, are the most service-intensive housing option, providing skilled nursing services and therapies as needed.

Decisions About Your Health

Begin by thinking about what would happen if you became seriously ill or disabled. Talk with your family and friends about who would provide care if you needed help for a long time.

You might delay or prevent the need for long-term care by staying healthy and independent. Talk to your doctor about your medical and family history and lifestyle. He or she may suggest actions you can take to improve your health.

Healthy eating, regular physical activity, not smoking, and limited drinking of alcohol can help you stay healthy. So can an active social life, a safe home, and regular healthcare.

Legal Decisions

Planning for long-term care includes legal planning. That means creating official documents—often called "advance directives"—that state your wishes for medical care in an emergency and at the end of life. You can also decide who will make healthcare decisions for you if you cannot make them yourself.

It is important to consider what you want before you need long-term care. Discuss the options with family members, a lawyer, and others. These discussions can be hard, but telling others your wishes ahead of time answers questions they might have later and takes the burden off your family.

Experts recommend creating three types of legal documents, or advance directives. These are:

- a healthcare power of attorney

- a living will

- a do-not-resuscitate order, if desired

Healthcare Power of Attorney

A healthcare power of attorney, also called a durable power of attorney for healthcare, is a legal document that names the person who will make medical decisions for you if you cannot make them yourself. This healthcare "agent" or "proxy" is your substitute decision maker. The person you choose should understand and respect your values and beliefs about healthcare. Talk with that person to make sure he or she is comfortable with this role.

Living Will

A living will, also called a healthcare directive, is a legal document that records your wishes for medical treatment near the end of life. It spells out what life-sustaining treatment you do or do not want if you are terminally ill, permanently unconscious, or in the final stage of a fatal illness. For example, the document can state whether or not you want to receive artificial breathing if you can no longer breathe on your own.

Do-Not-Resuscitate Order

A do-not-resuscitate (DNR) order tells healthcare providers not to perform cardiopulmonary resuscitation (CPR) or other life-support procedures if your heart stops or if you stop breathing. A DNR order is signed by a healthcare provider and put in your medical chart. Hospitals and long-term care facilities have DNR forms that a staff member can help you fill out. You do not have to have a DNR order.

Getting Expert Advice

Lawyers and other professionals can help you create legal documents to ensure that your healthcare wishes are expressed. These experts understand state laws and how changes, such as a divorce, move from your home, or death in the family, affect the way documents are prepared and maintained.

Be sure to discuss your preferences and give copies of your legal documents to family members, your healthcare proxy, and your doctor. It's important to review documents regularly and update them as needed.

Financial Decisions

Financial planning is another important part of long-term care planning. Government health insurance programs, including Medicare and Medicaid, pay for some long-term care services but not others. Most people do not have enough money to pay for all of their long-term care needs, especially if those needs are extensive or last a long time.

Reviewing Your Resources

Think about your financial resources and how you feel about using them to pay for long-term care. These resources may include:

• Social Security

• a pension or other retirement fund

• personal savings

• income from stocks and bonds

Your home is another type of asset that could be used if needed.

It's a good idea to review your insurance coverage, too. Many health insurance plans provide little, if any, coverage for long-term care. Review any private health insurance, Medicare, and Medigap policies to learn exactly what is covered and what is not.

Other Options

Consider other possible ways to pay for long-term care. An increasing number of private payment options are available. Two of the more common options are long-term care insurance and reverse mortgages.

The website www.LongTermCare.gov has information about long-term care planning and services. This website, run by the U.S. Administration on Aging (AOA), lists other sources of information and gives definitions of important terms.

To find out what long-term care services are in your community, call Eldercare Locator at 800-677-1116 or visit www.eldercare.gov

Paying for Long-Term Care

Long-term care involves a variety of services provided at home, in the community, and in facilities. These services include:

• home-based care such as home health aides

• community-based care such as adult day care

- facility-based care such as assisted living and nursing homes

Costs Can Be High

Long-term care can be expensive. Americans spend billions of dollars a year on various services. How people pay for long-term care depends on their financial situation and the kinds of services they use. Often, they rely on a variety of payment sources, including:

- personal funds

- government health insurance programs, such as Medicare and Medicaid

- private financing options, such as long-term care insurance

Personal Funds

At first, many people pay for long-term care services with their own money. They may use personal savings, a pension or other retirement fund, income from stocks and bonds, or proceeds from the sale of a home.

Much home-based care is paid for using personal funds ("out of pocket"). Initially, family and friends often provide personal care and other services, such as transportation, for free. But as a person's needs increase, paid services may be needed.

Many older adults also pay out-of-pocket to participate in adult day service programs, meals, and other community-based services provided by local governments and nonprofit groups, which help them remain in their homes.

Professional care given in assisted living facilities and continuing care retirement communities is almost always paid for out of pocket, though in some states Medicaid may pay some costs for people who meet financial and health requirements.

Medicare and Medicaid

Another source of funds for long-term care are government insurance programs like Medicare and Medicaid. Medicare is Federal health insurance for people age 65 and older, younger people with certain disabilities, and all people with late-stage kidney failure. Medicaid is a Federal and State health insurance program for people with limited income and resources. These programs have rules limiting who is eligible and what services are covered.

Medicare Coverage Is Limited

Contrary to what many people think, Medicare does not cover most long-term care costs. It does pay for some part-time services for people who are homebound and for short-term skilled nursing care, but it does not cover ongoing personal care at home, like help with bathing. It may cover part of the first 100 days in a nursing home.

"Medigap" policies, which supplement Medicare, are not designed to meet long-term care needs. But some policies cover copayments for nursing home stays that qualify for Medicare coverage.

Medicaid Coverage Is Broader

Medicaid pays for healthcare services for people with limited income, and it is an important source of payment for long-term care services. Personal care, home healthcare, adult day care, and nursing home care are examples of the types of Medicaid-covered services used by older adults. However, Medicaid is not available for everyone. To be eligible, you must meet certain financial and health requirements. People with financial resources above a certain limit will most likely not qualify unless they first use up their own resources to pay for care, which is called "spending down." Who is eligible and what services are covered vary from state to state.

Paying for Nursing Home Care

Nursing homes and 24-hour skilled care at home are the most expensive types of long-term care. Because nursing homes cost so much—thousands of dollars a month—most people who live in them for more than 6 months cannot pay the entire bill on their own. At first, many residents pay with their own money. They "spend down" their resources until they qualify for Medicaid. There are rules for spending down resources. Long-term care in facilities generally costs more than home-based care unless you need extensive services at home.

Veterans' Benefits

Veterans' benefits are another source of government funds, and they may help veterans with disabilities and their spouses pay for personal care and homemaker services provided at home. Disabled or aging veterans with long-term care needs may be able to get help from the U.S. Department of Veterans Affairs (VA). Its benefits pay for care in VA nursing homes and certain services at home.

Older Americans Act Programs

The Older Americans Act is a Federal program designed to organize, coordinate, and provide home- and community-based services to older adults and their families. A broad array of programs help older adults remain in the community as independently as possible.

Services under the Older Americans Act are provided by state and local agencies and other organizations. They include in-home personal care and homemaker services for frail older adults, meals in the community and for homebound elderly, local transportation services, respite care, and services for older Native Americans.

You do not have to have a certain income to use these programs, but they are targeted at low-income, frail, or disabled seniors over age 60; minority older adults; and older adults living in rural areas.

Private Financing Options

Most people don't have enough money to pay for all long-term care costs on their own, especially ongoing or expensive services like a nursing home. By planning ahead, they can use other private payment options, including:

- long-term care insurance

- reverse mortgages

- certain life insurance policies

- annuities

- trusts

Which private financing option is best for a person depends on many factors. These factors include the person's age, health status, personal finances, and risk of needing long-term care.

Long-Term Care Insurance

Long-term care insurance pays for many types of long-term care. The exact coverage depends on the type of policy you buy and what services are covered. You can purchase nursing home—only coverage or a comprehensive policy that includes both home care and facility care. Many companies sell long-term care insurance. It is a good idea to shop around and compare policies.

Buying long-term care insurance can be a good choice for younger, relatively healthy people at low risk of needing long-term care. Costs go up for people who are older, have health problems, or want more benefits.

Reverse Mortgages

A reverse mortgage is a special type of home loan that lets a homeowner convert part of the ownership value in his or her home into cash. Unlike a traditional home loan, no repayment is required until the borrower sells the home, no longer uses it as a main residence, or dies.

There are no income or medical requirements to get a reverse mortgage. The loan amount is tax-free and can be used for any expense, including long-term care. If long-term care costs are higher than the amount you borrow, selling your home is not required, but doing so may provide enough funds to repay the loan.

Life Settlements

Some life insurance policies can help pay for long-term care. Policies with an "accelerated death benefit" provide cash advances while you are still alive. The advance is subtracted from the amount your beneficiaries (the people who get the insurance proceeds) will receive when you die.

You can get an accelerated death benefit if you live permanently in a nursing home, need long-term care for an extended time, are terminally ill, or have a life-threatening diagnosis such as acquired immune deficiency syndrome (AIDS). Check your life insurance policy to see exactly what it covers.

You may be able to raise cash by selling your life insurance policy for its current value. This option, known as a "life settlement," is usually available only to people age 70 and older. The proceeds are taxable and can be used for any reason, including paying for long-term care.

A similar arrangement, called a "viatical settlement," allows a terminally ill person to sell his or her life insurance policy to an insurance company. This option is typically used by people who are expected to live 2 years or less. A viatical settlement provides immediate cash, but it can be hard to get.

Annuities

You may choose to enter into an annuity contract with an insurance company to help pay for long-term care services. In exchange for a single payment or a series of payments, the insurance company will send you an annuity, which is a series of regular payments over a specified and defined period of time. There are two types of annuities: immediate annuities and deferred long-term care annuities.

- If you have an immediate long-term care annuity, the insurance company will send you a specified monthly income in return for a single premium payment.

- Deferred long-term care annuities are available to people up to age 85. Similar to other annuities, in exchange for a single premium payment, you receive a stream of monthly income for a specified period of time.

Trusts

A trust is a legal entity that allows a person (the trustor) to transfer assets to another person (the trustee). Once the trustor establishes the trust, the trustee manages and controls the assets for the trustor or for another beneficiary.

You may choose to use a trust to provide flexible control of assets for the benefit of minor children. Another common use of a trust is to provide flexible control of assets for an older adult or a person with a disability, which could include yourself or your spouse. Two types of trusts can help pay for long-term care services: charitable remainder trusts and Medicaid disability trusts.

Section 55.2

Assisted Living

This section includes text excerpted from "Assisted Living,"
Eldercare Locator, U.S. Administration on Aging (AOA),
April 13, 2012. Reviewed April 2016.

Assisted living facilities offer a housing alternative for older adults who may need help with dressing, bathing, eating, and toileting, but do not require the intensive medical and nursing care provided in nursing homes.

Assisted living facilities may be part of a retirement community, nursing home, senior housing complex, or may stand-alone. Licensing requirements for assisted living facilities vary by state and can be known by as many as 26 different names including: residential care, board and care, congregate care, and personal care.

What Services are Provided?

Residents of assisted living facilities usually have their own units or apartment. In addition to having a support staff and providing meals, most assisted living facilities also offer at least some of the following services:

- Healthcare management and monitoring

- Help with activities of daily living such as bathing, dressing, and eating

- Housekeeping and laundry

- Medication reminders and/or help with medications

- Recreational activities

- Security

- Transportation

How to Choose a Facility?

The following suggestions can help you get started in your search for a safe, comfortable and appropriate assisted living facility:

- Think ahead. What will the resident's future needs be and how will the facility meet those needs?

- Is the facility close to family and friends? Are there any shopping centers or other businesses nearby (within walking distance)?

- Do admission and retention policies exclude people with severe cognitive impairments or severe physical disabilities?

- Does the facility provide a written statement of the philosophy of care?

- Visit each facility more than once, sometimes unannounced.

- Visit at mealtimes, sample the food, and observe the quality of mealtime and the service.

- Observe interactions among residents and staff.

- Check to see if the facility offers social, recreational, and spiritual activities.

- Talk to residents.

- Learn what types of training staff receive and how frequently they receive training.

- Review state licensing reports.

The following steps should also be considered:

- Contact your state's long-term care ombudsman to see if any complaints have recently been filed against the assisted living facility you are interested in. In many states, the ombudsman checks on conditions at assisted living units as well as nursing homes.

- Contact the local Better Business Bureau to see if that agency has received any complaints about the assisted living facility.

- If the assisted living facility is connected to a nursing home, ask for information about it, too.

What Is the Cost for Assisted Living?

Although assisted living costs less than nursing home care, it is still fairly expensive. Depending on the kind of assisted living facility and type of services an older person chooses, the price costs can range from less than $25,000 a year to more than $50,000 a year. Because there can be extra fees for additional services, it is very important for older persons to find out what is included in the basic rate and how much other services will cost.

Primarily, older persons or their families pay the cost of assisted living. Some health and long-term care insurance policies may cover some of the costs associated with assisted living. In addition, some residences have their own financial assistance programs.

The federal Medicare program does not cover the costs of assisted living facilities or the care they provide. In some states, Medicaid may pay for the service component of assisted living.

Where Can I Learn More About Assisted Living?

Older persons who want to find out more about the assisted living option can start by contacting their local Area Agency on Aging (AAA). Contact the U.S. Administration on Aging's (AOA) Eldercare Locator at 1-800-677-1116 or visit www.eldercare.gov to find the AAA office closest to you.

Chapter 56

Advance Care Planning

Advance care planning is not just about old age. At any age, a medical crisis could leave someone too ill to make his or her own healthcare decisions. Even if you are not sick now, making healthcare plans for the future is an important step toward making sure you get the medical care you would want, even when doctors and family members are making the decisions for you.

More than one out of four older Americans face questions about medical treatment near the end of life but are not capable of making those decisions. This tip sheet will discuss some questions you can think about now and describe ways to share your wishes with others. Write them down or at least talk about them with someone who would make the decisions for you. Knowing how you would decide might take some of the burden off family and friends.

What Is Advance Care Planning?

Advance care planning involves learning about the types of decisions that might need to be made, considering those decisions ahead of time, and then letting others know about your preferences, often by putting them into an advance directive. An advance directive is a legal document that goes into effect only if you are incapacitated and unable to speak for yourself. This could be the result of disease or

This chapter includes text excerpted from "Advance Care Planning," National Institute on Aging (NIA), National Institutes of Health (NIH), March 2014.

severe injury—no matter how old you are. It helps others know what type of medical care you want. It also allows you to express your values and desires related to end-of-life care. You might think of an advance directive as a living document—one that you can adjust as your situation changes because of new information or a change in your health.

Decisions That Could Come Up Near Death

Sometimes when doctors believe a cure is no longer possible and you are dying, decisions must be made about the use of emergency treatments to keep you alive. Doctors can use several artificial or mechanical ways to try to do this. Decisions that might come up at this time relate to:

- CPR (cardiopulmonary resuscitation)
- Ventilator use
- Artificial nutrition (tube feeding) or artificial hydration (intravenous fluids)
- Comfort care

CPR. CPR (cardiopulmonary resuscitation) might restore your heartbeat if your heart stops or is in a life-threatening abnormal rhythm. The heart of a young, otherwise healthy person might resume beating normally after CPR. An otherwise healthy older person, whose heart is beating erratically or not beating at all, might also be helped by CPR. CPR is less likely to work for an older person who is ill, can't be successfully treated, and is already close to death. It involves repeatedly pushing on the chest with force, while putting air into the lungs. This force has to be quite strong, and sometimes ribs are broken or a lung collapses. Electric shocks known as defibrillation and medicines might also be used as part of the process.

Ventilator use. Ventilators are machines that help you breathe. A tube connected to the ventilator is put through the throat into the trachea (windpipe) so the machine can force air into the lungs. Putting the tube down the throat is called intubation. Because the tube is uncomfortable, medicines are used to keep you sedated (unconscious) while on a ventilator. If you can't breathe on your own after a few days, a doctor may perform a tracheotomy or "trach" (rhymes with "make"). During this bedside surgery, the tube is inserted directly into the trachea through a hole in the neck. For long-term help with breathing, a trach is more comfortable, and sedation is not needed. People using such a breathing tube aren't able to speak without special help because exhaled air goes out of the trach rather than past their vocal cords.

Artificial nutrition or artificial hydration. A feeding tube and/ or intravenous (IV) liquids are sometimes used to provide nutrition when a person is not able to eat or drink. These measures can be helpful if you are recovering from an illness. However, if you are near death, these could actually make you more uncomfortable. For example, IV liquids, which are given through a plastic tube put into a vein, can increase the burden on failing kidneys. Or if the body is shutting down near death, it is not able to digest food properly, even when provided through a feeding tube. At first, the feeding tube is threaded through the nose down to the stomach. In time, if tube feeding is still needed, the tube is surgically inserted into the stomach.

Comfort care. Comfort care is anything that can be done to soothe you and relieve suffering while staying in line with your wishes. Comfort care includes managing shortness of breath; offering ice chips for dry mouth; limiting medical testing; providing spiritual and emotional counseling; and giving medication for pain, anxiety, nausea, or constipation. Often this is done through hospice, which may be offered in the home, in a hospice facility, in a skilled nursing facility, or in a hospital. With hospice, a team of healthcare providers works together to provide the best possible quality of life in a patient's final days, weeks, or months. After death, the hospice team continues to offer support to the family. Learn more about providing comfort at the end of life.

Getting Started

Start by thinking about what kind of treatment you do or do not want in a medical emergency. It might help to talk with your doctor about how your present health conditions might influence your health in the future. For example, what decisions would you or your family face if your high blood pressure leads to a stroke?

If you don't have any medical issues now, your family medical history might be a clue to thinking about the future. Talk to your doctor about decisions that might come up if you develop health problems similar to those of other family members.

In considering treatment decisions, your personal values are key. Is your main desire to have the most days of life, or to have the most life in your days? What if an illness leaves you paralyzed or in a permanent coma and you need to be on a ventilator? Would you want that?

561

What makes life meaningful to you? You might want doctors to try CPR if your heart stops or to try using a ventilator for a short time if you've had trouble breathing, if that means that, in the future, you could be well enough to spend time with your family. Even if the emergency leaves you simply able to spend your days listening to books on tape or gazing out the window watching the birds and squirrels compete for seeds in the bird feeder, you might be content with that.

But, there are many other scenarios. Here are a few. What would you decide?

- If a stroke leaves you paralyzed and then your heart stops, would you want CPR? What if you were also mentally impaired by a stroke—does your decision change?

- What if you develop dementia, don't recognize family and friends, and, in time, cannot feed yourself? Would you want a feeding tube used to give you nutrition?

- What if you are permanently unconscious and then develop pneumonia? Would you want antibiotics and a ventilator used?

For some people, staying alive as long as medically possible is the most important thing. An advance directive can help make sure that happens.

Your decisions about how to handle any of these situations could be different at age 40 than at age 85. Or they could be different if you have an incurable condition as opposed to being generally healthy. An advance directive allows you to provide instructions for these types of situations and then to change the instructions as you get older or if your viewpoint changes.

Making Your Wishes Known

There are two elements in an advance directive—a living will and a durable power of attorney for healthcare. There are also other documents that can supplement your advance directive or stand alone. You can choose which documents to create, depending on how you want decisions to be made. These documents include:

- living will

- durable power of attorney for healthcare

- other documents discussing DNR (do not resuscitate) orders, organ and tissue donation, dialysis, and blood transfusions

Living will. A living will is a written document that helps you tell doctors how you want to be treated if you are dying or permanently unconscious and cannot make decisions about emergency treatment. In a living will, you can say which of the procedures described above you would want, which ones you wouldn't want, and under which conditions each of your choices applies.

Durable power of attorney for healthcare. A durable power of attorney for healthcare is a legal document naming a healthcare proxy, someone to make medical decisions for you at times when you might not be able to do so. Your proxy, also known as a surrogate or agent, should be familiar with your values and wishes. This means that he or she will be able to decide as you would when treatment decisions need to be made. A proxy can be chosen in addition to or instead of a living will. Having a healthcare proxy helps you plan for situations that cannot be foreseen, like a serious auto accident.

A durable power of attorney for healthcare enables you to be more specific about your medical treatment than a living will.

Some people are reluctant to put specific health decisions in writing. For them, naming a healthcare agent might be a good approach, especially if there is someone they feel comfortable talking with about their values and preferences.

Other advance care planning documents. You might also want to prepare separate documents to express your wishes about a single medical issue or something not already covered in your advance directive. A living will usually covers only the specific life-sustaining treatments discussed earlier. You might want to give your healthcare proxy specific instructions about other issues, such as blood transfusion or kidney dialysis. This is especially important if your doctor suggests that, given your health condition, such treatments might be needed in the future.

Two medical issues that might arise at the end of life are DNR orders and organ and tissue donation.

A DNR (do not resuscitate) order tells medical staff in a hospital or nursing facility that you do not want them to try to return your heart to a normal rhythm if it stops or is beating unevenly. Even though a living will might say CPR is not wanted, it is helpful to have a DNR order as part of your medical file if you go to a hospital. Posting a DNR next to your bed might avoid confusion in an emergency situation. Without a DNR order, medical staff will make every effort to restore the normal rhythm of your heart. A non-hospital DNR will alert emergency medical personnel to your wishes regarding CPR and other measures to restore your heartbeat if you are not in the hospital. A similar document that is less familiar is called a DNI (do not intubate) order. A DNI tells medical staff in a hospital or nursing facility that you do not want to be put on a breathing machine.

Organ and tissue donation allows organs or body parts from a generally healthy person who has died to be transplanted into people who need them. Commonly, the heart, lungs, pancreas, kidneys, corneas, liver, and skin are donated. There is no age limit for organ and tissue donation. You can carry a donation card in your wallet. Some states allow you to add this decision to your driver's license. Some people also include organ donation in their advance care planning documents. At the time of death, family may be asked about organ donation. If those close to you, especially your proxy, know how you feel about organ donation, they will be ready to respond.

Selecting Your Healthcare Proxy

If you decide to choose a proxy, think about people you know who share your views and values about life and medical decisions. Your proxy might be a family member, a friend, your lawyer, or someone with whom you worship. It's a good idea to also name an alternate proxy. It is especially important to have a detailed living will if you choose not to name a proxy.

You can decide how much authority your proxy has over your medical care—whether he or she is entitled to make a wide range of decisions or only a few specific ones. Try not to include guidelines that make it impossible for the proxy to fulfill his or her duties. For example, it's probably not unusual for someone to say in conversation, "I don't want to go to a nursing home," but think carefully about whether you want a restriction like that in your advance directive. Sometimes, for financial or medical reasons, that may be the best choice for you.

Of course, check with those you choose as your healthcare proxy and alternate before you name them officially. Make sure they are comfortable with this responsibility.

Making It Official

Once you have talked with your doctor and have an idea of the types of decisions that could come up in the future and whom you would like as a proxy, if you want one at all, the next step is to fill out the legal forms detailing your wishes. A lawyer can help but is not required.

If you decide to use a lawyer, don't depend on him or her to help you understand different medical treatments. That's why you should start the planning process by talking with your doctor.

Many states have their own advance directive forms. Your local Area Agency on Aging can help you locate the right forms. You can find your area agency phone number by calling the Eldercare Locator toll-free at 1-800-677-1116 or going online at www.eldercare.gov.

Some states want your advance directive to be witnessed; some want your signature notarized. A notary is a person licensed by the state to witness signatures. You might find a notary at your bank, post office, or local library, or call your insurance agent. Some notaries charge a fee.

Some people spend a lot of time in more than one state—for example, visiting children and grandchildren. If that's your situation also, you might consider preparing an advance directive using forms for each state—and keep a copy in each place, too.

After You Set Up Your Advance Directive

There are key people who should be told that you have an advance directive. Give copies to your healthcare proxy and alternate proxy. Give your doctor a copy for your medical records. Tell key family members and friends where you keep a copy. If you have to go to the hospital, give staff there a copy to include in your records. Because you might change your advance directive in the future, it's a good idea to keep track of who receives a copy.

Review your advance care planning decisions from time to time—for example, every 10 years, if not more often. You might want to revise your preferences for care if your situation or your health changes. Or, you might want to make adjustments if you receive a serious diagnosis; if you get married, separated, or divorced; if your spouse dies; or if something happens to your proxy or alternate. If your preferences change, you will want to make sure your doctor, proxy, and family know about them.

Still Not Sure?

What happens if you have no advance directive or have made no plans and you become unable to speak for yourself? In such cases, the state where you live will assign someone to make medical decisions on your behalf. This will probably be your spouse, your parents if they are available, or your children if they are adults. If you have no family members, the state will choose someone to represent your best interests.

Always remember, an advance directive is only used if you are in danger of dying and need certain emergency or special measures to keep you alive but are not able to make those decisions on your own. An advance directive allows you to continue to make your wishes about medical treatment known.

Looking Toward the Future

Nobody can predict the future. You may never face a medical situation where you are unable to speak for yourself and make your wishes known. But having an advance directive may give you and those close to you some peace of mind.

Part Seven

Additional Help and Information

Chapter 57

Glossary of Terms Related to Stroke

acupuncture: A form of complementary and alternative medicine that involves inserting thin needles through the skin at specific points on the body to control pain and other symptoms.

acute stroke: A stage of stroke starting at the onset of symptoms and lasting for a few hours thereafter.

advance directive(s): Written instructions letting others know the type of care you want if you are seriously ill or dying. These include a living will and healthcare power of attorney.

agnosia: A cognitive disability characterized by ignorance of or inability to acknowledge one side of the body or one side of the visual field.

allergies: Disorders that involve an immune response in the body. Allergies are reactions to allergens such as plant pollen, other grasses and weeds, certain foods, rubber latex, insect bites, or certain drugs.

Alzheimer disease: A brain disease that cripples the brain's nerve cells over time and destroys memory and learning.

amputation: Removal of part or all of a body part, except for organs in the body.

This glossary contains terms excerpted from documents produced by several sources deemed reliable.

anemia: When the amount of red blood cells or hemoglobin (the substance in the blood that carries oxygen to organs) becomes reduced, causing fatigue that can be severe.

anesthesia: The use of medicine to prevent the feeling of pain or another sensation during surgery or other procedures that might be painful.

aneurysm: A weak or thin spot on an artery wall that has stretched or ballooned out from the wall and filled with blood, or damage to an artery leading to pooling of blood between the layers of the blood vessel walls.

angina: A recurring pain or discomfort in the chest that happens when some part of the heart does not receive enough blood. It is a common symptom of coronary heart disease, which occurs when vessels that carry blood to the heart become narrowed and blocked due to atherosclerosis. Angina feels like a pressing or squeezing pain, usually in the chest under the breast bone, but sometimes in the shoulders, arms, neck, jaws, or back. Angina is usually brought on by exertion, and relieved within a few minutes by resting or by taking prescribed angina medicine.

anoxia: A state of almost no oxygen delivery to a cell, resulting in low energy production and possible death of the cell.

antibiotics: Drugs used to fight many infections caused by bacteria. Some antibiotics are effective against only certain types of bacteria; others can effectively fight a wide range of bacteria. Antibiotics do not work against viral infections.

anticoagulants: A drug therapy used to prevent the formation of blood clots that can become lodged in cerebral arteries and cause strokes.

antidepressants: A name for a category of medications used to treat depression.

antiplatelet agents: A type of anticoagulant drug therapy that prevents the formation of blood clots by preventing the accumulation of platelets that form the basis of blood clots; some common antiplatelets include aspirin and ticlopidine.

antithrombotics: A type of anticoagulant drug therapy that prevents the formation of blood clots by inhibiting the coagulating actions of the blood protein thrombin; some common antithrombotics include warfarin and heparin.

anus: The body opening from which stool passes from the lower end of the intestine and out of the body.

anxiety disorder: Serious medical illness that fills people's lives with anxiety and fear. Some anxiety disorders include panic disorder, obsessive-compulsive disorder, posttraumatic stress disorder, social phobia (or social anxiety disorder), specific phobias, and generalized anxiety disorder.

aphasia: Total or partial loss of the ability to use or understand language; usually caused by stroke, brain disease, or injury.

apraxia: A movement disorder characterized by the inability to perform skilled or purposeful voluntary movements, generally caused by damage to the areas of the brain responsible for voluntary movement.

arteries: Blood vessels that carry oxygen and blood to the heart, brain and other parts of the body.

arteriography: An X-ray of the carotid artery taken when a special dye is injected into the artery.

arteriovenous malformation (AVM): A congenital disorder characterized by a complex tangled web of arteries and veins.

arthritis: Swelling, redness, warmth, and pain of the joints, the places where two bones meet, such as the elbow or knee. There are more than 100 types of arthritis. The two most common types of arthritis are osteoarthritis and rheumatoid arthritis.

asthma: A chronic disease of the lungs. Symptoms include cough, wheezing, a tight feeling in the chest, and trouble breathing.

atherosclerosis: A blood vessel disease characterized by deposits of lipid material on the inside of the walls of large to medium-sized arteries which make the artery walls thick, hard, brittle, and prone to breaking.

atrial fibrillation: Irregular beating of the left atrium, or left upper chamber, of the heart.

autoimmune: Individual's immune system produces abnormal antibodies that react against the body's healthy tissues.

autoimmune disease: Disease caused by an immune response against foreign substances in the tissues of one's own body.

bacteria: Microorganisms that can cause infections.

beta blockers: A type of medication that reduces nerve impulses to the heart and blood vessels. This makes the heart beat slower and with less force. Blood pressure drops and the heart works less hard.

bile: A brown liquid made by the liver. It contains some substances that break up fat for digestion, while other substances are waste products.

biological: Having to do with, or related to, living things.

biopsy: Removal of a small piece of tissue for testing or examination under a microscope.

bladder: The organ in the human body that stores urine. It is found in the lower part of the abdomen.

blood: Fluid in the body made up of plasma, red and white blood cells, and platelets. Blood carries oxygen and nutrients to and waste materials away from all body tissues. In the breast, blood nourishes the breast tissue and provides nutrients needed for milk production.

blood glucose level: Also called blood sugar level, it is the amount of glucose, or sugar, in the blood. Too much glucose in the blood for a long time can cause diabetes and damage many parts of the body, such as the heart, blood vessels, eyes, and kidneys.

blood pressure: Blood pressure is the force of blood against the walls of arteries. Blood pressure is noted as two numbers—the systolic pressure (as the heart beats) over the diastolic pressure (as the heart relaxes between beats). The numbers are written one above or before the other, with the systolic number on top and the diastolic number on the bottom.

blood transfusion: The transfer of blood or blood products from one person (donor) into another person's bloodstream (recipient). Most times, it is done to replace blood cells or blood products lost through severe bleeding. Blood can be given from two sources, your own blood (autologous blood) or from someone else (donor blood).

body mass index: A measure of body fat based on a person's height and weight.

bowels: Also known as the intestine, which is a long tube-like organ in the human body that completes digestion or the breaking down of food. The small bowel is the small intestine and the large bowel is the large intestine.

calorie: A unit of energy-producing potential in food.

carbohydrates: Compounds such as sugars and starches that occur in food and are broken down to release energy in the body.

cardiovascular diseases: Disease of the heart and blood vessels.

carotid artery: An artery, located on either side of the neck, that supplies the brain with blood.

carotid endarterectomy: Surgery used to remove fatty deposits from the carotid arteries.

central stroke pain (central pain syndrome): Pain caused by damage to an area in the thalamus. The pain is a mixture of sensations, including heat and cold, burning, tingling, numbness, and sharp stabbing and underlying aching pain.

cerebrospinal fluid (CSF): Clear fluid that bathes the brain and spinal cord.

cerebrovascular disease: A reduction in the supply of blood to the brain either by narrowing of the arteries through the buildup of plaque on the inside walls of the arteries, called stenosis, or through blockage of an artery due to a blood clot.

cholesterol: A waxy substance, produced naturally by the liver and also found in foods, that circulates in the blood and helps maintain tissues and cell membranes. Excess cholesterol in the body can contribute to atherosclerosis and high blood pressure.

clipping: Surgical procedure for treatment of brain aneurysms, involving clamping an aneurysm from a blood vessel, surgically removing this ballooned part of the blood vessel, and closing the opening in the artery wall.

computed tomography (CT) scan: A series of cross-sectional X-rays of the brain and head; also called computerized axial tomography or CAT scan.

convulsion: Also known as a seizure. An uncontrollable contraction of muscles that can result in sudden movement or loss of control.

Coumadin: A commonly used anticoagulant, also known as warfarin.

dehydration: Excessive loss of body water that the body needs to carry on normal functions at an optimal level. Signs include increasing thirst, dry mouth, weakness or lightheadedness (particularly if worse on standing), and a darkening of the urine or a decrease in urination.

delusion: When a person believes something that is not true and that person keeps the belief even though there is strong evidence against it. Delusions can be the result of brain injury or mental illness.

dementia: A group of symptoms caused by disorders that affect the brain. Symptoms may include memory loss, confusion, personality changes, and difficulty with normal activities like eating or dressing. Dementia has many causes, including Alzheimer disease and stroke.

depression: Term used to describe an emotional state involving sadness, lack of energy and low self-esteem.

detachable coil: A platinum coil that is inserted into an artery in the thigh and strung through the arteries to the site of an aneurysm. The coil is released into the aneurysm creating an immune response from the body. The body produces a blood clot inside the aneurysm, strengthening the artery walls and reducing the risk of rupture.

dialysis: Medical treatment used when kidneys fail. Special equipment filters the blood to rid the body of harmful wastes, salt, and extra water.

dysarthria: Of speech disorders caused by disturbances in the strength or coordination of the muscles of the speech mechanism as a result of damage to the brain or nerves.

dysphagia: Trouble swallowing.

edema: The swelling of a cell that results from the influx of large amounts of water or fluid into the cell.

embolic stroke: A stroke caused by an embolus.

embolus: A free-roaming clot that usually forms in the heart.

endoscopy: A diagnostic procedure in which a thin, flexible tube is introduced through the mouth or rectum to view parts of the digestive tract.

esophagus: Tube that connects the throat with the stomach.

estrogen: A group of female hormones that are responsible for the development of breasts and other secondary sex characteristics in women. Estrogen is produced by the ovaries and other body tissues. Estrogen, along with progesterone, is important in preparing a woman's body for pregnancy.

fat: A source of energy used by the body to make substances it needs. Fat helps your body absorb certain vitamins from food. Some fats are better for your health than others. To help prevent heart disease and stroke, most of the fats you eat should be monounsaturated and polyunsaturated fats.

fatigue: A feeling of lack of energy, weariness or tiredness.

fatty tissue: Connective tissue that contains stored fat. Also referred to as adipose tissue. Fatty tissue in the breast protects the breast from injury.

gastrointestinal: A term that refers to the stomach and the intestines or bowels.

gene: The functional and physical unit of heredity made up of DNA, which has a specific function and is passed from parent to offspring.

global aphasia: Loss of speech caused by a serious injury to the region of the brain that controls speech and language.

heart disease: A number of abnormal conditions affecting the heart and the blood vessels in the heart. The most common type of heart disease is coronary artery disease, which is the gradual buildup of plaques in the coronary arteries, the blood vessels that bring blood to the heart. This disease develops slowly and silently, over decades. It can go virtually unnoticed until it produces a heart attack.

hemiparesis: Weakness on one side of the body.

hemiplegia: Complete paralysis on one side of the body.

hemorrhagic stroke: Sudden bleeding into or around the brain.

heparin: A type of anticoagulant.

high-density lipoprotein (HDL): Also known as the good cholesterol; a compound consisting of a lipid and a protein that carries a small percentage of the total cholesterol in the blood and deposits it in the liver.

hypertension (high blood pressure): Characterized by persistently high arterial blood pressure defined as a measurement greater than or equal to 140 mm/Hg systolic pressure over 90 mm/Hg diastolic pressure.

infarct: An area of tissue that is dead or dying because of a loss of blood supply.

infarction: A sudden loss of blood supply to tissue, causing the formation of an infarct.

intracerebral hemorrhage: Occurs when a vessel within the brain leaks blood into the brain.

ischemia: A loss of blood flow to tissue, caused by an obstruction of the blood vessel, usually in the form of plaque stenosis or a blood clot.

ischemic stroke: A blockage of blood vessels supplying blood to the brain, causing a decrease in blood supply.

menopausal hormone therapy (MHT): Replaces the hormones that a woman's ovaries stop making at the time of menopause, easing symptoms like hot flashes and vaginal dryness. MHT is associated with serious risks, including breast cancer, heart disease and stroke. Women who choose to use MHT should use the lowest dose that helps for the shortest time needed.

neuron: The main functional cell of the brain and nervous system, consisting of a cell body, an axon, and dendrites.

plaque: Fatty cholesterol deposits found along the inside of artery walls that lead to atherosclerosis and stenosis of the arteries.

plasticity: The ability to be formed or molded; in reference to the brain, the ability to adapt to deficits and injury.

platelets: Structures found in blood that are known primarily for their role in blood coagulation.

recombinant tissue plasminogen activator (r-tPA): A genetically engineered form of tPA, a thrombolytic, anti-clotting substance made naturally by the body.

small vessel disease: A cerebrovascular disease defined by stenosis in small arteries of the brain.

speech disorder: Any defect or abnormality that prevents an individual from communicating by means of spoken words. Speech disorders may develop from nerve injury to the brain, muscular paralysis, structural defects, hysteria, or mental retardation.

stenosis: Narrowing of an artery due to the buildup of plaque on the inside wall of the artery.

stroke belt: An area of the southeastern United States with the highest stroke mortality rate in the country.

subarachnoid hemorrhage: Bleeding within the meninges, or outer membranes, of the brain into the clear fluid that surrounds the brain.

thrombolytics: Drugs used to treat an ongoing, acute ischemic stroke by dissolving the blood clot causing the stroke and thereby restoring blood flow through the artery.

thrombosis: The formation of a blood clot in one of the cerebral arteries of the head or neck that stays attached to the artery wall until it grows large enough to block blood flow.

thrombotic stroke: A stroke caused by thrombosis.

transcranial magnetic stimulation (TMS): A small magnetic current delivered to an area of the brain to promote plasticity and healing.

transient ischemic attack (TIA): A short-lived stroke that lasts from a few minutes up to 24 hours; often called a mini-stroke.

traumatic brain injury (TBI): A brain injury that results from a sudden blow to the head. Symptoms may be mild, moderate or serious, depending on the extent of damage.

vasodilators: Medications that increase blood flow to the brain by expanding or dilating blood vessels.

vasospasm: A dangerous side effect of subarachnoid hemorrhage in which the blood vessels in the subarachnoid space constrict erratically, cutting off blood flow.

vertebral artery: An artery on either side of the neck; see carotid artery.

warfarin: A commonly used anticoagulant, also known as Coumadin.

Chapter 58

Directory of Organizations That Help Stroke Patients and Their Families

Government Agencies That Provide Information about Stroke

*Administration on
Aging (AoA)*
Administration for Community
Living (ACL)
330 C St. S.W.
Washington, DC 20201
Toll-Free: 800-677-1116
Phone: 202-401-4634
Fax: 202-357-3555
Website: www.aoa.acl.gov
E-mail: aoainfo@aoa.hhs.gov

*Agency for Healthcare
Research and Quality (AHRQ)*
5600 Fishers Ln.
Rockville, MD 20857
Phone: 301-427-1364
Website: www.ahrq.gov

*Centers for Medicare and
Medicaid Services (CMS)*
7500 Security Blvd.
Baltimore, MD 21244
Toll-Free: 877-267-2323
Phone: 410-786-3000
TTY: 410-786-0727
Toll-Free TTY: 866-226-1819
Website: www.cms.gov

Resources in this chapter were compiled from several sources deemed reliable; all contact information was verified and updated in April 2017.

Centers for Disease Control and Prevention (CDC)
1600 Clifton Rd.
Atlanta, GA 30329-4027
Toll-Free: 800-CDC-INFO
(800-232-4636)
TTY: 888-232-6348
Website: www.cdc.gov

Eldercare Locator
Toll-Free: 800-677-1116
Website: www.eldercare.gov
E-mail: eldercarelocator@n4a.org

Eunice Kennedy Shriver
National Institute of Child Health and Human Development (NICHD)
Information Resource Center
P.O. Box 3006
Rockville, MD 20847
Toll-Free: 800-370-2943
Toll-Free TTY: 888-320-6942
Toll-Free Fax: 866-760-5947
Website: www.nichd.nih.gov
E-mail:
NICHDInformationResource
Center@mail.nih.gov

Healthfinder®
National Health Information Center
1101 Wootton Pkwy
Rockville, MD 20852
Website: www.healthfinder.gov
E-mail: healthfinder@hhs.gov

National Cancer Institute (NCI)
9609 Medical Center Dr.
Bldg. 9609 MSC 9760
Bethesda, MD 20892-9760
Toll-Free: 800-4-CANCER
(800-422-6237)
Website: www.cancer.gov

National Center for Complementary and Integrative Health (NCCIH)
National Institutes of Health (NIH)
9000 Rockville Pike
Bethesda, Maryland 20892
Toll-Free: 888-644-6226
Toll-Free TTY: 866-464-3615
Toll-Free Fax: 866-464-3616
Website: www.nccih.nih.gov
E-mail: info@nccih.nih.gov

National Center for Health Statistics (NCHS)
3311 Toledo Rd.
Hyattsville, MD 20782-2064
Toll-Free: 800-CDC-INFO
(800-232-4636)
Website: www.cdc.gov/nchs
E-mail: cdcinfo@cdc.gov

National Heart, Lung, and Blood Institute (NHLBI)
NHLBI Health Information Center
P.O. Box 30105
Bethesda, MD 20824-0105
Phone: 301-592-8573
TTY: 240-629-3255
Fax: 240-629-3246
Website: www.nhlbi.nih.gov
E-mail: nhlbiinfo@nhlbi.nih.gov

National Highway Traffic Safety Administration (NHTSA)
1200 New Jersey Ave. S.E.
Washington, DC 20590
Toll-Free: 888-327-4236
Toll-Free TTY: 800-424-9153
Website: www.nhtsa.gov

National Institute of Neurological Disorders and Stroke (NINDS)
P.O. Box 5801
Bethesda, MD 20824
Toll-Free: 800-352-9424
Phone: 301-496-5751
TTY: 301-468-5981
Website: www.ninds.nih.gov

National Institute on Aging (NIA)
31 Center Dr.
MSC 2292
Bethesda, MD 20892
Toll-Free: 800-222-2225
Phone: 301-496-1752
Toll-Free TTY: 800-222-4225
Website: www.nia.nih.gov
E-mail: niaic@nia.nih.gov

National Institute on Alcohol Abuse and Alcoholism (NIAAA)
Toll-Free: 888-MY-NIAAA
(888-69-64222)
Website: www.niaaa.nih.gov
E-mail: niaaaweb-r@exchange.nih.gov

National Institutes of Health (NIH)
9000 Rockville Pike
Bethesda, MD 20892
Phone: 301-496-4000
TTY: 301-402-9612
Website: www.nih.gov
E-mail: NIHinfo@od.nih.gov

National Women's Health Information Center (NWHIC)
Office on Women's Health (OWH)
200 Independence Ave. S.W.
Rm. 712E
Washington, DC 20201
Toll-Free: 800-994-9662
Phone: 202-690-7650
Toll-Free TDD: 888-220-5446
Fax: 202-205-2631
Website: www.womenshealth.gov

Office of Extramural Research (OER)
Phone: 301-945-7573
Website: grants.nih.gov
E-mail: grantsinfo@od.nih.gov

Office of Minority Health (OMH)
Tower Oaks Bldg.
1101 Wootton Pwky
Ste. 600
Rockville, MD 20852
Toll-Free: 800-444-6472
Phone: 240-453-2882
Fax: 240-453-2883
Website: minorityhealth.hhs.gov
E-mail: info@minorityhealth.hhs.gov

Smokefree.gov
Toll-Free: 800-QUIT-NOW
(800-784-8669)
Website: www.smokefree.gov
E-mail: NCISmokefreeTeam@
mail.nih.gov

*U.S. Department of Health
and Human Services (HHS)*
200 Independence Ave. S.W.
Washington, DC 20201
Toll-Free: 877-696-6775
Website: www.hhs.gov

*U.S. Department of Veterans
Affairs (VA)*
810 Vermont Ave. N.W.
Washington, DC 20420
Toll-Free: 877-222-VETS
(877-222-8387)
Website: www.va.gov

*U.S. Equal Employment
Opportunity Commission
(EEOC)*
131 M St. N.E.
Washington, DC 20507
Phone: 202-663-4900
TTY: 202-663-4494
Website: www.eeoc.gov
E-mail: info@eeoc.gov

*U.S. National Library of
Medicine (NLM)*
8600 Rockville Pike
Bethesda, MD 20894
Toll-Free: 888-FIND-NLM
(888-346-3656)
Phone: 301-594-5983
Website: www.nlm.nih.gov

*U.S. Social Security
Administration (SSA)*
Office of Public Inquiries
1100 West High Rise
6401 Security Blvd.
Baltimore, MD 21235
Toll-Free: 800-772-1213
Toll-Free TTY: 800-325-0778
Website: www.ssa.gov

Private Agencies That Provide Information about Stroke

*American Academy of Family
Physicians (AAFP)*
11400 Tomahawk Creek Pkwy
Leawood, KS 66211-2680
Toll-Free: 800-274-2237
Phone: 913-906-6000
Fax: 913-906-6075
Website: www.aafp.org
E-mail: aafp@aafp.org

*American Academy of
Neurology (AAN)*
201 Chicago Ave.
Minneapolis, MN 55415
Toll-Free: 800-879-1960
Phone: 612-928-6000
Fax: 612-454-2746
Website: www.aan.com
E-mail: memberservices@aan.
com

**American Academy of
Pediatrics (AAP)**
141 N.W. Point Blvd.
Elk Grove Village, IL
60007-1098
Toll-Free: 800-433-9016
Phone: 847-434-4000
Fax: 847-434-8000
Website: www.aap.org
E-mail: kidsdocs@aap.org

**American Academy of
Physical Medicine and
Rehabilitation (AAPM&R)**
9700 W. Bryn Mawr Ave.
Ste. 200
Rosemont, IL 60018
Phone: 847-737-6000
Website: www.aapmr.org
E-mail: info@aapmr.org

**American Association of
Neurological Surgeons
(AANS)**
5550 Meadowbrook Dr.
Rolling Meadows, IL 60008-3852
Toll-Free: 888-566-AANS
(888-566-2267)
Phone: 847-378-0500
Fax: 847-378-0600
Website: www.aans.org
E-mail: info@aans.org

**American Congress
of Obstetricians and
Gynecologists (ACOG)**
409 12th St. S.W.
Washington, DC 20024-2188
Toll-Free: 800-673-8444
Phone: 202-638-5577
Website: www.acog.org
E-mail: resources@acog.org

**American College of
Radiology (ACR)**
1891 Preston White Dr.
Reston, VA 20191
Phone: 703-648-8900
Website: www.acr.org
E-mail: info@acr.org

**American Congress of
Rehabilitation Medicine
(ACRM)**
11654 Plaza America Dr.
Ste. 535
Reston, VA 20190-4700
Phone: 703-435-5335
Toll-Free Fax: 866-692-1619
Website: www.acrm.org
E-mail: info@ACRM.org

**American Heart Association
(AHA)/American Stroke
Association**
National Center
7272 Greenville Ave.
Dallas, TX 75231
Toll-Free: 800-AHA-USA-1
(800-242-8721) / 888-4-STROKE
(888-478-7653)
Websites: www.heart.org; www.
strokeassociation.org

**American Medical
Association (AMA)**
AMA Plaza
330 N. Wabash Ave.
Ste. 39300
Chicago, IL 60611-5885
Toll-Free: 800-621-8335
Website: www.ama-assn.org

American Migraine Foundation (AMF)
19 Mantua Rd.
Mount Royal, NJ 08061
Phone: 856-423-0043
Fax: 856-423-0082
Website:
americanmigrainefoundation.org
E-mail: amf@talley.com

American Occupational Therapy Association (AOTA)
4720 Montgomery Ln.
Ste. 200
Bethesda, MD 20814-3449
Toll-Free: 800-SAY-AOTA
(800-729-2682)
Phone: 301-652-6611
Fax: 301-652-7711
Website: www.aota.org

American Physical Therapy Association (APTA)
1111 N. Fairfax St.
Alexandria, VA 22314-1488
Toll-Free: 800-999-2782
Phone: 703-684-2782
TDD: 703-683-6748
Fax: 703-684-7343
Website: www.apta.org

American Society of Neurorehabilitation (ASNR)
5841 Cedar Lake Rd.
Ste. 204
Minneapolis, MN 55416
Phone: 952-545-6324
Fax: 952-545-6073
Website: www.asnr.com
E-mail: asnr@llmsi.com

American Speech-Language-Hearing Association (ASHA)
2200 Research Blvd.
Rockville, MD 20850-3289
Toll-Free: 800-638-8255
Phone: 301-296-5700
TTY: 301-296-5650
Fax: 301-296-8580
Website: www.asha.org

Brain Aneurysm Foundation, Inc.
269 Hanover St.
Hanover, MA 02339
Toll-Free: 888-272-4602
Phone: 781-826-5556
Fax: 781-826-5566
Website: www.bafound.org
E-mail: office@bafound.org

Brain Injury Association of America (BIAA)
1608 Spring Hill Rd.
Ste. 110
Vienna, VA 22182
Toll-Free: 800-444-6443
Phone: 703-761-0750
Fax: 703-761-0755
Website: www.biausa.org

Brain Injury Recovery Network
840 Central Ave.
Carlisle, OH 45005
Toll-Free: 877-810-2100
Fax: 877-810-2100
Website: www.tbirecovery.org
E-mail: help@tbirecovery.org

Caring.com
2600 S. El Camino Real, Ste. 300
San Mateo, CA 94403
Phone: 650-312-7100
Website: www.caring.com

*Children's Hemiplegia and
Stroke Association (CHASA)*
4101 W. Green Oaks
Ste. 305-149
Arlington, TX 76016
Websites: www.chasa.org; www.
pediatricstroke.org

Cleveland Clinic
9500 Euclid Ave.
Cleveland, OH 44195
Toll-Free: 800-223-CARE
(800-223-2273)
Phone: 216-444-2200
Website: my.clevelandclinic.org

*Family Caregiver Alliance
(FCA)*
235 Montgomery St., Ste. 950
San Francisco, CA 94104
Toll-Free: 800-445-8106
Phone: 415-434-3388
Fax: 415-434-3508
Website: www.caregiver.org
E-mail: info@caregiver.org

*Hazel K. Goddess Fund for
Stroke Research in Women*
785 Park Ave., Ste. 3E
New York, NY 10021
Phone: 561-623-0504
Fax: 561-623-0502
Website: www.thegoddessfund.
org
E-mail: officemanager@
thegoddessfund.org

HeartHealthyWomen.org
Cardiovascular Research
Foundation (CRF)
111 East 59th St.
New York, NY 10022-1122
Phone: 212-851-9300
Website: www.
hearthealthywomen.org
E-mail: hhw@crf.org

Internet Stroke Center
Department of Neurology and
Neurotherapeutics
5323 Harry Hines Blvd.
Dallas, TX 75390
Phone: 214-648-3111
Website: www.strokecenter.org
E-mail: neuroInfo@
utsouthwestern.edu

*Job Accommodation Network
(JAN)*
West Virginia University
P.O. Box 6080
Morgantown, WV 26506-6080
Toll-Free: 800-526-7234
Toll-Free TTY: 877-781-9403
Fax: 304-293-5407
Website: askjan.org
E-mail: jan@askjan.org

*National Alliance for
Caregiving*
4720 Montgomery Ln.
Ste. 205
Bethesda, MD 20814
Phone: 301-718-8444
Fax: 301-951-9067
Website: www.caregiving.org
E-mail: info@caregiving.org

National Aphasia Association (NAA)
P.O. Box 87
Scarsdale, NY 10583
Website: www.aphasia.org
E-mail: naa@aphasia.org

National Brain Tumor Society (NBTS)
55 Chapel St.
Ste. 200
Newton, MA 02458
Phone: 617-924-9997
Fax: 617-924-9998
Website: www.braintumor.org

National Center for Learning Disabilities (NCLD)
32 Laight St. 2nd Fl.
New York, NY 10013
Phone: 212-545-7510
Fax: 212-545-9665
Website: www.ncld.org

National Information Center for Children and Youth with Disabilities (NICHCY)
1825 Connecticut Ave. N.W.
Washington, DC 20009
Toll-Free: 800-695-0285 (Voice and TTY)
Phone: 202-884-8200 (Voice and TTY)
Website: www.parentcenterhub.org

National Rehabilitation Information Center (NARIC)
8400 Corporate Dr.
Ste. 500
Landover, MD 20785
Toll-Free: 800-346-2742
Phone: 301-459-5900
TTY: 301-459-5984
Fax: 301-459-4263
Website: www.naric.com
E-mail: naricinfo@
heitechservices.com

National Stroke Association
9707 E. Easter Ln.
Ste. B
Centennial, CO 80112
Toll-Free: 800-STROKES
(800-787-6537)
Fax: 303-649-1328
Website: www.stroke.org
E-mail: info@stroke.org

Neuro-Patient Resource Center
Montreal Neurological Institute and Hospital
3801 Rue University
Rm. 354
Montréal, QC H3A 2B4
Phone: 514-398-5358
Website: www.mcgill.
ca/neuro/patients/
neuro-patient-resource-centre

Shirley Ryan AbilityLab
(formerly known as
Rehabilitation Institute of
Chicago)
355 E. Erie
Chicago, IL 60611
Toll-Free: 800-354-REHAB
(800-354-7342)
Phone: 312-238-LIFE
(312-238-5433)
Website: www.sralab.org

*Society for Vascular Surgery
(SVS)*
633 North Saint Clair St. 22nd Fl.
Chicago, IL 60611
Toll-Free: 800-258-7188
Phone: 312-334-2300
Fax: 312-334-2320
Website: www.vascularweb.org
E-mail: vascular@
vascularsociety.org

Stroke Association
Stroke Association House
240 City Rd.
London, EC1V 2PR
Phone: 207-566-0300
Fax: 207-490-2686
Website: www.stroke.org.uk
E-mail: info@stroke.org.uk

*Stroke Awareness
Foundation*
51 E. Campbell Ave.
Ste. 106-M
Campbell, CA 95008
Phone: 408-370-5282
Website: www.strokeinfo.org
E-mail: noemi@strokeinfo.org

Well Spouse Association
63 West Main St.
Ste. H
Freehold, NJ 07728
Toll-Free: 800-838-0879
Phone: 732-577-8899
Fax: 732-577-8644
Website: www.wellspouse.org
E-mail: info@wellspouse.org

Index

Index

Page numbers followed by 'n' indicate a footnote. Page numbers in *italics* indicate a table or illustration.

A

"A New Rehabilitation Treatment Following Stroke" (ClinicalTrials .gov) 83n
A1C test, diabetes 183
AAN *see* American Academy of Neurology
abdominal obesity
  metabolic syndrome 146
  weight management 210
ABI *see* ankle-brachial index
ACA *see* Affordable Care Act
ACE inhibitors *see* angiotensin-converting enzyme inhibitors
aCL *see* anticardiolipin antibody
activities of daily living, rehabilitation 453
acupuncture, defined 569
acute stroke, defined 569
Adalat (nifedipine), tabulated *361*
Administration for Community Living (ACL)
  publications
    long-term care insurance 526n
    state Medicaid programs 526n

Administration on Aging (AoA), contact 579
"Advance Care Planning" (NIA) 559n
advance directives
  defined 569
  long-term care 548
advocate, legal decisions 548
AF *see* atrial fibrillation
Affordable Care Act (ACA)
  overview 524–5
  rehabilitation 374
"Affordable Care Act (ACA)" (CMS) 524n
"African-American Men and Stroke" (CDC) 51n
"African-American Women and Stroke" (CDC) 51n
African Americans, stroke disparities 52
Agency for Healthcare Research and Quality (AHRQ)
  contact 579
  publication
    acute ischemic stroke patients 352n
agnosia
  defined 569
  overview 380–2
"Agnosia" (GARD) 380n
AHA *see* American Heart Association

591

Alaska Natives, stroke disparities 53
alcohol use
  dementia 388
  recurrent stroke 120
  traumatic brain injury 260
  see also lifestyle changes
alcoholic cardiomyopathy, risk
  factors 249
allergic reactions
  CT scans 315
  percutaneous coronary
    intervention 345
allergies
  defined 569
  sleep apnea 240
allodynia, central poststroke pain 426
alpha-adrenergic blockers, drugs 441
alpha-beta blockers, high blood
  pressure 199
alpha blockers, high blood pressure 199
Alzheimer disease
  agnosia 381
  aphasia 396
  caregiver stress 514
  defined 569
  dementia 386
  neurologists 292
  traumatic brain injury 265
American Academy of Family
  Physicians (AAFP), contact 582
American Academy of Neurology
  (AAN), contact 582
American Academy of Pediatrics
  (AAP), contact 583
American Academy of Physical
  Medicine and Rehabilitation
  (AAPM&R), contact 583
American Association of Neurological
  Surgeons (AANS), contact 583
American College of Radiology (ACR),
  contact 583
American Congress of Obstetricians
  and Gynecologists (ACOG),
  contact 583
American Congress of Rehabilitation
  Medicine (ACRM), contact 583
American Heart Association (AHA)/
  American Stroke Association,
  contact 583

"American Indian and Alaska Native
  Heart Disease and Stroke Fact
  Sheet" (CDC) 51n
American Indians, stroke
  disparities 53
American Medical Association (AMA),
  contact 583
American Migraine Foundation (AMF)
  contact 584
  publication
    migraine, stroke, and heart
      disease 235n
American Occupational Therapy
  Association (AOTA), contact 584
American Physical Therapy
  Association (APTA), contact 584
American Society of
  Neurorehabilitation (ASNR),
  contact 584
American Speech-Language-Hearing
  Association (ASHA)
  contact 584
  publication
    brain damage 382n
Americans with Disabilities Act of
  1990, vocational therapists 455
amphetamines, risk factors 8
amputation, defined 569
amyotrophic lateral sclerosis (ALS)
  dysphagia 406
  foot drop 413
  neurologists 292
anabolic steroids, described 256
anemia, defined 570
anesthesia, defined 570
aneurysm
  computed tomography 111
  defined 570
  hemorrhagic stroke 6
  high blood pressure 195
  magnetic resonance imaging 317
  stent procedure 343
  see also cerebral aneurysm
aneurysm clipping, coil
  embolization 325
angina
  coronary heart disease 133
  defined 570
  heart attack signs 186

angiography
  atherosclerosis 140
  described 111
  see also magnetic resonance
      angiography
angioplasty, blocked artery 178
angiotensin-converting enzyme (ACE)
  inhibitors, high blood pressure 199
angiotensin II receptor blockers,
  recurrent stroke prevention 121
ankle-brachial index (ABI)
  atherosclerosis 139
  peripheral artery disease 179
anosognosia
  right hemisphere brain damage 382
  stroke survivors 451
anoxia
  defined 570
  traumatic brain injury 258
antibiotics, defined 570
anticardiolipin antibody (aCL), blood
  clotting problems 169
anticoagulants
  defined 570
  described 355
  intracerebral hemorrhagic strokes 104
  neurological disorders 293
  rehabilitation 28
"Anticoagulants" (NIH) 355n
antidepressant medication,
  menopausal hormone therapy 36
antidepressants
  defined 570
  depression 517
  traumatic brain injury 263
antiplatelet agents
  defined 570
  described 355
  stroke treatment 34
antithrombotics
  defined 570
  stroke medications 47
anxiety disorder, defined 571
aorta
  described 12
  depicted *160*
  echocardiography 300
aortic aneurysm or tear, stent
  procedure 343

aphasia
  defined 571
  overview 395–9
  speech problems 44
"Aphasia" (NIDCD) 395n
apnea *see* sleep apnea
apraxia
  defined 571
  described 401
apraxia of speech, aphasia 395
arrhythmia
  atherosclerosis 136
  atrial fibrillation 157
  described 249
  percutaneous coronary
      intervention 344
arteries, defined 571
arteriography
  carotid artery disease 350
  defined 571
arteriosclerosis *see* atherosclerosis
arteriovenous malformation
  cerebral aneurysms 108
  defined 571
  hemorrhagic stroke 6
  repair 325
artery wall, depicted *132*
arthritis, defined 571
ASHA *see* American Speech-
  Language-Hearing Association
Asian Americans, stroke disparities 54
aspiration pneumonia, dysphagia 405
aspirin
  antiplatelet drugs 356
  carotid artery dissection 101
  cerebral aneurysm 113
  heart disease prevention 253
  recurrent stroke 121
  stroke prevention 15
  stroke treatment 34
"Assisted Living" (AOA) 555n
asthma, defined 571
Asymptomatic Carotid Atherosclerosis
  Study (ACAS), carotid
  endarterectomy 347
ataxia, described 450
atherosclerosis
  childhood stroke 26
  defined 571

atherosclerosis, *continued*
  dementia risk factors 388
  hemorrhagic stroke 104
  obesity 281
  overview 132–44
  peripheral artery disease 171
"Atherosclerosis" (NHLBI) 132n
atrial fibrillation (AF)
  defined 571
  electrocardiogram 300
  overview 157–66
  sleep apnea 241
  vascular dementia 387
"Atrial Fibrillation" (NHLBI) 157n
aura, migraine 236
autoimmune disease, defined 571
AVM *see* arteriovenous malformation

B

baclofen, spasticity 410
bad cholesterol *see* low-density
  lipoprotein (LDL)
balance problems, overview 417–21
"Balance Problems after Stroke"
  (Omnigraphics) 417n
Balloon Assisted Coiling (BAC),
  described 330
balloon catheters, self-expanding
  stents 332
bariatric surgery, overweight and
  obesity 225
basic metabolic panel (BMP),
  described 303
Benefits of Quitting (CDC) 277n
beta blockers
  defined 572
  high blood pressure 199
  recurrent stroke 121
bile, defined 572
bile acid sequestrants, cholesterol-
  lowering medicines 211
Binswanger disease *see* multi-infarct
  dementia
"Binswanger's Disease"
  (GARD) 391n
biofeedback, Kegel exercises 440
biological, defined 572
biopsy, defined 572

birth control
  blood clotting problems 168
  stroke risk 7, 33
birth control methods, described 33
bladder, defined 572
bladder control problems
  overview 435–42
  see also bladder training; overactive
    bladder
bladder training, treatment 438
blood, defined 572
blood chemistry tests, described 303
blood clots
  antithrombotics 47
  coronary heart disease 133
  CT scans 314
  echocardiography 308
  ischemic stroke 96
  multi-infarct dementia 392
  stent procedures 342
  stroke complications 9
  transient ischemic attack 323
blood clotting disorders,
  overview 167–9
"Blood Clotting Problems and Stroke
  Risk" (OWH) 167n
blood glucose level, defined 572
blood oxygen levels, neurologists 293
blood pressure
  defined 572
  high blood pressure
    management 270
  overview 190–202
  Stroke Belt 57
  stroke prevention 39
  stroke risk factors 23
  see also high blood pressure
blood tests
  complete blood count 301
  heart disease risk 304
  stroke 45, 301
"Blood Tests—Types of Blood Tests"
  (NHLBI) 301n
blood thinners *see* anticoagulants
blood transfusion, defined 572
body mass index (BMI)
  defined 572
  diagnosis of overweight and
    obesity 221

body mass index (BMI), *continued*
　healthy weight 276
　obesity 218
bone marrow disorder, hematocrit 302
Botox (botulinum toxin), facial
　wrinkles 441
botulinum toxin *see* Botox
"Bowel Control Problems"
　(NIDDK) 431n
bowel problems
　overview 431–3
　sensory disturbances 450
　stroke complications 10
bowels, defined 572
brachial artery, depicted *176*
brain
　aneurysms 110
　carotid artery disease 144
　computed tomography 10
　depicted *4*
　hemorrhagic stroke 4
　magnetic resonance imaging 317
　speech problems 44
　traumatic brain injury 257
brain aneurysm *see* cerebral
　aneurysm
Brain Aneurysm Foundation, Inc.,
　contact 584
brain attack *see* stroke
brain damage
　agnosia 380
　aphasia 395
　cerebral aneurysms 113
　memory problems 509
　right hemisphere brain damage 382
　speech therapy 49
　symptoms of stroke 21
　vascular dementia 391
brain injury
　aphasia 396
　choosing a rehabilitation facility 461
　stroke recovery 373
　see also traumatic brain injury
Brain Injury Association of America
　(BIAA), contact 584
Brain Injury Recovery Network,
　contact 584
"Brain Mapping of Language
　Impairments" (NIH) 395n

brain scans
　diagnosing dementia 390
　stroke treatment 288
brainstem stroke
　balance problems after stroke 418
　strokes in older adults 45
Broca aphasia 397
bruit, diagnose stroke 10
bupropion, overweight and
　obesity 224
"Buying Long-Term Care Insurance"
　(ACL) 526n

C

CABG *see* coronary artery bypass
　graft
CADASIL *see* cerebral autosomal
　dominant arteriopathy with
　subcortical infarcts and
　leukoencephalopathy
Caduet, combination medicines 371
calcium channel blockers
　blood pressure treatment 199, *365*
　recurrent stroke 121
caloric intake, weight loss 282
calorie, defined 573
cancer
　blood clotting problems 168
　obesity 221
　physical activity benefits 231
　quitting smoking 278
carbohydrates, defined 573
cardiac arrest
　arrhythmias 249
　cocaine 255
　hypothermia 48
cardiologist, peripheral artery
　disease 174
cardiopulmonary resuscitation (CPR)
　described 560
　do-not-resuscitate order 549
cardiovascular diseases, defined 573
"Caregiver Stress" (OWH) 513n
"Caregiver Stress and Depression"
　(VA) 513n
caregivers
　assistive technology 479
　healthcare team 506

caregivers, *continued*
  home-based services 541
  overview 513–8
  rehabilitation nurses 453
  sexuality after stroke 502
  stroke rehabilitation 374
  stroke support group 520
  traumatic brain injury 261
Caring.com, contact 585
carotid angiography
  described 11
  diagnostic tests 149
carotid arteries
  carotid angiography 11
  carotid endarterectomy 346
  carotid ultrasound 11
  defined 573
  depicted *145*
  described 137
  heart-healthy lifestyle 150
  ischemic stroke 6
carotid artery disease
  high blood cholesterol 203
  overview 144–55
"Carotid Artery Disease"
  (NHLBI) 144n
carotid artery dissection,
  overview 98–102
"Carotid Artery Dissection"
  (Omnigraphics) 98n
carotid endarterectomy
  atherosclerosis treatment 142
  defined 573
  ischemic stroke treatment 117
  overview 346–50
"Carotid Plaque Imaging in Acute
  Stroke (CAPIAS)" (ClinicalTrials.
  gov) 89n
carotid ultrasound
  described 11
  diagnostic tests 149
  see also ultrasound
catheter
  angioplasty and stent
    placement 178
  arteriogram 177
  atherectomy 178
  carotid angiography 299

catheter, *continued*
  cerebral angiography 305
  depicted *153*
  stents 340
  urine retention treatment 441
catheterization, overactive
  bladder 439
Centers for Disease Control and
  Prevention (CDC)
  contact 580
  publications
    African-American men and
      stroke 51n
    African-American women and
      stroke 51n
    American Indian and Alaska
      Native heart disease and
      stroke 51n
    benefits of quitting
      smoking 277n
    healthy living and stroke
      prevention 276n
    heart disease and stroke
      prevention 41n
    Hispanic men and stroke 51n
    Hispanic women and
      stroke 51n
    men and stroke 38n
    physical activity and
      health 230n
    preventing diabetes 268n
    stroke and smoking and heart
      disease 251n, 277n
    stroke mortality among
      adults 63n
    stroke recovery 467n
    stroke risk 125n
    stroke signs and
      symptoms 21n, 63n
    stroke treatment 287n
    stroke types 96n
    weight loss 281n
    women and stroke 30n
Centers for Medicare and Medicaid
  Services (CMS)
  contact 579
  publication
    Affordable Care Act
      (ACA) 524n

central pain syndrome (CPS), stroke
   effects 44
"Central Post-Stroke Pain"
   (GARD) 424n
central stroke pain (central pain
   syndrome), defined 573
central stroke pain *see* central pain
   syndrome (CPS)
centrally-acting alpha adrenergics *365*
cerebral aneurysm, overview 108–14
"Cerebral Aneurysms Fact Sheet"
   (NINDS) 108n
"Cerebral Aneurysms Information
   Page" (NINDS) 108n
cerebral angiography, overview 305–7
"Cerebral Angiography"
   (Omnigraphics) 305n
cerebral arteries, depicted *97*
cerebral autosomal dominant
   arteriopathy with subcortical
   infarcts and leukoencephalopathy
   (CADASIL), described 387
cerebrospinal fluid (CSF), defined 573
cerebrospinal fluid (CSF) analysis,
   described 112
cerebrovascular accident (CVA) *see*
   stroke
cerebrovascular disease
   defined 573
   prehospital emergency care 27
   vascular dementia 387
CHD *see* coronary heart disease
childbirth, bowel control problems 431
childhood stroke, described 26
children
   high blood pressure 194
   obesity 214
   traumatic brain injury 260
Children's Hemiplegia and Stroke
   Association (CHASA), contact 585
cholesterol
   defined 573
   see also high cholesterol
cholesterol levels
   atherosclerosis 134
   obesity 127
   recurrent stroke 121
   stroke risk 8
cigarette smoking *see* smoking

CIMT *see* constraint-induced
   movement therapy
Cleveland Clinic
   contact 585
   publications
      choosing a rehabilitation
         facility 461n
      stress at work and stroke 246n
clinical trials
   overview 78–83
   tissue plasminogen activator 352
clipping
   aneurysm repair 328
   defined 573
clonazepam
   pharmacologic approaches 412
   spasticity 410
clopidogrel
   blood thinners 16
   carotid artery disease 150
   stents 346
CMS *see* Centers for Medicare and
   Medicaid Services
CNS *see* central nervous system
coagulation panel, blood clotting
   tests 305
cocaine
   cerebral aneurysm causes 109
   described 255
   stroke risk factors 8
cognitive problems
   overview 379–93
   traumatic brain injury 262
coil embolization
   hemorrhagic stroke 324
   see also detachable coil
coma, traumatic brain injury 257
comfort care, described 561
communication problems
   overview 395–401
   right hemisphere brain damage 382
"Compassionate Allowances" (SSA) 529n
complementary or alternative
   therapies, defined 427
complete blood count (CBC),
   described 301
computed tomography (CT)
   defined 573
   overview 313–5
   tissue plasminogen activator 353

"Computed Tomography (CT)"
(NIBIB) 313n
computed tomography angiogram
(CTA), stroke diagnosis 11
computer-assisted tomography,
defined 292
concussion, traumatic brain
injury 258
congenital heart defects,
echocardiography 309
consciousness
intracerebral hemorrhagic
stroke 105
stroke symptoms 9
traumatic brain injury 258
constipation, bowel control
problems 432
constraint-induced movement therapy
(CIMT), overview 414–6
"Constraint-Induced Movement
Therapy" (Omnigraphics) 414n
continuous positive airway pressure
(CPAP), sleep disorders 243
contraception *see* birth control
contractures, spasticity symptoms 410
contrast dye
carotid angiography 300
cerebral angiography 305
computed tomography 111
magnetic resonance
angiography 149
"Controlling Cholesterol with Statins"
(FDA) 369n
contusion, brain trauma 258
convulsion, defined 573
coronary artery, depicted *345*
coronary artery bypass graft 142
coronary heart disease (CHD)
atrial fibrillation risk factors 158
carotid artery disease risk factor 146
high blood cholesterol 203
smoking 251
stents 338
coronary microvascular disease
(MVD), coronary arteries 137
Coumadin, defined 573
counselor, presymptomatic tests 390
CPS *see* central pain syndrome
CPSP *see* central poststroke pain

creatine kinase (CK) tests, blood
enzyme tests 304
creatinine
acute ischemic stroke 87
blood chemistry tests 303
carotid plaque imaging 91
CSF *see* cerebrospinal fluid
CT scan *see* computed tomography
CTA *see* computed tomography
angiogram

D

dabigatran (Pradaxa), anticoagulants
48, 355
dalteparin (Fragmin), injectable
anticoagulant 48, 355
DASH *see* Dietary Approaches to Stop
Hypertension
deep brain stimulators, MRI scan
considerations 317
dehydration, defined 573
delusion, defined 574
dementia
defined 574
described 385
see also multi-infarct dementia;
vascular dementia
"Dementia: Hope through Research"
(NINDS) 385n
Department of Veterans Affairs
see U.S. Department of Veterans
Affairs
depression
antidepressants 263
atherosclerosis 143
caregiver stress 515
clinical depression 452
defined 574
dementia risk factor 388
long-term stress 245
obesity 221
overview 505–7
poststroke pain effect 425
sleep problem 498
stroke effects 468, 501
traumatic brain injury 265
see also poststroke depression
"Depression after Stroke" (VA) 505n

detachable coil
  defined 574
  endovascular embolization 113
  research 330
diabetes
  ACE inhibitors warnings 359
  atrial fibrillation risk factor 157
  carotid artery disease risk factor 146
  dementia risk factors 388, 392
  described 7
  incidence among men/women 38, 52
  insulin resistance 135
  long-term stress 245
  obesity complications 281, 516
  overview 181–7
  peripheral artery disease
    causes 172
  prevention and management
    45, 233, 268
  recurrent stroke risk factors 120
  risk calculator, tabulated *207*
  statin treatment 17, 141, 150
  stent procedure consideration 342
  stroke risk 126
"Diabetes, Heart Disease, and Stroke"
  (NIDDK) 181n
diagnostic tests
  atherosclerosis 138
  atrial fibrillation 162
  blood tests for stroke 301
  carotid artery disease 149, 350
  carotid artery dissection 100
  central poststroke pain 425
  cerebral aneurysm 110
  dementia 389, 392
  described 12
  heart disease 186
  high blood cholesterol 205
  neurological exam 292
  overweight/obesity 222
  peripheral artery disease 175
  stroke 297
  traumatic brain injury 261
dialysis, defined 574
diarrhea
  angiotension II antagonists side
    effects 364
  beta blockers side effects 360
  described 432
  renin inhibitors side effects 366

diazepam
  muscle relaxant / bladder
    control 441
  spasticity treatment 410
diet and nutrition *see* nutrition
Dietary Approaches to Stop
  Hypertension (DASH)
  carotid artery disease 152
  high blood pressure 165
"Differences in Stroke Mortality among
  Adults Aged 45 and Over: United
  States, 2010–2013" (CDC) 63n
diplopia *see* double vision
dipyridamole
  antiplatelet drugs 48, 355
  recurrent stroke prevention 121
disabilities
  assistive technologies 476
  categories 478
  disability benefits 529
  stroke effects 43, 449
"Disability Benefits" (SSA) 529n
diuretics
  hypertension management 121, 199
  tabulated *368*
  traumatic brain injury treatment
    263
do not resuscitate (DNR),
  described 549
Doppler ultrasound
  carotid artery disease 154
  carotid ultrasound 11, 299
  described 176, 321
double vision
  birth control pills 34
  cerebral aneurysms 109
  stroke complications 418, 444
  traumatic brain injury 265
driver rehabilitation specialist,
  described 482
"Driving after You Have a Stroke"
  (NHTSA) 481n
drug abuse
  cerebral aneurysms causes 108
  stroke risk 254
Drug Enforcement Administration
  (DEA)
  publication
    drug 254n

durable power of attorney for
healthcare, described 549, 563
dysarthria
defined 574
described 400
speech problems after stroke 44
dysesthesia, poststroke pain 426
dysphagia
defined 574
overview 403–7
rehabilitation 264
special diets 487
"Dysphagia" (NIDCD) 403n, 486n

E

ECG *see* electrocardiogram
echo *see* echocardiography
echocardiography (echo)
described 12, 139, 163, 300
overview 308–12
"Echocardiography" (NHLBI) 308n
edema, defined 574
EEG *see* electroencephalogram
"The Effect of Aerobic Exercise
in Patients with Minor Stroke
(HITPALS)" (ClinicalTrials.gov) 91n
EKG *see* electrocardiogram
Eldercare Locator, contact 580
electrocardiogram (ECG; EKG)
described 11, 139, 162, 300
overview 312–3
"Electrocardiogram" (NHLBI) 312n
electroencephalogram (EEG),
described 292
electrolytes, described 303
electromyogram (EMG), described
292, 437
embolic stroke
defined 574
described 4, 96
embolus
defined 574
depicted *97*
ischemic stroke 4
emergency care
cerebrovascular disorders in
children 27
stroke 3
traumatic brain injury 263

EMG *see* electromyogram
emotional problems
atherosclerosis 143
caregiver stress 514
obesity complication 282
poststroke 44, 452
endoscopy, defined 574
endovascular embolization, cerebral
aneurysm 113
energy balance
fat tissue types 214
maintain healthy weight 223
obesity 215
enoxaparin, anticoagulants 48, 355
environmental factors, obesity 217
esophagus
defined 574
depicted *404*
estrogen, defined 574
Eunice Kennedy Shriver National
Institute of Child Health and
Human Development (NICHD)
contact 580
publications
rehabilitative and assistive
technology 475n
traumatic brain injury (TBI) 257n
exercise
carotid artery dissection cause 99
healthy lifestyle changes 223, 253
hypertension control 120
Kegel exercises 440
obesity/weight loss 121
overview 230–5
physical therapy 48, 122, 468
poststroke balance problems
treatment 418
strengthening muscles 427
see also lifestyle changes; physical
activity
"Exercise after Stroke" (VA) 488n
expressive aphasia *see* Broca aphasia
eye patches, vision aid 445
ezetimibe, cholesterol-lowering
medicines 211

F

falls, prevention 420

familial hypercholesterolemia, described 204
Family Caregiver Alliance (FCA), contact 585
family history
  atherosclerosis 135, 146
  dementia 389
  heart disease 183
  high blood pressure 195
  high cholesterol 273
  obesity 217
  sleep apnea 240
  stroke risk 7, 128
  see also genetics
F.A.S.T. warning signs of stroke 22
fat, defined 574
fatigue
  atrial fibrillation symptoms 160
  cardiomyopathy signs 249
  defined 575
  poststroke 429
fatty tissue, defined 575
"FDA Approves New Device for Prevention of Recurrent Strokes in Certain Patients" (FDA) 74n
"FDA Executive Summary" (FDA) 328n
fecal incontinence *see* bowel control problem
feeding tubes, artificial nutrition 561
FEESST *see* Flexible Endoscopic Evaluation of Swallowing with Sensory Testing
FES *see* Functional electrical stimulation
fetal echocardiography, described 310
fibrates, cholesterol-lowering medicine 211
fMRI *see* functional magnetic resonance imaging
"Focus on Stem Cell Research" (NINDS) 72n
foot drop
  functional electrical stimulation 420
  overview 413–4
"Foot Drop Information Page" (NINDS) 413n
Fragmin (dalteparin), injectable anticoagulant 48

functional electrical stimulation (FES), described 420
functional magnetic resonance imaging (fMRI), described 317

G

gabapentin, antispasmodic drug 412
gastrointestinal, defined 575
gender
  clinical trials 80
  high blood pressure risk 194
  long-term care 541
  nutrition 489
  recurrent stroke 119
  stroke facts 43
  stroke risk 7
gene, defined 575
Genetic and Rare Diseases Information Center (GARD) publications
    agnosia 380n
    Binswanger disease 391n
    poststroke pain 424n
genetics
  atherosclerosis 135
  cerebral aneurysm 108
  dementia 389
  factor V Leiden 163
  high blood pressure 193
  obesity 215
  stroke risk 128
"Geography and Stroke: The Stroke Belt" (Omnigraphics) 57n
Glasgow coma scale (GCS), traumatic brain injury 261
global aphasia
  defined 575
  measuring stroke severity 46
  traumatic brain injury 261
good cholesterol *see* high-density lipoprotein (HDL)

H

hand, paralysis 3
hardening of the arteries *see* atherosclerosis; peripheral artery disease

Hazel K. Goddess Fund for Stroke
Research in Women, contact 585
HDL *see* high-density lipoprotein
head injuries, subarachnoid
hemorrhagic stroke risk 106
headache
intracerebral hemorrhagic stroke
symptom 104
menopausal hormone therapy side
effects 37
stroke symptoms 9
transient ischemic attack
symptom 147
health insurance, overview 528–30
healthcare power of attorney, types of
legal documents 548
healthcare proxy, advance care
planning 565
healthcare specialists, described 138
Healthfinder®, contact 580
"HEart and BRain Interfaces in
Acute Ischemic Stroke (HEBRAS)"
(ClinicalTrials.gov) 86n
heart attack
omega-3 fatty acids 210
sleep apnea 136
heart disease
blood test 308
cholesterol 374
defined 575
depression 518
hormone therapy 35
obesity 213
pediatric stroke 27
smoking 277
statistics 248
"Heart Disease and Stroke—Stroke
Recovery Steps" (OWH) 373n
heart murmurs, echo 308
heart valves, echo 313
HeartHealthyWomen.org, contact 585
hematoma
defined 575
traumatic brain injury 258
hemiplegia
defined 575
movement problems 43
hemorrhagic stroke
amphetamine abuse 8
children 25

hemorrhagic stroke, *continued*
defined 575
described 42
intracerebral and subarachnoid
104–7
treatment 13
hemorrhoids, bowel control
problem 436
heparin
antithrombotics 572
blood clot prevention 293
defined 575
injectable anticoagulants 48
heredity *see* family history; genetics
high blood cholesterol *see* cholesterol
levels
"High Blood Cholesterol"
(NHLBI) 202n
high blood pressure
atherosclerosis 134
carotid artery disease 145
described 125
genetic factors 128
hemorrhagic stroke 6
metabolic syndrome 146
Stroke Belt 59
stroke risk 30
transient ischemic attack 23
"High Blood Pressure" (NHLBI) 190n
"High Blood Pressure—Medicines to
Help You" (FDA) 357n
high cholesterol, overview 273–5
high-density lipoprotein (HDL)
abnormal cholesterol 269
atherosclerosis 134
defined 575
described 370
tests 304
Hispanic Americans, stroke
disparities 55
"Hispanic Men and Stroke" (CDC) 51n
"Hispanic Women and Stroke"
(CDC) 51n
Holter and event monitors,
described 162
home-based rehabilitation,
programs 457
home healthcare, Medicare
coverage 552

home modification, overview 471–4
home rehabilitation, described 457
hormonal fluctuations, women 31
hormone replacement therapy (HRT),
   described 36
hospice, stroke rehabilitation 374
hospitalization, poststroke
   rehabilitation 452
"How Do You Manage Spasticity?"
   (VA) 410n
"How to Choose a Rehabilitation
   Facility" (Omnigraphics) 458n
HRT *see* hormone replacement
   therapy
humanitarian device exemption
   (HDE) process, stent-assisted coiling
   (SAC) 332
hydrocephalus, subarachnoid
   hemorrhage 110
hygiene, skin care 494
hypercoagulable state, described 167
hypertension *see* high blood pressure
hypertonicity, spasticity 410
hypothermia, brain function 48
hypothyroidism, obesity 215

I

ICP *see* intracranial pressure
imaging techniques, stroke
   diagnosis 46
immune system disorders, complete
   blood count 301
implantable cardioverter-
   defibrillators, MRI scan 317
incontinence
   bowel 431
   poststroke 501
   subcortical vascular dementia 388
   urine retention 436
infarction
   defined 575
   perinatal stroke 25
infections
   managing spasticity 411
   traumatic brain injury 265
inflammation, stress 247
inpatient rehabilitation, described 457
insomnia, cocaine 255

insulin
   defined 126
   production 269
insulin resistance
   atherosclerosis 134
   carotid artery disease 145
insurance *see* health insurance
"Intensive Physical Therapy Boosts
   Stroke Recovery" (VA) 467n
intermittent claudication, peripheral
   artery disease 173
internal carotid artery (ICA),
   coiling 329
International Subarachnoid
   Aneurysm Trial (ISAT), surgical
   clipping 328
Internet Stroke Center, contact 585
"Intracerebral and Subarachnoid
   Hemorrhagic Stroke"
   (Omnigraphics) 104n
intracerebral hemorrhage
   defined 576
   hemorrhagic stroke type 4
intracranial pressure (ICP), traumatic
   brain injury 262
intravenous (IV) contrast agents, soft
   tissues 315
ischemia
   CT scan 46
   defined 576
ischemic stroke
   defined 576
   depicted *97*
   hospital 288
   migraine 236
   overview 96–8
   sickle cell disease 126
   thrombolytic drugs 47
   treatment 116
   treatment options 324

J

Job Accommodation Network (JAN),
   contact 585

K

kidney disease, atherosclerosis 133

L

laboratory tests *see* diagnostic tests
language problems *see* communication
    problems
LDL *see* low-density lipoprotein
learned non-use, postsurgery 414
legal issues, rehabilitation 547
life expectancy, foot drop 414
lifestyle changes
    atherosclerosis 140
    carotid artery disease 149
    high blood pressure 197
    high cholesterol 206
    obesity/weight control 216
    recurrent stroke 121
    risk factor control 15
    stroke risk factor 98
lipoprotein
    described 370
    desirable levels 205
    see also high-density lipoprotein;
        low-density lipoprotein
lipoprotein panel, described 205
LiverTox®, National Institutes of
    Health (NIH)
    publication
        anticoagulants 355n
living will, described 549
long-term care
    overview 540–55
    rehabilitation services 374
"Long-Term Care: What Is Long-Term
    Care?" (NIA) 540n
Lovenox (enoxaparin), injectable
    anticoagulants 48
low blood glucose levels, stroke
    diagnosis 12
low-density lipoprotein (LDL),
    described 182
lumbar puncture *see* cerebrospinal
    fluid (CSF) analysis

M

magnetic resonance angiogram
    (MRA), described 177
magnetic resonance angiography,
    carotid artery dissection 100
magnetic resonance imaging (MRI)
    aphasia 397
    brain scans 390
    central poststroke pain
        diagnosis 425
    described 47
    overview 316–9
"Magnetic Resonance Imaging (MRI)"
    (NIBIB) 316n
magnifiers, vision aids 445
malnutrition, abnormal calcium
    levels 303
Marfan syndrome, carotid artery
    dissection 99
marijuana, neurological
    problems 254
mean corpuscular volume (MCV),
    complete blood count 303
mechanical clot removal in cerebral
    ischemia (MERCI), ischemic stroke
    treatment 324
Medicaid and Medicare coverage,
    long-term care 552
medications
    carotid artery disease 101
    pain 44
    recurrent stroke 121
    side effects
        balance problems 418
        headache 368
        high blood pressure 359
        weight gain 215
    spasticity 410
    subarachnoid hemorrhagic
        strokes 107
    transient ischemic attack 324
    weight loss 197
memory, rehabilitation therapies 264
memory loss
    dementia 385
    methamphetamine 256
    traumatic brain injury 261
    types 510
"Memory Problems" (VA) 509n
men
    stroke risks 38
    see also gender
menopausal hormone therapy (MHT),
    defined 576

menopause
  stroke risk 32
  see also hormone replacement
    therapy
MERCI *see* mechanical clot removal in
  cerebral ischemia
metabolic syndrome
  atrial fibrillation 159
  carotid artery disease 146
  described 146
  obesity 213
  peripheral artery disease 172
  weight management 210
meth *see* methamphetamine
methamphetamine, neurological
  problems 255
MHT *see* menopausal hormone
  therapy
MID *see* multi-infarct dementia
migraine, stroke risk 235
migraine with aura, stroke risk 236
Million Hearts® initiative, stroke
  prevention 253
mini-stroke *see* transient ischemic
  attack (TIA)
mood changes, mild TBI 259
"More Sensitive Stroke Detection"
  (NIH) 316n
movement disorders, surgery 445
MRA *see* magnetic resonance
  angiogram
MRI *see* magnetic resonance imaging
multi-infarct dementia (MID),
  described 387
"Multi-Infarct Dementia Information
  Page" (NINDS) 391n
muscle spasticity, overview 410–3
muscular dystrophy, foot drop 413
myositis, foot drop 413

N

narcotics, pain medicines 427
National Alliance for Caregiving,
  contact 585
National Aphasia Association (NAA),
  contact 586
National Brain Tumor Society
  (NBTS), contact 586

National Cancer Institute (NCI)
  contact 580
  publication
    MHT and cancer 35n
National Center for Complementary
  and Integrative Health (NCCIH),
  contact 580
National Center for Health Statistics
  (NCHS), contact 580
National Center for Learning
  Disabilities (NCLD), contact 586
National Heart, Lung, and Blood
  Institute (NHLBI)
  contact 580
  publications
    atherosclerosis 132n
    atrial fibrillation 157n
    blood tests 301n
    carotid artery disease 144n
    echocardiography 308n
    electrocardiogram 312n
    high blood cholesterol 202n
    high blood pressure 190n
    overweight and obesity
      213n, 281n
    peripheral artery disease 171n
    quit smoking 277n
    sleep apnea and stroke 239n
    stents 337n
    stroke 3n, 96n
    stroke diagnosis 298n, 301n
    stroke treatment 115n, 323n
National Highway Traffic Safety
  Administration (NHTSA)
  contact 581
  publication
    driving after stroke 481n
National Information Center
  for Children and Youth with
  Disabilities (NICHCY), contact 586
National Institute of Biomedical
  Imaging and Bioengineering
  (NIBIB)
  publications
    computed tomography
      (CT) 313n
    magnetic resonance imaging
      (MRI) 316n
    ultrasound 319n

National Institute of Diabetes and
Digestive and Kidney Diseases
(NIDDK)
publications
    bladder control problems and
    nerve disease 435n
    bowel control problems 431n
    diabetes, heart disease, and
    stroke 181n, 268n
National Institute of Neurological
Disorders and Stroke (NINDS)
contact 581
publications
    carotid endarterectomy 346n
    cerebral aneurysms 108n
    childhood stroke 25n
    dementia 385n
    foot drop 413n
    multi-infarct dementia 391n
    poststroke rehabilitation 448n
    spasticity 410n
    stem cell research 72n
    stroke 3n, 21n
    stroke research 30n
    transient ischemic
    attack 115n
National Institutes of Health (NIH)
contact 581
publications
    brain mapping of language
    impairments 395n
    brain repair after stroke 70n
    exercise and stroke prevention
    230n
    perinatal stroke 25n
    sensitive stroke
    detection 316n
    stem cell therapy 72n
National Institute on Aging (NIA)
contact 581
publications
    advance care planning 559n
    long-term care 540n
    stroke 41n, 287n
National Institute on Alcohol Abuse
and Alcoholism (NIAAA)
contact 581
publication
    alcohol and stroke 248n

National Institute on Deafness and
Other Communication Disorders
(NIDCD)
publications
    aphasia 395n
    dysphagia 403n, 486n
National Institute on Drug Abuse
(NIDA)
publication
    drug misuse and neurological
    effects 254n
National Rehabilitation Information
Center (NARIC), contact 586
National Stroke Association,
contact 586
National Women's Health Information
Center (NWHIC), contact 581
nausea, drug therapy 439
NCCAM *see* National Center for
Complementary and Alternative
Medicine
neglect syndrome
defined 43
thinking problems 43
nephrologist, defined 138
neurectomy, muscle spasticity 413
neurological disorders, stem cell
therapy 72
neurological examination, multi-
infarct dementia 392
neurologist
described 138
working with 291
neurons
brain repair 70
defined 576
stem cell therapy 72
neuropathic pain, described 450
Neuro-Patient Resource Center,
contact 586
neuroprotectants, defined 48
neuropsychologist, defined 510
neurosonography, described 292
NHLBI *see* National Heart, Lung, and
Blood Institute
NIA *see* National Institute on Aging
nicotinic acid, cholesterol levels 211
nifedipine, calcium channel
blockers 361

NIH *see* National Institutes of Health

"NIH Clinical Research Trials and You—The Basics" (NIH) 78n

NIH Stroke Scale, stroke severity measure 46

NINDS *see* National Institute of neurological Disorders and Stroke

nonsteroidal anti-inflammatory drugs (NSAIDs), stroke risk 8

North American Symptomatic Carotid Endarterectomy Trial (NASCET)

notary, defined 565

NSAIDs *see* nonsteroidal anti-inflammatory drugs

nutrition
 advance care planning 561
 poststroke 489
 salt 490
 skin care 494

O

obesity
 diabetes 182
 race and ethnicity 52
 recurrent stroke 121
 see also overweight and obesity

obesity hypoventilation syndrome 220, 281

obstructive sleep apnea *see* sleep apnea

occlusion, described 112

occupational therapists, rehabilitation 18

occupational therapy
 described 48
 rehabilitation 295
 subarachnoid hemorrhage 113

Office of Extramural Research (OER), contact 581

Office of Minority Health (OMH)
 contact 581
 publications
  Asian Americans and stroke 51n
  stroke recovery 373n

Office on Women's Health (OWH)
 publications
  birth control methods 33n

Office on Women's Health (OWH) publications, *continued*
  blood clotting problems and stroke risk 167n
  caregiver stress 513n
  menopausal hormone therapy 35n
  stroke 33n

older adults
 atherosclerosis 135
 bowel control problems 431
 dysphagia 486
 overview 41–9
 sleep apnea 241

Omnigraphics
 publications
  balance problems after stroke 417n
  carotid artery dissection 98n
  cerebral angiography 305n
  constraint-induced movement therapy 414n
  intracerebral and subarachnoid hemorrhagic stroke 104n
  neurologist 291n
  recurrent stroke 119n
  rehabilitation facility 458n
  stress and stroke risk 244n
  Stroke Belt 57n
  vision problems after stroke 443n

organ and tissue donation, end of life 562

orthoses, spasticity 411

OSA *see* obstructive sleep apnea

osteoarthritis, obesity 281

OT *see* occupational therapy

outpatient rehabilitation, described 457

overactive bladder, treatments 438

over-the-counter (OTC) pain medicines 427

overweight and obesity
 high blood pressure 193
 overview 213–27
 sleep apnea 243
 triglyceride level 206

"Overweight and Obesity" (NHLBI) 213n

P

PAD *see* peripheral artery disease
pain
  aneurysms 106
  atrial fibrillation 157
  carotid artery dissection 100
  coronary heart disease 133
  heart attack 186
  overview 424–9
  peripheral artery disease 173, 179
  stress testing 140
  see also central stroke pain
"Pain after Stroke" (VA) 424n
paralysis
  Broca aphasia 397
  carotid artery disease 144
  cerebral aneurysms 109
  foot drop 413
  high blood pressure 195
  intracerebral hemorrhagic stroke 105
  stroke 449
paresthesias, defined 454
Parkinson disease, traumatic brain
  injury 265
partial thromboplastin time (PTT),
  blood clot 12, 301
patent foramen ovale (PFO), stroke
  risk 169
PCOS *see* polycystic ovary syndrome
pericardium, echocardiography 308
peripheral artery disease (PAD)
  atherosclerosis 138
  overview 171–80
  statins 141
"Peripheral Artery Disease"
  (NHLBI) 171n
perinatal stroke, overview 25–6
"Perinatal Stroke" (NIH) 25n
peripherally acting alpha-adrenergic
  blockers *362*
personality changes, brain damage 452
PET scan *see* positron emission
  tomography scan
PFO *see* patent foramen ovale
physiatrists, spasticity 411
physical activity
  atherosclerosis 135
  carotid artery disease 146

physical activity, *continued*
  cholesterol levels 121
  diabetes 184
  high blood pressure 193
  obesity 216
  peripheral artery disease 174
  transient ischemic attack 15, 117
  see also exercise; lifestyle changes;
    therapeutic lifestyle changes
"Physical Activity and Health"
  (CDC) 230n
physical examination
  bladder problem 441
  carotid artery dissection 100
physical inactivity
  atherosclerosis 135
  carotid artery disease 146
  high blood pressure 193
  obesity 216
  triglyceride levels 206
  weight gain 204
physical therapists, rehabilitation
  48, 453
physical therapy (PT)
  goals 454
  neurologists 291
  recurrent stroke 122
  spasticity 410
physicians, dysphagia 406
pins and needles, central poststroke
  pain 425
plaque
  atherosclerosis 6
  carotid artery disease 10
  defined 576
  depicted *97*
  embolic stroke 4
  hemorrhagic stroke 42
  ischemic stroke 96
  smoking 120
plasticity
  defined 576
  speech therapy 49
platelets
  antithrombotics 48
  atherosclerosis 134
  defined 12
polycystic ovary syndrome (PCOS),
  obesity 218

polysomnogram, sleep apnea 241
positron emission tomography (PET) scan
  atherosclerosis 140
  dementia 390
poststroke depression, defined 44
"Post-Stroke Rehabilitation" (NINDS) 448n
potassium, high blood pressure 192
power of attorney *see* healthcare power of attorney
Pradaxa (dabigatran) 48
prediabetes
  blood tests 227
  described 269
pregnancy
  echocardiography 309
  FVL mutation 168
  high blood pressure 201
  hormonal fluctuations 31
  perinatal stroke 26
  smoking 278
prehypertension
  obesity 194
  stages *191*
"Preventing Stroke: Healthy Living" (CDC) 276n
prothrombin, blood clotting problems 169
prothrombin time 12, 301
psychological or psychiatric therapy, depression 49
PT *see* physical therapy

Q

"Quality of Life after Stroke Using a Telemedicine-Based Stroke Network (STROKE TeleQOL)" (ClinicalTrials.gov) 88n
"Questions and Answers about Carotid Endarterectomy" (NINDS) 346n
"Questions and Answers about Stroke" (NINDS) 3n, 21n

R

racial and ethnic factors
  atrial fibrillation 158
  diabetes 269

racial and ethnic factors, *continued*
  factor V Leiden 168
  high blood pressure 194
  overview 51–6
  overweight and obesity 218
  pediatric stroke 27
  peripheral artery disease 173
  recurrent stroke 119
  stroke risk 7
range of motion, spasticity 410
receptive aphasia *see* Wernicke aphasia
"Recognition and Treatment of Stroke in Children" (NINDS) 25n
recombinant tissue plasminogen activator (r-tPA)
  acute ischemic stroke 352
  defined 576
  see also tissue plasminogen activator
recurrent stroke
  overview 119–22
  patent foramen ovale 74
  statistics 42
rehab *see* rehabilitation
rehabilitation
  defined 18
  overview 447–63
  poststroke 48
rehabilitation facilities, overview 447–63
Rehabilitation Institute of Chicago (renamed as Shirley Ryan AbilityLab)
  publication
    skin care after stroke 493n
rehabilitation team, long-term care 452
"Rehabilitative and Assistive Technology" (NICHD) 475n
renin inhibitors
  recurrent stroke 121
  tabulated *365*
"RESCUE Fact Sheet—Feeling Tired after Stroke" (VA) 429n
"RESCUE Fact Sheet—Healthy Eating" (VA) 488n
research
  birth control patch 34
  ischemic stroke 13

research, *continued*
  menopausal hormone therapy 36
  overview 70–6
  pregnancy and childbirth 31
  Stroke Belt 57
"Right Hemisphere Brain Damage"
  (American Speech-Language-
  Hearing Association) 382n
risk factors
  medical history 10
  stroke 7, 23
  see also lifestyle changes
rivaroxaban (Xarelto) 48
r-tPA *see* recombinant tissue
  plasminogen activator

S

"Safe Swallowing" (VA) 486n
saturated fat
  atrial fibrillation 165
  lifestyle changes 121
  source 204
  Stroke Belt 59
"Scientists Identify Main Component
  of Brain Repair after Stroke"
  (NIH) 70n
secondary prevention, antiplatelet
  agents 356
secondhand smoke
  atherosclerosis 143
  blood pressure 7
  coronary heart disease 252
  obesity 212
  stroke 128
seizures
  addictive drugs 254
  anticonvulsants 106
  traumatic brain injury 263
sensory disturbances, described 450
septum, sleep apnea 240
"Sex after Stroke" (VA) 501n
shaken baby syndrome, traumatic
  brain injury 258
SHHS *see* Sleep Heart Health Study
Shirley Ryan AbilityLab, contact 587
sick sinus syndrome, defined 159
sickle cell disease, defined 126
silent strokes, defined 391

single-infarct dementia, defined 387
single photon emission computed
  tomography (SPECT), dementia 390
sinus problems, angiotension II
  antagonists 364
"Skin Care after a Stroke" (Shirley
  Ryan AbilityLab (formerly
  Rehabilitation Institute of
  Chicago)) 493n
skull fracture, traumatic brain
  injury 258
sleep apnea
  atrial fibrillation 159
  defined 136
  overview 239–43
sleep disorders, obesity 213
Sleep Heart Health Study (SHHS),
  sleep apnea 241
sleep problems
  causes 497
  coronary microvascular disease 137
sleep studies, defined 293
sleep-wake cycle disorders, defined 498
"Sleeping Problems" (VA) 497n
SLP *see* speech-language pathologist
slurred speech, traumatic brain
  injury 259
small vessel disease, defined 576
Smokefree.gov, contact 582
smoking
  cerebral aneurysms 108
  quitting 15
  statistics 54
  stroke risk 7
  transient ischemic attack 117
  see also lifestyle changes
Smoking and Heart Disease and
  Stroke (CDC) 277n
social support *see* support group
social worker
  depression 430
  rehabilitation 456
Society for Vascular Surgery (SVS),
  contact 587
socioeconomic status, obesity 217
sodium, lifestyle changes 32, 39
sonography *see* ultrasound
spasticity, overview 409–16
"Spasticity Information Page"
  (NINDS) 410n

SPECT *see* single photon emission computed tomography
"Speech and Communication (Aphasia, Dysarthria, and Apraxia)" (VA) 395n
speech disorder, defined 576
speech-language pathologist (SLP), described 454
speech problems *see* communication problems
spinal tap *see* cerebrospinal fluid (CSF) analysis
"State Medicaid Programs" (ACL) 526n
statin drugs
  high cholesterol 17
  stroke treatment 48
statistics, overview 63–7
stem cell therapy, overview 72–4
"Stem Cell Therapy Heals Injured Mouse Brain" (NIH) 72n
stenosis
  defined 576
  ischemic stroke 42
stents
  atherosclerosis 142
  carotid artery dissection 101
"Stents" (NHLBI) 337n
steppage gait, foot drop 413
steroids, spasticity 427
"Strategies to Quit Smoking" (NHLBI) 277n
stress
  atherosclerosis 136
  overview 244–6
stress echocardiography, described 310
stress testing, described 140
stretching exercises, physical therapist 427
"Stroke" (NHLBI) 3n, 96n
"Stroke" (NIA) 41n
"Stroke and Asian Americans" (OMH) 51n
Stroke Association, contact 587
Stroke Awareness Foundation, contact 587
Stroke Belt
  defined 576
  overview 57–61

"Stroke Fact Sheet" (CDC) 41n
"Stroke—Frequently Asked Questions" (NIA) 287n
"Stroke—How Is a Stroke Diagnosed?" (NHLBI) 298n, 301n
"Stroke—How Is a Stroke Treated?" (NHLBI) 115n, 323n
"Stroke: Percent of Acute Ischemic Stroke Patients for Whom IV T-PA Was Initiated at the Hospital within 3 Hours (Less than or Equal to 180 Minutes) of Time Last Known Well" (AHRQ) 352n
stroke recovery, overview 373–5
"Stroke—Recovering from Stroke" (CDC) 467n
"Stroke Risk" (CDC) 125n
"Stroke—Signs and Symptoms" (CDC) 21n
"Stroke—Stroke Treatment" (CDC) 352n
"Stroke Support Group" (VA) 519n
stroke survivor
  pain 424
  rehabilitation 374
"Stroke Treatment" (CDC) 287n
"Stroke—Types of Stroke" (CDC) 96n
subarachnoid hemorrhage
  cerebral aneurysm 110
  defined 576
  hemorrhagic stroke 4
  surgical clipping 328
support group
  aphasia 398
  overview 519–21
surgical procedures
  carotid artery dissection 101
  obesity 224
swallowing
  overview 403–7
  paralysis 449
  see also dysphagia
synthetic stimulants (bath salts) 255

T

talk therapy
  depression 506
  mental health 49

talk therapy, *continued*
  tips for caregivers 517
TBI *see* traumatic brain injury
TEE *see* transesophageal
  echocardiography
teens
  healthy living 276
  high blood pressure 190
  traumatic brain injury (TBI) 262
"10 Tips for Choosing a Rehab
  Facility" (Cleveland Clinic) 461n
tenotomy, spasticity 413
TENS *see* transcutaneous electrical
  nerve stimulation
thalamic pain syndrome, stroke
  survivors 450
therapeutic lifestyle changes (TLC),
  cholesterol 208
therapeutic ultrasound, described 320
thinking problems *see* cognitive
  problems
three-dimensional echocardiography,
  diagnosing stroke 310
thrombolytic
  antiplatelets and
    anticoagulants 355
  defined 577
  described 47
  overview 352–4
  stroke treatment and
    rehabilitation 28
thrombosis, defined 577
thrombotic stroke
  defined 577
  described 4
thrombus, depicted *160*
TIA *see* transient ischemic attack
ticlopidine
  antiplatelet drugs 48
  recurrent stroke 121
timed voiding
tissue plasminogen activator (tPA)
  overview 352–4
  stroke treatment 34, 288
  thrombolytics 47
  see also recombinant tissue
    plasminogen activator
tizanidine, spasticity treatment 410
TLC *see* therapeutic lifestyle changes

TMS *see* transcranial magnetic
  stimulation
tobacco use *see* smoking
tPA *see* tissue plasminogen activator
trans fats
  atherosclerosis 135
  healthy diet 60
  high blood cholesterol 204
  obesity 216
transcranial Doppler (TCD),
  neurologists 292
transcranial magnetic stimulation
  (TMS)
  defined 577
  rehabilitative technologies 477
transducer
  diagnostic ultrasound 163
  transthoracic echocardiography 309
  ultrasound 320
transesophageal echocardiography
  (TEE), stroke diagnosis 163, 310
transient ischemic attack (TIA)
  defined 577
  overview 115–7
  peripheral artery disease 174
  stroke treatment 323
"Transient Ischemic Attack
  Information Page" (NINDS) 115n
transthoracic echocardiography,
  stroke diagnosis 163, 309
traumatic brain injury (TBI)
  agnosia 380
  brain damage 383
  defined 577
  overview 257–65
  Social Security Administration
    (SSA) 538
treatment plans
  high blood pressure 197
  rehabilitation facility 460
  working with a neurologist 294
trouble speaking
  carotid arteries 137
  heart disease and stroke 252
  high blood pressure 195
  signs and symptoms of stroke 9
triglycerides
  atrial fibrillation 165
  blood tests 304

triglycerides, *continued*
  high blood cholesterol 205
  overweight and obesity 214
  risk factors for diabetes 182
  smoking 252, 277
  stroke risks 126
typoscope, vision aids 445

U

ultrasound
  carotid artery disease 349
  carotid ultrasound 299
  diagnostic tests 149
  overview 319–22
  see also Doppler ultrasound
"Ultrasound" (NIBIB) 319n
United States
  statistics 63–7
  stroke 19
  Stroke Belt 57
urethral stent, urine retention 441
urinary incontinence
  overweight and obesity 220, 281
  vascular dementia 388
urine retention
  bladder control problems 436
  treatments 441
"Urologic Diseases—Bladder Control
  Problems and Nerve Disease"
  (NIDDK) 435n
U.S. Administration on Aging (AOA)
  publication
    assisted living 555n
U.S. Department of Health
  and Human Services (HHS),
  contact 582
U.S. Department of Veterans Affairs
  (VA)
  contact 582
  publications
    communication problems after
      stroke 395n
    depression after stroke 505n
    electrocardiogram (EKG) 312n
    exercise after stroke 488n
    fatigue after stroke 429n
    healthy eating 488n
    high blood pressure 270n

U.S. Department of Veterans Affairs
  (VA)
  publications, *continued*
    high cholesterol 273n
    home modification 471n
    memory problems 509n
    pain after stroke 424n
    physical therapy for stroke
      recovery 467n
    safe swallowing 486n
    sexuality after stroke 501n
    sleeping problems 497n
    spasticity 410n
    stroke support group 519n
    tips for caregivers 513n
U.S. Equal Employment
  Opportunity Commission (EEOC),
  contact 582
U.S. Food and Drug Administration
  (FDA)
  publications
    Amplatzer PFO Occluder
      device 74n
    cholesterol and statins 369n
    high blood pressure
      medicines 357n
    sleep apnea 239n
U.S. National Institutes of Health
  (NIH)
  publications
    acute ischemic stroke 86n
    aerobic exercise for minor
      stroke 91n
    carotid plaque imaging in acute
      stroke 89n
    life after stroke 88n
    NIH clinical research 78n
    stroke rehabilitation
      treatment 83n
    vitamin D and stroke 85n
U.S. National Library of Medicine
  (NLM), contact 582
U.S. Social Security Administration
  (SSA)
  contact 582
  publications
    compassionate
      allowances 529n
    disability benefits 529n

613

V

VA *see* U.S. Department of Veterans Affairs
"VA Electrocardiogram (EKG) Learn More" (VA) 312n
vaccines
  caregiver stress 516
  high blood pressure 199
vascular dementia
  overview 385–91
  treatment 391
vascular specialist
  atherosclerosis 138
  carotid artery dissection 102
  peripheral artery disease 174
vasodilators
  blood pressure medicines 199
  defined 577
vasospasm
  cerebral aneurysms 110
  defined 577
ventilator use, advance care planning 560
ventricular tachycardia 249
vertebral artery, defined 577
vision problems
  neurologist 295
  overview 443–6
  subarachnoid hemorrhagic stroke 106
"Vision Problems after Stroke" (Omnigraphics) 443n
visual field loss 443
"Vitamin D and Stroke" (ClinicalTrials.gov) 85n
vitamin K, anticoagulants 355
vocational therapists
  described 455
  poststroke rehabilitation 452

W

warfarin (Coumadin®)
  anticoagulants 48
  blood clotting tests 305
  defined 577
  recurrent stroke 121
  stroke treatment 34

"Ways to Make the Home Safer (Home Modification)" (VA) 471n
weight
  atrial fibrillation 165
  body mass index 121
  complications of obesity 281
  heart-healthy lifestyle changes 141, 150
  see also lifestyle changes; overweight and obesity
weight loss
  behavioral weight-loss programs 223
  high blood pressure 197
  poststroke rehabilitation 452
  preventing diabetes 268
Well Spouse Association, contact 587
Wernicke aphasia, aphasia 396
"What Is Recurrent Stroke?" (Omnigraphics) 119n
wheelchairs, stroke survivors 472
white coat hypertension 197
women
  blood clotting problems 169
  high blood cholesterol 204
  long-term care 541
  menopausal hormone therapy 35
  obesity 218
  racial and ethnic disparities 51
  risk of stroke with migraine 236
  sleep apnea and stroke 242
  stress at work 246
  stroke in women 20
  stroke risks 129
  see also gender
"Working up a Sweat May Help Reduce Stroke Risk" (NIH) 230n
"Working with a Neurologist" (Omnigraphics) 291n

X

Xarelto (rivaroxaban), anticoagulants 48
X-rays
  angiography 140
  carotid angiography 11
  computed tomography (CT) scan 313
  computed tomography angiography 149

X-rays, *continued*
   diagnose intracerebral hemorrhagic
      stroke 105

Y

yoga
   carotid artery dissection 99

yoga, *continued*
   complementary or alternative
      therapies 427
   poststroke balance problems 419
   tips for caregivers 518
   stress management 185, 245